Unified Airway Disease

Editors

DEVYANI LAL
ANGELA M. DONALDSON
DAVID W. JANG

OTOLARYNGOLOGIC CLINICS OF NORTH AMERICA

www.oto.theclinics.com

Consulting Editor
SUJANA S. CHANDRASEKHAR

February 2023 • Volume 56 • Number 1

ELSEVIER

1600 John F. Kennedy Boulevard • Suite 1800 • Philadelphia, Pennsylvania, 19103-2899

http://www.oto.theclinics.com

OTOLARYNGOLOGIC CLINICS OF NORTH AMERICA Volume 56, Number 1
February 2023 ISSN 0030-6665, ISBN-13: 978-0-323-93914-0

Editor: Stacy Eastman
Developmental Editor: Diana Grace Ang

Photocopying
Single photocopies of single articles may be made for personal use as allowed by national copyright laws. Permission of the Publisher and payment of a fee is required for all other photocopying, including multiple or systematic copying, copying for advertising or promotional purposes, resale, and all forms of document delivery. Special rates are available for educational institutions that wish to make photocopies for non-profit educational classroom use. For information on how to seek permission visit www.elsevier.com/permissions or call: (+44) 1865 843830 (UK)/(+1) 215 239 3804 (USA).

Derivative Works
Subscribers may reproduce tables of contents or prepare lists of articles including abstracts for internal circulation within their institutions. Permission of the Publisher is required for resale or distribution outside the institution. Permission of the Publisher is required for all other derivative works, including compilations and translations (please consult www.elsevier. com/permissions).

Electronic Storage or Usage
Permission of the Publisher is required to store or use electronically any material contained in this periodical, including any article or part of an article (please consult www.elsevier.com/permissions). Except as outlined above, no part of this publication may be reproduced, stored in a retrieval system or transmitted in any form or by any means, electronic, mechanical, photocopying, recording or otherwise, without prior written permission of the Publisher.

Notice
No responsibility is assumed by the Publisher for any injury and/or damage to persons or property as a matter of products liability, negligence or otherwise, or from any use or operation of any methods, products, instructions or ideas contained in the material herein. Because of rapid advances in the medical sciences, in particular, independent verification of diagnoses and drug dosages should be made.

Although all advertising material is expected to conform to ethical (medical) standards, inclusion in this publication does not constitute a guarantee or endorsement of the quality or value of such product or of the claims made of it by its manufacturer.

Otolaryngologic Clinics of North America (ISSN 0030-6665) is published bimonthly by Elsevier, Inc., 360 Park Avenue South, New York, NY 10010-1710. Months of issue are February, April, June, August, October, and December. Business and Editorial Offices: 1600 John F. Kennedy Blvd., Suite 1800, Philadelphia, PA 19103-2899. Customer Service Office: 6277 Sea Harbor Drive, Orlando, FL 32887-4800. Periodicals postage paid at New York, NY and additional mailing offices. Subscription prices are $468.00 per year (US individuals), $1117.00 per year (US institutions), $100.00 per year (US & Canadian student/resident), $599.00 per year (Canadian individuals), $1416.00 per year (Canadian institutions), $653.00 per year (international individuals), $1416.00 per year (international institutions), $270.00 per year (international student/resident). Foreign air speed delivery is included in all *Clinics'* subscription prices. All prices are subject to change without notice. **POSTMASTER:** Send address changes to *Otolaryngologic Clinics of North America*, Elsevier Health Sciences Division, Subscription Customer Service, 3251 Riverport Lane, Maryland Heights, MO 63043. **Telephone: 1-800-654-2452 (U.S. and Canada); 314-447-8871 (outside U.S. and Canada). Fax: 314-447-8029. E-mail: journalscustomerservice-usa@elsevier.com (for print support); journalsonlinesupport-usa@elsevier.com (for online support).**

Reprints. For copies of 100 or more of articles in this publication, please contact the Commercial Reprints Department, Elsevier Inc., 360 Park Avenue South, New York, NY 10010-1710. Tel.: 212-633-3874; Fax: 212-633-3820; E-mail: reprints@ elsevier.com.

Otolaryngologic Clinics of North America is also published in Spanish by McGraw-Hill Interamericana Editores S.A., P.O. Box 5-237, 06500 Mexico D.F., Mexico.

Otolaryngologic Clinics of North America is covered in *MEDLINE/PubMed (Index Medicus), Current Contents/Clinical Medicine, Excerpta Medica, BIOSIS, Science Citation Index,* and *ISI/BIOMED.*

Contributors

CONSULTING EDITOR

SUJANA S. CHANDRASEKHAR, MD, FACS, FAAOHNS
Past President, American Academy of Otolaryngology–Head and Neck Surgery, Secretary-Treasurer, and President-Elect, American Otological Society, Eastern Section Vice President, Triological Society, Partner, ENT & Allergy Associates, LLP, Clinical Professor, Department of Otolaryngology–Head and Neck Surgery, Zucker School of Medicine at Hofstra–Northwell, Hempstead, New York, USA; Clinical Associate Professor, Department of Otolaryngology–Head and Neck Surgery, Icahn School of Medicine at Mount Sinai, New York, New York, USA

EDITORS

DEVYANI LAL, MD, FARS
Professor of Otolaryngology, Consultant, Otolaryngology–Head and Neck Surgery, Chair, Division of Rhinology, Dean of Education, Mayo Clinic, Phoenix, Arizona, USA

ANGELA M. DONALDSON, MD, FARS
Department of Otolaryngology Head and Neck Surgery, Mayo Clinic, Jacksonville, Florida, USA

DAVID W. JANG, MD
Associate Professor, Division of Rhinology and Endoscopic Skull Base Surgery, Duke Endoscopic Skull Base Surgery Program, Rhinology Clinical Research Program, Department of Head and Neck Surgery and Communication Sciences, Duke University, Durham, North Carolina, USA

AUTHORS

JUMAH G. AHMAD, MD
Department of Otorhinolaryngology–Head and Neck Surgery, University of Texas Health Science Center, Houston, Texas, USA

TRIPTI K. BRAR, MBBS, MD
Department of Otolaryngology–Head and Neck Surgery, Mayo Clinic, Phoenix, Arizona, USA

DO-YEON CHO, MD
Associate Professor, Department of Otolaryngology–Head and Neck Surgery, Gregory Fleming James Cystic Fibrosis Research Center, University of Alabama at Birmingham, Division of Otolaryngology, Department of Surgery, Veteran Affairs Medical Center, Birmingham, Alabama, USA

GARRET CHOBY, MD
Associate Professor, Rhinology and Endoscopic Skull Base Surgery, Chair of Quality, Department of Otorhinolaryngology - Head and Neck Surgery, Joint Appointment; Department of Neurologic Surgery, Mayo Clinic, Rochester, Minnesota, USA

ROHIT D. DIVEKAR, MBBS, PhD
Assistant Professor of Medicine, Division of Allergic Diseases, Mayo Clinic Rochester, Minnesota, USA

ANGELA M. DONALDSON, MD, FARS
Department of Otolaryngology Head and Neck Surgery, Mayo Clinic Florida, Jacksonville, Florida, USA

WYTSKE FOKKENS, MD, PhD
Professor, Department of Otorhinolaryngology, Amsterdam University Medical Centres, Location AMC, Amsterdam, the Netherlands

NAVROOP GILL, MD
Department of General Surgery, Loyola University Medical Center, Maywood, Illinois, USA

JESSICA W. GRAYSON, MD
Assistant Professor, Department of Otolaryngology–Head and Neck Surgery, University of Alabama at Birmingham, Birmingham, Alabama, USA

DAVID A. GUDIS, MD
Department of Otolaryngology–Head and Neck Surgery, Columbia University Irving Medical Center, New York-Presbyterian Hospital, New York, New York, USA

JOHN B. HAGAN, MD
Department of Allergic Diseases, Mayo Clinic College of Medicine, Rochester, Minnesota, USA

CLAIRE HOPKINS, DM, FRCS (ORL-HNS)
Professor, Consultant ENT Surgeon, Guy's and St Thomas' NHS Foundation Trust, Professor of Rhinology, King's College London, United Kingdom

DAVID W. JANG, MD
Associate Professor, Division of Rhinology and Endoscopic Skull Base Surgery, Duke Endoscopic Skull Base Surgery Program, Rhinology Clinical Research Program, Department of Head and Neck Surgery and Communication Sciences, Duke University, Durham, North Carolina, USA

DEVYANI LAL, MD, FARS
Professor of Otolaryngology, Consultant, Otolaryngology–Head and Neck Surgery, Chair, Division of Rhinology, Dean of Education, Mayo Clinic, Phoenix, Arizona, USA

MACKENZIE LATOUR, MD
Department of Otolaryngology–Head and Neck Surgery, Louisiana State University Health, Shreveport, Louisiana, USA

PATRICIA LUGAR, MD
Division of Allergy and Immunology, Department of Medicine, Duke University, Durham, North Carolina, USA

VALERIE J. LUND, MBBS, MS, FRCS, FRCSED, DMHON, FACSHON, CBE
Professor, Royal National Ear, Nose and Throat and Eastman Dental Hospitals, University College London Hospital, Ear Institute, University College London, London, United Kingdom

AMBER U. LUONG, MD, PhD
Department of Otorhinolaryngology–Head and Neck Surgery, University of Texas Health Science Center, Center for Immunology and Autoimmune Diseases, Institute of Molecular Medicine, McGovern Medical School at The University of Texas Health Science Center, Houston, Texas, USA

CHADI A. MAKARY, MD
Department of Otolaryngology–Head and Neck Surgery, West Virginia University, Morgantown, West Virginia, USA

MICHAEL J. MARINO, MD
Department of Otolaryngology–Head and Neck Surgery, Mayo Clinic, Phoenix, Arizona, USA

MITESH P. MEHTA, MD
Resident Physician, Department of Otolaryngology–Head and Neck Surgery, Emory University School of Medicine, Atlanta, Georgia, USA

AMAR MIGLANI, MD
Assistant Professor of Otolaryngology and Associate Program Director, Department of Otolaryngology–Head and Neck Surgery, Mayo Clinic, Phoenix, Arizona, USA

CARLY MULINDA, BA
Department of Otolaryngology–Head and Neck Surgery, Columbia University Irving Medical Center, New York–Presbyterian Hospital, New York, New York, USA

ERIN K. O'BRIEN, MD
Department of Otolaryngology–Head and Neck Surgery, Mayo Clinic College of Medicine, Rochester, Minnesota, USA

MONICA PATADIA, MD
Department of Otolaryngology, Head and Neck Surgery, Loyola University Medical Center, Maywood, Illinois, USA

CARLOS D. PINHEIRO-NETO, MD, PhD
Department of Otolaryngology–Head and Neck Surgery, Mayo Clinic College of Medicine, Rochester, Minnesota, USA

MURUGAPPAN RAMANATHAN, Jr, MD
Department of Otolaryngology–Head and Neck Surgery, Johns Hopkins Medical Institutions, Baltimore, Maryland, USA

SIETZE REITSMA, MD, PhD
Medical Doctor, Department of Otorhinolaryngology, Amsterdam University Medical Centres, Location AMC, Amsterdam, the Netherlands

JOANNE RIMMER, MBBS, MA, FRCS(ORL-HNS), FRACS
Associate Professor, Department of Surgery, Monash University, Department of Otolaryngology Head and Neck Surgery, Monash Health, Department of Otolaryngology Head and Neck Surgery, St Vincent's Hospital, Melbourne, Australia

EAMON SHAMIL, MBBS, MRES, FRCS (ORL-HNS)
Specialist Registrar (ST8) in ENT Surgery, Guy's and St Thomas' NHS Foundation Trust, ENT Department, Great Maze Pond, Guy's Hospital, London, United Kingdom

JESSE SIEGEL, MD
Department of Otolaryngology, Head and Neck Surgery, Loyola University Medical Center, Maywood, Illinois, USA

JANALEE K. STOKKEN, MD
Department of Otolaryngology–Head and Neck Surgery, Mayo Clinic College of Medicine, Rochester, Minnesota, USA

BENJAMIN K. WALTERS, MD
Department of Otolaryngology, San Antonio Military Medical Center, San Antonio, Texas, USA

THOMAS J. WILLSON, MD
Department of Otolaryngology, San Antonio Military Medical Center, San Antonio, Texas, USA

SARAH K. WISE, MD, MSCR
Professor, Department of Otolaryngology–Head and Neck Surgery, Emory University School of Medicine, Atlanta, Georgia, USA

BRADFORD A. WOODWORTH, MD, FACS
James J. Hicks Endowed Professor, Department of Otolaryngology–Head and Neck Surgery, Gregory Fleming James Cystic Fibrosis Research Center, University of Alabama at Birmingham, Birmingham, Alabama, USA

NATHAN YANG, MD
Department of Otolaryngology–Head and Neck Surgery, Columbia University Irving Medical Center, New York–Presbyterian Hospital, New York, New York, USA

MICHAEL T. YIM, MD
Department of Otolaryngology–Head and Neck Surgery, Louisiana State University Health, Shreveport, Louisiana, USA

Contents

> Upper and lower airways diseases are very common, with population prevalence of 10% to 40%. The conditions are usually interlinked and referred to as "unified airway disease" or "the united airways." Especially in phenotypes with more severe disease, type 2 immunologic endotype is often noted. Comorbid upper and lower airway diseases are usually caused by similar underlying immunologic response. Any patient with rhinitis or rhinosinusitis should have their lower respiratory tract evaluated. A multidisciplinary approach in the diagnosis and treatment of airway disease is advised, especially, for more severe phenotypes.

> The concept of a unified airway posits that pathology affects the respiratory tract in a continuum and that disease in one part of the respiratory tract may be associated with or directly or indirectly affect the function of a different part. Transcriptomic analysis has shown 91% homology between the genes expressed in the upper and the lower airway. Approaching inflammatory airway disorders using the unified airway hypothesis allows for a better clarification of disease process and provides a detailed and a high-level overview of dysfunction. There are several tools available to the clinician to use to subtype and diagnose accurately the abnormal pathways operating in inflammatory airway disorders. These tools include clinical history, physical examination findings, imaging (computed tomography and MRI), allergy and laboratory testing, pulmonary function testing (PFT), and tissue histopathology. Tests can be categorized based on platform, by specimen, or the marker being studied.

> Although unified airway disease (UAD) may have heritable components, genetic changes involving coexistent chronic rhinosinusitis (CRS) are not well understood. Genetic predisposition is stronger in patients with CRS with nasal polyps compared with those without nasal polyps (CRSsNP). Genetic factors account for 25% to 80% of asthma risk and 90% of allergic rhinitis risk but risk contributions are not well described for CRS.

Susceptibility genes identified in coexistent CRS-asthma relate to innate and adaptive immunity, cytokine signaling, tissue remodeling, arachidonic acid metabolism, and other proinflammatory pathways. Non-type 2 UAD such as CRS-bronchitis/bronchiectasis and CRSsNP are currently inadequately characterized.

associated with better long-term outcomes, so a high index of suspicion is required. Bloody nasal discharge and crusting are highly suspicious for granulomatous disease, which should also be considered in atypical or recalcitrant disease. A combination of clinical findings, serologic tests, imaging, and histology may be required to confirm the diagnosis.

Primary Ig deficiencies are a heterogeneous group of disorders with widespread implications for the unified airway. Manifestations can vary greatly, with some patients being asymptomatic, whereas others suffering from acute and chronic life-threatening pathologic conditions of the upper and lower airways. Although the diagnosis of PIDs can be complex, the onus of early diagnosis and initiation of treatment will often fall on the shoulders of the otolaryngologist.

Aspirin-exacerbated respiratory disease (AERD) is characterized by abnormal arachidonic acid metabolism leading to chronic rhinosinusitis with nasal polyposis (CRSwNP), asthma, and upper and/or lower respiratory symptoms after ingestion of cyclooxygenase-1 inhibiting nonsteroidal antiinflammatory drugs. Diagnosis is clinical and may involve an aspirin challenge. Inflammatory biomarkers may be useful for diagnosis and treatment monitoring. Conventional medical management for asthma and CRSwNP is often inadequate. Endoscopic sinus surgery followed by continued medical management with or without aspirin desensitization frequently improves symptoms and objective disease measures. Biological agents targeting eosinophilic inflammation are promising alternatives to conventional management.

Cystic fibrosis (CF) is a genetic disease caused by mutations in the cystic fibrosis transmembrane conductance regulator (CFTR) gene. The CFTR channel is responsible for the transport of the anions (chloride and bicarbonate) across airway epithelia. Patients with CF have thick mucus, disrupted mucociliary transport, and chronic bacterial infections in the upper and lower airways. In this article, the pathophysiology of CFTR dysfunction and its impact on the united airway are reviewed as well as the treatment strategies for patients with chronic rhinosinusitis–related CF and acquired CFTR dysfunction.

The unified airway concept is a framework for the understanding and management of the upper and lower airways as one integrated physiologic unit. The sinonasal and bronchopulmonary systems have an interdependent physiologic function, and inflammatory conditions that impact one system tend to impact the other similarly. The application of the unified airway concept in the pediatric population is not well described. This study identifies and characterizes the common manifestations of the pediatric unified airway, including pediatric chronic rhinosinusitis, adenoid disease, asthma, cystic fibrosis, and primary ciliary dyskinesia.

Angela M. Donaldson

Upper airway cough syndrome (UACS), formerly known as postnasal drip syndrome, is one of the most common causes of chronic cough. UACS, asthma, and gastroesophageal reflux make up 90% of the cause of chronic cough. UACS is a clinical diagnosis of exclusion with no diagnostic testing or objective findings. UACS can be present with or without associated rhinitis and chronic rhinosinusitis. Treatment includes dual therapy with H1 receptor antihistamines and decongestants. Diagnosis is confirmed when therapeutic intervention results in symptom resolution.

Eamon Shamil and Claire Hopkins

Concurrent chronic rhinosinusitis with nasal polyps (CRSwNP) in the upper airway, and asthma in the lower airway, often have a shared underlying pathophysiology, namely type 2 inflammation; hence, the term "unified airway disease." The combination of CRSwNP and asthma is associated with uncontrolled disease. The range of treatment of CRSwNP includes intranasal corticosteroids, nasal saline irrigation, oral corticosteroids, antibiotics, and biologics. A combined clinical algorithm for the management of the upper and lower airways in type 2 inflammation will be beneficial, especially for patients with uncontrolled disease who may benefit from biologics.

Amar Miglani, Tripti K. Brar, and Devyani Lal

Support for the unified airway hypothesis is embedded in similarities in upper and lower airway structure, function, and cellular/extracellular compositions. The impact of endoscopic sinus surgery (ESS) on the unified airway is influenced by multiple factors including the underlying upper and lower airway condition(s) present and severity of pathology. Beyond improvements in subjective and objective CRS outcomes, ESS also improves clinical asthma outcomes and measures of asthma control. Emerging evidence suggests that early ESS may mitigate the risk of developing asthma in CRS patients without asthma. Comprehensive management of upper and lower airways is paramount to optimize patient outcomes.

Jumah G. Ahmad, Michael J. Marino, and Amber U. Luong

Unified airway disease describes the shared epidemiologic and pathophysiologic relationship among the chronic inflammatory diseases of the upper and lower airways including allergic rhinitis, chronic rhinosinusitis, asthma, and chronic otitis media. This concept proposes that these diseases are manifestations of a single inflammatory process and require an integrated diagnostic and therapeutic approach to achieve global disease control. Future directions to further establish this entity should focus on pathophysiology, diagnostic markers, flora microbes with particular emphasis on fungi, the role of type 3 inflammation, and targeted therapeutics including biologics, JAK inhibitors, and synthetic peptides.

Unified Airway Disease

OTOLARYNGOLOGIC CLINICS OF NORTH AMERICA

SERIES OF RELATED INTEREST

Facial Plastic Surgery Clinics
Available at: https://www.facialplastic.theclinics.com/

THE CLINICS ARE AVAILABLE ONLINE!
Access your subscription at:
www.theclinics.com

Foreword

Eliminating Artificial Airway Divisions Enhances Patient Outcomes

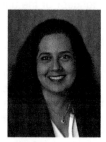

Sujana S. Chandrasekhar, MD, FACS, FAAOHNS
Consulting Editor

In medical school, there are artificial divisions drawn between the upper airway—nose, paranasal sinuses, pharynx, and larynx, and the lower airway—trachea, bronchi, and lungs. Material relating to these organ systems is taught in individual silos of otolaryngology and pulmonology. This separation continues on in the way medicine is practiced. However, patients experience disease that affects both upper and lower airways, and it behooves the astute clinician to understand the airway as a unified phenomenon.

The concept of a unified airway is based on long-standing clinical observations that patients with lower airway disease have a high incidence of upper airway disease as well. In the last two decades, interest has increased in the relationship between the lower and the upper airways and the shared inflammation between the two. Dr Jack Krouse proposed three criteria in support of the theory of the unified airway[1]:

1. Patients with upper airway disease, such as rhinitis and rhinosinusitis, should have a higher prevalence of lower respiratory diseases, such as asthma; the corollary, increased prevalence of upper respiratory disease among patients with lower respiratory diseases, also should be present.
2. Interrelated pathophysiologic mechanisms between upper and lower airway diseases should exist to explain the interaction of these two disease processes.
3. Treatment of one portion of the unified airway should improve symptoms in a separate portion of the respiratory system.

www.ears.nyc

Otolaryngol Clin N Am 56 (2023) xiii–xiv
https://doi.org/10.1016/j.otc.2022.10.001
0030-6665/23/© 2022 Published by Elsevier Inc.

oto.theclinics.com

Drs Devyani Lal, Angela M. Donaldson, and David W. Jang took on the challenge of updating the 2008 issue of *Otolaryngologic Clinics of North America* on the Unified Airway with aplomb. As the original concept is now well-recognized, these Guest Editors selected topics and authors to highlight the advances in knowledge of inflammation and targeted therapies. This 2023 issue explores topics such as diagnosis, why some get airways disease and others do not, including genetics, epigenetics, environmental factors, and sex differences, and various specific airways diseases, and concludes with medical and surgical treatments. I hope that once you read this issue you will feel inclined to share it with your colleagues in pulmonary medicine and allergy/immunology and continue to promote the concept of the unified airway to enhance patient care.

Sujana S. Chandrasekhar, MD, FACS, FAAOHNS
Consulting Editor
Otolaryngologic Clinics of North America
Past President
American Academy of Otolaryngology–
Head and Neck Surgery
Secretary-Treasurer and President-Elect
American Otological Society
Eastern Section Vice President
Triological Society
Partner, ENT & Allergy Associates LLP
18 East 48th Street, 2nd Floor
New York, NY 10017, USA

Clinical Professor
Department of Otolaryngology, Head and Neck Surgery
Zucker School of Medicine at Hofstra–Northwell
Hempstead, NY, USA

Clinical Associate Professor
Department of Otolaryngology, Head and Neck Surgery
Icahn School of Medicine at Mount Sinai
New York, NY, USA

E-mail address:
ssc@nyotology.com

REFERENCES

1. Krouse JH, Brown RW, Fineman SM, et al. Asthma and the unified airway. Otolaryngol Head Neck Surg 2007;136:S75–106.

Preface

The Unified Airway: From Concept to Practice

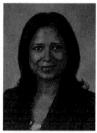 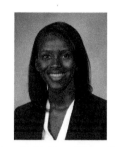 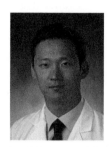

Devyani Lal, MD, FARS   Angela M. Donaldson, MD   David W. Jang, MD
Editors

While the close relationship between upper- and lower-airway disease has been known for centuries, the concept of the unified airway has come to the forefront in the last few decades. The April 2008 issue of *Otolaryngologic Clinics of North America* was dedicated to the unified airway and provided for the otolaryngologist a comprehensive review of the knowledge available at that time on this important concept. A common theme of the issue was the frequent co-occurrence of upper- and lower-airway disease and the need to recognize and treat these conditions concurrently. The concepts discussed highlighted the growing importance of multidisciplinary collaboration for the optimization of patient care.

Nearly fifteen years later, advances in our understanding of airway inflammation have further refined the concept of the unified airway and have led to more targeted medical therapies. With a greater understanding of type 2 inflammation, we have seen the development and widespread use of biologics for the treatment of nasal polyps and asthma. We have also seen the impact of translational medicine on cystic fibrosis patients. The advent of CFTR modulators has transformed the way we manage the unified airway and has improved the quality of life and morbidity of these patients. With these new advances, close collaboration between otolaryngologists, allergists, pulmonologists, and other specialists has become critical for patient care.

This issue of *Otolaryngologic Clinics of North America* provides an updated review of the pathophysiology underlying unified airway disease, specifically, the role of intrinsic factors, such as genetics/epigenetics, age (namely the pediatric population), and sex differences, and extrinsic factors, such as microbial infection and inhalants. Other sections are dedicated to the concept of classification and subtyping, which are now important aspects in the management of chronic rhinosinusitis and asthma. Two articles are dedicated to medical and surgical management of airway disease. Finally,

Otolaryngol Clin N Am 56 (2023) xv–xvi
https://doi.org/10.1016/j.otc.2022.09.017
0030-6665/23/© 2022 Published by Elsevier Inc.

oto.theclinics.com

several articles focus on specific conditions, such as autoimmune granulomatous disease, immunoglobulin deficiency, aspirin-exacerbated respiratory disease, and cystic fibrosis, all of which are conditions that highlight the centrality of the unified airway.

While important themes are repeated throughout this issue, we believe that each set of expert authors presents their ideas from a unique perspective. A new issue dedicated to the unified airway is long overdue, and we hope that the articles can provide the otolaryngologist with a greater appreciation of important concepts as well as real, practical ways to advance everyday patient care.

Devyani Lal, MD, FARS
Otolaryngology–Head & Neck Surgery
Division of Rhinology
Mayo Clinic
Scottsdale, AZ 85259, USA

Angela M. Donaldson, MD
Department of Otolaryngology Head and Neck Surgery
Mayo Clinic
4500 San Pablo Road
Davis 3 East
Jacksonville, FL 32224, USA

David W. Jang, MD
Division of Rhinology and
Endoscopic Skull Base Surgery
Department of Head and Neck Surgery &
Communication Sciences
Duke University
200 Trent Drive, Box 3805
Durham, NC 27710, USA

E-mail addresses:
Lal.Devyani@mayo.edu (D. Lal)
Donaldson.Angela@mayo.edu (A.M. Donaldson)
David.jang@duke.edu (D.W. Jang)

Unified Airway Disease

A Contemporary Review and Introduction

Wytske Fokkens, MD, PhD*, Sietze Reitsma, MD, PhD

KEYWORDS

- Allergic rhinitis • Chronic rhinosinusitis • Asthma • Care-pathways • United airways

KEY POINTS

- Inflammatory diseases of upper and lower airways usually occur together: the "united airways" or "unified airway."
- Allergic rhinitis, chronic rhinosinusitis, and asthma are conditions with high prevalence and significant impact on quality of life.
- Upper and lower airway diseases have similarities in phenotypes and endotypes.
- Treatment should depend on phenotype/endotype.
- The cornerstone of treatment is appropriate medical treatment, which usually consists of at least topical/inhaled corticosteroids.

INTRODUCTION

The upper and lower airways are linked from anatomical, histological, and immunological perspectives and form a united airways system with inflammation in one part of the airways influencing the other part.[1] Various international guidelines such as the Allergic Rhinitis and its Impact on Asthma (ARIA), the International Consensus Statement On Allergy And Rhinology: Allergic Rhinitis And Rhinosinusitis, and the European Position Paper on Rhinosinusitis and Nasal Polyps (EPOS), examine the interaction between the upper and lower airways. The mucosa and submucosa of the upper and lower airways are similar, with differentiators being absence of smooth muscles in the upper airways and the lack of extensive subepithelial capillaries, arterial systems, and venous cavernous sinusoids in the lower airways. Although differing in presenting symptoms, diseases in the upper and lower airways are usually linked with similar immunologic response, with type 2 immunologic endotype being dominant, especially in phenotypes with more severe disease. The development of novel systemic treatments that target specific immune pathways (biologicals) necessitates a contemporaneous, nuanced and thorough understanding of the relationship between upper and lower airways.[2-5]

Department of Otorhinolaryngology, Amsterdam University Medical Centres, Location AMC, Amsterdam, the Netherlands
* Corresponding author.
E-mail address: w.j.fokkens@amsterdamumc.nl

Otolaryngol Clin N Am 56 (2023) 1–10
https://doi.org/10.1016/j.otc.2022.09.001
0030-6665/23/© 2022 Elsevier Inc. All rights reserved.

Due to the systemic nature of these biological treatments, it has become possible to treat multiple affected organs that result from the same underlying inflammatory disease with a single therapeutic agent.

In this article, the inflammatory diseases of the upper and lower airways are discussed. Other syndromes involving both the upper and lower airways such as obstructive sleep apnea syndrome and cystic fibrosis are not considered.

EPIDEMIOLOGY

Both upper and lower airways diseases are extremely common with prevalences of 10% to 40% depending on the diagnosis. Upper airway involvement occurs in 80% to 100% of asthma patients, and 40% (allergic rhinitis [AR]) to 70% (chronic rhinosinusitis [CRS]) of patients with chronic upper airway problems have lower airway involvement. Most studies have reported a link between the severity and/or control of upper and lower airway diseases, and find that asthma is more common in patients with moderate-to-severe persistent rhinitis compared with those with mild rhinitis, and more common in type 2 dominated CRS than in rhinitis. Both chronic upper and lower airway problems have a significant and comparable impact on quality of life[6,7] and patients having both upper and lower airway disease usually have the lowest quality of life[7-9] and are likely to experience higher rates of surgery and more secondary care visits.[10]

PHENOTYPES

The characterization of rhinitis and asthma phenotypes is very similar, with emphasis on the presence or absence of allergy and eosinophilia. Both upper and lower airway phenotypes may show a considerable overlap but in general AR is more associated with allergic and exercise induced asthma, whereas CRS (especially with nasal polyps) associates more with late onset asthma (**Fig. 1**).[11-13] Both AR and asthma are characterized by hyperreactivity that is not correlated to the atopic state.[14-16] Furthermore, nonallergic phenotypes exist in both upper and lower airways.[17]

ENDOTYPES

Although conventionally endotyping with emphasis on type 2 versus nontype 2 immune responses has been used, we must realize that in reality, multiple clusters with more or less type 2-like profiles can be distinguished.[18,19] In allergic disease, but also in a considerable part of the more severe nonallergic airway inflammation, the prominent

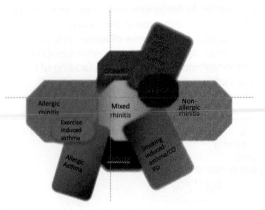

Fig. 1. Phenotypes in upper and lower airways.

endotype is type 2 (Th2 cells, type2 B-cells, IL-4 producing NK(T) cells, basophils, eosinophils, mast cells, ILC2, IL4, IL5, IL13, IL-25, IL-31, IL-33).[20–23] Similarities between upper and lower airways cannot only be found in the acquired immune response[18,24] but also in the role of innate immunity[25] such as epithelial barrier function[26] and innate lymphoid cells (ILCs).[27,28]

The pathophysiological mechanisms of inflammatory airway diseases are connected to large biological networks involving the environment and the host. On the host side of AR, the nasal epithelium is the first to encounter aeroallergens.[29] However, disruption of the passive structural barrier function of the epithelium by intrinsic proteolytic activity of allergens may facilitate allergen penetration into local tissues and lead to chronic and ongoing inflammatory processes.[30] Recent data provided evidence that also intrinsic barrier dysfunction contributes to the development of inflammatory diseases such as AR, CRS, and asthma.[31–34] Yet, it remains to be elucidated to what extent primary (genetic) versus secondary (inflammatory) mechanisms drive barrier dysfunction. However, epithelial cells do not only act as a physical barrier toward inhaled allergens but are shown to also contribute to airway inflammation actively by detecting and responding to environmental factors. The nasal epithelium expresses pattern recognition receptors in the form of toll-like receptors[35,36] that after activation by allergens or pathogens lead to the production of different mediators. These mediators affect recruitment of inflammatory cells to local tissues and create a microenvironment that affects the function of immune cells, thereby propagating local inflammatory processes.[37] In allergic disease, the nasal epithelium seems to be in a permanently activated state,[38] potentially as a consequence of the inability to switch off the activation response.[39]

An exciting recent development was the discovery of ILCs as potential key players in the pathogenesis of Th2 type diseases, such as AR, CRS with nasal polyps, and asthma.[27,40,41] ILCs are a family of effector cells that are important for protection against infiltrating pathogens and restoration of tissue integrity. ILCs do not express antigen-specific T cell receptors but can react promptly to "danger signals" and produce an array of cytokines that direct ensuing immune responses. Three major subsets have been defined based on their phenotype and functional similarities to Th1 (ILC1), Th2 (ILC2), and Th17 (ILC3) cells. On exposure to environmental antigens, including viruses and allergens, airway epithelial cells rapidly release the cytokines IL-25, IL-33, and TSLP. These so-called alarmins directly activate ILC2s, which then produce the prototypical type 2 cytokines IL-5 and IL-13.[42] As such, blocking epithelial factors of the innate immune system, such as anti-TSLP, may be more effective than the more downstream monoclonal antibodies available at the moment.

PATHOPHYSIOLOGICAL MECHANISMS BETWEEN UPPER AND LOWER AIRWAYS

The mucosa of the upper and lower airways is similar, with pseudostratified epithelium with columnar, ciliated cells located on a basement membrane. In the submucosa, there are vessels, mucus glands, fibroblasts, and some inflammatory cells.

Significant differences include the absence of smooth muscles in the upper airways as compared with the lower airways, and the lack of extensive subepithelial capillaries, arterial systems, and venous cavernous sinusoids in the lower airways as compared with the upper airways.

Several mechanisms may explain the influence of the diseased nose on the lower airways, that is, altered breathing pattern, pulmonary aspiration of nasal contents, the nasal–bronchial reflex, and the uptake of inflammatory mediators in the systemic circulation.[43]

The nose acts as a filter and air conditioner, thereby protecting the lower airways. The reduced filter and air-conditioning function of the nose may lead to increased exposure of the lower airways to allergens. Mouth breathing is independently associated with asthma morbidity[44] indicating that air conditioning can be of major importance. The efficacy of the nose filter depends on the size of the inhaled particles. Small molecules, such as molds and cat dander, are more associated with an increased risk for asthma, whereas larger molecules, such as tree and grass pollen, are primarily associated with upper airway symptoms. Therefore, the role of preferential mouth breathing in the development of asthma is unclear.[45]

Although there is a clear relationship between postnasal drip and coughing, no direct contact has been proven between nasal secretions and bronchial mucosa. In contrast, after nasal application, deposits of radioactive labeled allergen can be found in the digestive tract but not in the respiratory tract. Stimulation of pharyngolaryngeal receptors is more likely to be responsible for a postnasal drip–related cough.[45] Interestingly, cough is not induced in rhinitis subjects or healthy controls when artificial postnasal drip was created.[46]

There is not much evidence supporting the nasobronchial reflex as an important contributor to the unified airways. A nasal allergen challenge can be blocked with a vasoconstrictor but not with lidocaine; moreover, the lower airway responses after allergen challenge are in general more delayed than would be expected following a nasobronchial reflex.[45]

Allergen provocation studies are a good model to study nasobronchial cross talk in allergic airway disease. In patients with AR, segmental bronchial provocation, as well as nasal provocation, induced allergic inflammation in both the nasal and bronchial mucosa.[47–49] Presumably, absorption of inflammatory mediators (eg, IL-5 and eotaxin) from sites of inflammation into the systemic circulation results in the release of eosinophils, basophils, and their progenitor cells from the bone marrow.[50] The systemic allergic response is further characterized by increased expression of adhesion molecules, such as vascular cell adhesion molecule 1 and E-selectin, on nasal and bronchial endothelium, which facilitates the migration of inflammatory cells into the tissue.[49]

Increases in CD34+ cells capable of eosinophil differentiation, as well as other circulatory mediators (IL-5, eotaxin, and cysteinyl leukotrienes), are associated with impaired lung function parameters and enhanced mucosal inflammation in asthmatic patients[50] and react to local corticosteroids in rhinitis patients.[51] In conclusion, these studies demonstrate that AR is not a local disease but that the complete respiratory tract is involved, even in the absence of clinical asthma. Systemic factors, such as the number of blood eosinophils and atopy severity, are indicative of more extensive airway disease.

There are very few studies evaluating the mechanistic aspects of this influence of CRS on the lower airways. Frequent severe exacerbations in patients with eosinophilic asthma are independently associated with high Lund-Mackay scores on CT.[52] The presence of specific IgE to Staphylococcal enterotoxins is associated with severe asthma defined by hospitalizations, oral steroid use and decrease in lung function, and even associated with the development into severe asthma with exacerbations.[53] The exact mechanism of these associations in the development of (severe) asthma needs further evaluation.

DIAGNOSIS

The united airways concept has important implications for the diagnosis and treatment of disorders of the upper and lower airways. In the diagnosis, continuous attention to the complete airway (and sometimes to all manifestations of the atopic syndrome) is important. Any patient with rhinitis or rhinosinusitis should have their lower respiratory tract evaluated. It is also important to pay attention to good treatment, adequate use of medication, and compliance with known asthma. Conversely, it can be assumed that every patient with asthma also has at least rhinitis and in late-onset asthma usually rhinosinusitis.

The use of standardized questionnaires (such as SNOT-22 for CRS, and ACQ for asthma) in the doctor's office optimizes attention for the united airways.

A multidisciplinary approach in the diagnosis and treatment of airway disease is advised.

BIOMARKERS

The cellular, biochemical, or molecular changes in patients that are measurable in secretions, sputum and/or blood, can be considered as biomarkers.[54] These biomarkers are used for disease diagnosis, selection of targeted therapy, disease monitoring, and prediction of prognosis.[55] Often used biomarkers to identify type 2 disease are IgE, eosinophilia, and in the lower airways fractional exhaled nitric oxide (FeNO). Unfortunately, nasal NO is not reliable to identify inflammatory upper airway disease,[56,57] probably because of the interaction between NO production in the sinuses and the closure of their ostia in disease. It is important to realize that biomarkers measured in blood are dependent on the size of the shock organ and thus are often more reliable for asthma than for diseases of the upper airways. The measurement of local biomarkers is the most reliable. Research focusing on proinflammatory mediators, genes, the epithelial barrier, and microbiomes is now emerging. Some of the biomarkers showing a strong ability to identify disease endotypes or phenotypes may also act as therapeutic targets.

TREATMENT

Various international guidelines have emphasized the use of integrated care pathways and the importance of the united airways when considering treatment.

To arrive at an optimal personalized treatment, good coordination between the specialisms involved is essential. This can be done in various ways: by doing a joint outpatient clinic in which several specialists see a patient together, or by discussing it in a multidisciplinary meeting. Several aspects need to be addressed in this regard.

ASPECTS TO BE ADDRESSED WHEN TREATING THE UNITED AIRWAYS

- Determining the nature and seriousness of the respiratory complaints
- Relevant comorbidity
- Illness insight (adherence to treatment/treatment willingness)
- Lifestyle (smoking, overweight, exercise pattern)
- Therapeutic options (local vs systemic)
- Personal wishes of the patient

The ARIA, EPOS2020, and GINA guidelines can help with the choice of treatment if necessary. ENT specialists and pulmonologists can be expected to have at least a general practitioner's command of the treatment of the part of the airways that is not their primary expertise. For pulmonologists, this means that in all patients with asthma, a proper history of the upper airways is considered. Moreover, nasal corticosteroids are to be prescribed whenever type 2 disease is likely. When there is evidence of CRS, patients should in addition to the nasal corticosteroids be advised to rinse the nose with NaCl. If this has insufficient effect, consultation/referral to an ENT specialist is necessary.

For otorhinolaryngologists, this means that awareness of asthma, appropriate diagnosis (or referral) with peak flow measurements, spirometry and/or FeNO, and first-line treatment with inhaled corticosteroids combined with (long-acting) broncho dilatators as needed is recommended (GINA).[58]

TREATMENT EFFECTS ON THE UNITED AIRWAYS

Data on the effect of treating the upper airways on the lower airways are limited.

Intranasal corticosteroids (INCS) significantly improve some asthma-specific outcome measures in patients suffering from both AR and asthma.[59] This effect was most pronounced with INCS sprays when patients were not on orally inhaled corticosteroids, or when corticosteroid medications were inhaled through the nose into the lungs.

A systemic review evaluated the prevention of asthma by allergen immunotherapy (AIT).[60] The review supported a possible preventive effect of AIT in asthma onset and suggested an enhanced effect when administered in children, monosensitized, and for at least 3 years, independent of allergen type.

Endoscopic sinus surgery in CRS patients with concomitant bronchial asthma improves clinical asthma outcome measures,[61] and lung function testing (forced expiratory volume at 1 second and peak expiratory flow). However, the quality of the evidence is low.[62] There is some indication that early sinus surgery may prevent the development and severity of asthma.[63] Data on the effect of nasal corticosteroid treatment of CRS on asthma are limited but do not seem to have a positive effect.[64]

Systemic treatment such as systemic corticosteroids and biologicals has positive effects on symptoms of upper and lower airways.[65–69] However, they either have significant side effects or high costs and are therefore only appropriate for a limited group of patients.

SUMMARY

- Inflammatory diseases of upper and lower airways usually occur together: the united airways.
- AR, CRS, and asthma are conditions with high prevalence and significant impact on quality of life.
- Upper and lower airway diseases have similar phenotypes and endotypes.
- Comorbid upper and lower airway diseases are usually caused by similar underlying immunologic response.
- Any patient with rhinitis or rhinosinusitis should have their lower respiratory tract evaluated. Conversely, every patient with asthma also has at least rhinitis and in late-onset asthma usually rhinosinusitis.
- Treatment should depend on phenotype/endotype.
- The cornerstone of treatment is appropriate medical treatment that usually consists of at least topical/inhaled corticosteroids.
- (Timely) treatment of the upper airways reduces asthma symptoms and may prevent asthma to develop.

DISCLOSURE

The Department of Otorhinolaryngology of the Amsterdam University Medical centers, location AMC received grants for research in Rhinology from: ALK, AllergyTherapeutics, Chordate, Novartis, EU, GSK, MYLAN, Sanofi-Aventis, and Zon-MW; Prof Dr Wytske Fokkens received consultation and/or speaker fees from Bioinspire, GSK, Novartis, and Sanofi-Aventis/Regeneron. Dr. Sietze Reitsma: received consultation and/or speaker fees from GSK, Novartis, and Sanofi-Aventis/Regeneron.

ACKNOWLEDGMENTS

The authors than the Amsterdam Rhino Team for their help in research.

REFERENCES

1. Genuneit J, Seibold AM, Apfelbacher CJ, et al. Overview of systematic reviews in allergy epidemiology. Allergy 2017;7:12. https://doi.org/10.1186/s13601-017-0146-y.
2. Hellings PW, Verhoeven E, Fokkens WJ. State-of-the-art overview on biological treatment for CRSwNP. Rhinology 2021;59(2):151–63.
3. Agache I, Beltran J, Akdis C, et al. Efficacy and safety of treatment with biologicals (benralizumab, dupilumab, mepolizumab, omalizumab and reslizumab) for severe eosinophilic asthma. A systematic review for the EAACI Guidelines - recommendations on the use of biologicals in severe asthma. Allergy 2020; 75(5):1023–42.
4. Shamji MH, Palmer E, Layhadi JA, et al. Biological treatment in allergic disease. Allergy 2021;76(9):2934–7.
5. Desrosiers M, Mannent LP, Amin N, et al. Dupilumab reduces systemic corticosteroid use and sinonasal surgery rate in CRSwNP. Rhinology 2021;59(3):301–11.
6. Leynaert B, Neukirch C, Liard R, et al. Quality of life in allergic rhinitis and asthma. A population-based study of young adults. Am J Respir Crit Care Med 2000; 162(4 Pt 1):1391–6.
7. Fokkens WJ, Lund VJ, Hopkins C, et al. European position paper on rhinosinusitis and nasal polyps 2020. Rhinology 2020;58(Suppl S29):1–464.
8. Linneberg A, Dam Petersen K, Hahn-Pedersen J, et al. Burden of allergic respiratory disease: a systematic review. Clin Mol Allergy 2016;14:12.
9. Khan A, Huynh TMT, Vandeplas G, et al. The GALEN rhinosinusitis cohort: chronic rhinosinusitis with nasal polyps affects health-related quality of life. Rhinology 2019;57(5):343–51.
10. Hopkins C, Conlon S, Chavda S, et al. Investigating the secondary care system burden of CRSwNP in sinus surgery patients with clinically relevant comorbidities using the HES database. Rhinology 2022;60(4):252–60.
11. Akdis CA, Bachert C, Cingi C, et al. Endotypes and phenotypes of chronic rhinosinusitis: a PRACTALL document of the European Academy of Allergy and Clinical Immunology and the American Academy of Allergy, Asthma & Immunology. J Allergy Clin Immunol 2013;131(6):1479–90.
12. Asano K, Ueki S, Tamari M, et al. Adult-onset eosinophilic airway diseases. Allergy 2020;75(12):3087–99.
13. Kanda A, Kobayashi Y, Asako M, et al. Regulation of interaction between the upper and lower airways in united airway disease. Med Sci (Basel) 2019;7(2):27. https://doi.org/10.3390/medsci7020027.
14. Backaert W, Steelant B, Jorissen M, et al. Self-reported nasal hyperreactivity is common in all chronic upper airway inflammatory phenotypes and not related to general well-being. Allergy 2021;76(12):3806–9.
15. Feijen J, Seys SF, Steelant B, et al. Prevalence and triggers of self-reported nasal hyperreactivity in adults with asthma. World Allergy Organ J 2020;13(6):100132.
16. Doulaptsi M, Steelant B, Prokopakis E, et al. Prevalence and impact of nasal hyperreactivity in chronic rhinosinusitis. Allergy 2020;75(7):1768–71.
17. Avdeeva KS, Fokkens WJ, Reitsma S. Towards a new epidemiological definition of chronic rhinitis: prevalence of nasal complaints in the general population. Rhinology 2021;59(3):258–66.

18. Tomassen P, Vandeplas G, Van Zele T, et al. Inflammatory endotypes of chronic rhinosinusitis based on cluster analysis of biomarkers. J Allergy Clin Immunol 2016;137(5):1449–56, e4.
19. Stevens WW, Peters AT, Tan BK, et al. Associations between inflammatory endotypes and clinical presentations in chronic rhinosinusitis. J Allergy Clin Immunol Pract 2019;7(8):2812–20.e3.
20. Agache I, Sugita K, Morita H, et al. The Complex type 2 endotype in allergy and asthma: from laboratory to bedside. Curr Allergy Asthma Rep 2015;15(6):29.
21. Papadopoulos NG, Bernstein JA, Demoly P, et al. Phenotypes and endotypes of rhinitis and their impact on management: a PRACTALL report. Allergy 2015;70(5):474–94.
22. Viiu B, Christer J, Fredrik S, et al. Asthma in combination with rhinitis and eczema is associated with a higher degree of type-2 inflammation and symptom burden than asthma alone. Allergy 2021;76(12):3827–9.
23. Hong H, Liao S, Chen F, et al. Role of IL-25, IL-33, and TSLP in triggering united airway diseases toward type 2 inflammation. Allergy 2020;75(11):2794–804.
24. Kato A, Peters AT, Stevens WW, et al. Endotypes of chronic rhinosinusitis: Relationships to disease phenotypes, pathogenesis, clinical findings, and treatment approaches. Allergy 2022;77(3):812–26.
25. Cho HJ, Ha JG, Lee SN, et al. Differences and similarities between the upper and lower airway: focusing on innate immunity. Rhinology 2021;59(5):441–50.
26. Steelant B, Seys SF, Boeckxstaens G, et al. Restoring airway epithelial barrier dysfunction: a new therapeutic challenge in allergic airway disease. Rhinology 2016;54(3):195–205.
27. Scadding GK, Scadding GW. Innate and adaptive immunity: ILC2 and Th2 Cells in upper and lower airway allergic diseases. J Allergy Clin Immunol Pract 2021;9(5):1851–7.
28. van der Ploeg EK, Golebski K, van Nimwegen M, et al. Steroid-resistant human inflammatory ILC2s are marked by CD45RO and elevated in type 2 respiratory diseases. Sci Immunol 2021;6(55):eabd3489.
29. Stamataki S, Papadopoulos NG, Lakoumentas J, et al. Nasal epithelium: new insights and differences of the cytokine profile between normal subjects and subjects with allergic rhinitis. Rhinology Online 2021;4:223–32.
30. Bashir ME, Ward JM, Cummings M, et al. Dual function of novel pollen coat (surface) proteins: IgE-binding capacity and proteolytic activity disrupting the airway epithelial barrier. PLoS One 2013;8(1):e53337.
31. Steelant B, Farre R, Wawrzyniak P, et al. Impaired barrier function in patients with house dust mite-induced allergic rhinitis is accompanied by decreased occludin and zonula occludens-1 expression. J Allergy Clin Immunol 2016;137(4):1043–53.e1-5.
32. Hellings PW, Steelant B. Epithelial barriers in allergy and asthma. J Allergy Clin Immunol 2020;145(6):1499–509.
33. Tuli JF, Ramezanpour M, Cooksley C, et al. Association between mucosal barrier disruption by Pseudomonas aeruginosa exoproteins and asthma in patients with chronic rhinosinusitis. Allergy 2021;76(11):3459–69.
34. Kao SS, Ramezanpour M, Bassiouni A, et al. Barrier disruptive effects of mucus isolated from chronic rhinosinusitis patients. Allergy 2020;75(1):200–3.
35. van Tongeren J, Golebski K, Van Egmond D, et al. Synergy between TLR-2 and TLR-3 signaling in primary human nasal epithelial cells. Immunobiology 2015;220(4):445–51.

36. Radman M, Golshiri A, Shamsizadeh A, et al. Toll-like receptor 4 plays significant roles during allergic rhinitis. Allergologia et Immunopathologia 2015;43(4): 416–20.
37. van Tongeren J, Roschmann KI, Reinartz SM, et al. Expression profiling and functional analysis of Toll-like receptors in primary healthy human nasal epithelial cells shows no correlation and a refractory LPS response. Clin Translational Allergy 2015;5:42.
38. Vroling AB, Jonker MJ, Luiten S, et al. Primary nasal epithelium exposed to house dust mite extract shows activated expression in allergic individuals. Am J Respir Cell Mol Biol 2008;38(3):293–9.
39. Golebski K, van Egmond D, de Groot EJ, et al. EGR-1 and DUSP-1 are important negative regulators of pro-allergic responses in airway epithelium. Mol Immunol 2015;65(1):43–50.
40. Mjosberg JM, Trifari S, Crellin NK, et al. Human IL-25- and IL-33-responsive type 2 innate lymphoid cells are defined by expression of CRTH2 and CD161. Nat Immunol 2011;12(11):1055–62.
41. Kortekaas Krohn I, Shikhagaie MM, Golebski K, et al. Emerging roles of innate lymphoid cells in inflammatory diseases: Clinical implications. Allergy 2018; 73(4):837–50.
42. Karta MR, Broide DH, Doherty TA. Insights into group 2 innate lymphoid cells in human airway disease. Curr Allergy Asthma Rep 2016;16(1):8.
43. Braunstahl GJ, Fokkens W. Nasal involvement in allergic asthma. Allergy 2003; 58(12):1235–43.
44. Izuhara Y, Matsumoto H, Nagasaki T, et al. Mouth breathing, another risk factor for asthma: the Nagahama Study. Allergy 2016;71(7):1031–6.
45. Braunstahl GJ. United airways concept: what does it teach us about systemic inflammation in airways disease? Proc Am Thorac Soc 2009;6(8):652–4.
46. Rimmer J, Hellgren J, Harvey RJ. Simulated postnasal mucus fails to reproduce the symptoms of postnasal drip in rhinitics but only in healthy subjects. Rhinology 2015;53(2):129–34.
47. Braunstahl GJ, Kleinjan A, Overbeek SE, et al. Segmental bronchial provocation induces nasal inflammation in allergic rhinitis patients. Am J Respir Crit Care Med 2000;161(6):2051–7.
48. Braunstahl GJ, Overbeek SE, Fokkens WJ, et al. Segmental bronchoprovocation in allergic rhinitis patients affects mast cell and basophil numbers in nasal and bronchial mucosa. Am J Respir Crit Care Med 2001;164(5):858–65.
49. Braunstahl GJ, Overbeek SE, Kleinjan A, et al. Nasal allergen provocation induces adhesion molecule expression and tissue eosinophilia in upper and lower airways. J Allergy Clin Immunol 2001;107(3):469–76.
50. Allakhverdi Z, Comeau MR, Smith DE, et al. CD34+ hemopoietic progenitor cells are potent effectors of allergic inflammation. J Allergy Clin Immunol 2009;123(2): 472–8.
51. Sergejeva S, Malmhall C, Lotvall J, et al. Increased number of CD34+ cells in nasal mucosa of allergic rhinitis patients: inhibition by a local corticosteroid. Clin Exp Allergy 2005;35(1):34–8.
52. de Groot JC, Amelink M, de Nijs SB, et al. Risk factors for frequent severe exacerbations in late-onset eosinophilic asthma. Am J Respir Crit Care Med 2015; 192(7):899–902.
53. Bachert C, Humbert M, Hanania NA, et al. Staphylococcus aureus and its IgE-inducing enterotoxins in asthma: current knowledge. Eur Respir J 2020;55(4): 1901592.

54. Breiteneder H, Peng YQ, Agache I, et al. Biomarkers for diagnosis and prediction of therapy responses in allergic diseases and asthma. Allergy 2020;75(12): 3039–68.

55. Ogulur I, Pat Y, Ardicli O, et al. Advances and highlights in biomarkers of allergic diseases. Allergy 2021;76(12):3659–86.

56. Ambrosino P, Molino A, Spedicato GA, et al. Nasal nitric oxide in chronic rhinosinusitis with or without nasal polyps: a systematic review with meta-analysis. J Clin Med 2020;9(1):200.

57. Rimmer J, Hellings P, Lund VJ, et al. European position paper on diagnostic tools in rhinology. Rhinology 2019;57(Suppl S28):1–41.

58. Reddel HK, Bacharier LB, Bateman ED, et al. Global initiative for asthma strategy 2021: executive summary and rationale for key changes. Eur Respir J 2022;59(1): 2102730.

59. Lohia S, Schlosser RJ, Soler ZM. Impact of intranasal corticosteroids on asthma outcomes in allergic rhinitis: a meta-analysis. Allergy 2013;68(5):569–79.

60. Farraia M, Paciência I, Castro Mendes F, et al. Allergen immunotherapy for asthma prevention: A systematic review and meta-analysis of randomized and non-randomized controlled studies. Allergy 2022;77(6):1719–35.

61. Vashishta R, Soler ZM, Nguyen SA, et al. A systematic review and meta-analysis of asthma outcomes following endoscopic sinus surgery for chronic rhinosinusitis. Int Forum Allergy Rhinology 2013;3(10):788–94.

62. Cao Y, Hong H, Sun Y, et al. The effects of endoscopic sinus surgery on pulmonary function in chronic rhinosinusitis patients with asthma: a systematic review and meta-analysis. Eur Arch Otorhinolaryngol 2019;276(5):1405–11.

63. Hopkins C, Rimmer J, Lund VJ. Does time to endoscopic sinus surgery impact outcomes in Chronic Rhinosinusitis? Prospective findings from the National Comparative Audit of Surgery for Nasal Polyposis and Chronic Rhinosinusitis. Rhinology 2015;53(1):10–7.

64. Dixon AE, Castro M, Cohen RI, et al. Efficacy of nasal mometasone for the treatment of chronic sinonasal disease in patients with inadequately controlled asthma. J Allergy Clin Immunol 2015;135(3):701–9.e5.

65. Agache I, Song Y, Alonso-Coello P, et al. Efficacy and safety of treatment with biologicals for severe chronic rhinosinusitis with nasal polyps: a systematic review for the EAACI guidelines. Allergy 2021;76(8):2337–53.

66. Maspero JF, FitzGerald JM, Pavord ID, et al. Dupilumab efficacy in adolescents with uncontrolled, moderate-to-severe asthma: LIBERTY ASTHMA QUEST. Allergy 2021;76(8):2621–4.

67. Mullol J, Laidlaw TM, Bachert C, et al. Efficacy and safety of dupilumab in patients with uncontrolled severe chronic rhinosinusitis with nasal polyps and a clinical diagnosis of NSAID-ERD: Results from two randomized placebo-controlled phase 3 trials. Allergy 2022;77(4):1231–44.

68. van der Lans RJL, Fokkens WJ, Adriaensen G, et al. Real-life observational cohort verifies high efficacy of dupilumab for chronic rhinosinusitis with nasal polyps. Allergy 2022;77(2):670–4.

69. Hox V, Lourijsen E, Jordens A, et al. Benefits and harm of systemic steroids for short- and long-term use in rhinitis and rhinosinusitis: an EAACI position paper. Clin Translational Allergy 2020;10:1.

Unified Airway Disease
Diagnosis and Subtyping

Amar Miglani, MD[a], Devyani Lal, MD[a],
Rohit D. Divekar, MBBS PhD[b],*

KEYWORDS

- Unified airway • Unified airway disease • Chronic rhinosinusitis
- Aspirin exacerbated respiratory disease • Asthma • Nasal polyps

KEY POINTS

- Diagnostic tests in chronic rhinosinusitis can benefit from a frame work of unified airways approach.
- Unified airways approach to chronic rhinosinusitis, allows for possible characterization of underlying pathology.
- Unified approach can be applied to a diagnostic tests on variety of biospecimens as well as functional and imaging studies.

Approaching inflammatory airway disorders with a conceptual framework of the unified airway allows the diagnostician to complement the patient history and physical examination with a set of diagnostic tests and tools to better characterize the underlying pathology. Illumination of underlying mechanisms allows for a personalized approach with targeted or biomarker-based therapy to ameliorate symptoms. This especially is true with regard to biologic therapy, which have precise inhibitory effects on the inflammatory pathways.[2] Several biologicals that have been used in asthma have found application to the management of chronic sinusitis.[3] The underlying immune signatures that are common to these diseases also underlie the foundation of the unified airway hypothesis. The approach (**Fig. 1**) to diagnosis and appropriate subtyping of unified airway disease should include clinical history, physical examination, and appropriate clinical testing that may include imaging, allergy testing, PFT, laboratory testing, and genetics.

Clinical history: Clinical history provides valuable information and is the first step in directing subsequent workups. Relevant history that can guide upper and lower airway disease subtyping includes the age of onset, presence of unified airway symptoms (ie,

Disclosures: None.
[a] Department of Otolaryngology-Head & Neck Surgery, Mayo Clinic Arizona, USA; [b] Division of Allergic Diseases, Mayo Clinic Rochester, 200 1st Street, MN 55905, USA
* Corresponding author.
E-mail address: Divekar.Rohit@mayo.edu

Otolaryngol Clin N Am 56 (2023) 11–22
https://doi.org/10.1016/j.otc.2022.09.015
0030-6665/23/© 2022 Elsevier Inc. All rights reserved.

oto.theclinics.com

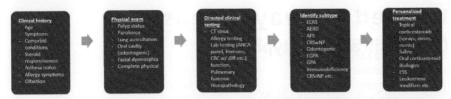

Fig. 1. Approach to personalized management. CBC w/diff, complete blood count with differential; CRSsNP, chronic rhinosinusitis without nasal polyps; ESS, endoscopic sinus surgery.

chronic rhinosinusitis [CRS] and asthma symptoms), laterality of symptoms in regards to sinus disease, the trajectory of disease course (progressive vs chronic with acute flares), presence of olfactory impairment, presence of comorbid atopic conditions, and responsive to medications (particularly steroids).[4,5] A prototypical example is the eosinophilic unified airway disease patient that presents in their 40s to 50s with new-onset asthma and CRS symptoms. Olfactory dysfunction is a common complaint, and these patients tend to be very steroid responsive with improvements in asthma and upper airway symptoms (olfaction and congestion). This subtype of unified airway disease tends to present with chronic symptoms with periodic acute flares. A subset of these patients may have aspirin sensitivity or note nasal congestion with certain foods or alcohol. A distinct unified airway subtype that is also type 2 inflammation dominant are patients with allergic asthma and CRS that is immunoglobulin E (IgE) mediated—these patients are referred to as having central compartment atopic disease (CCAD). These patients present much younger in (youth/teens/20s) with allergic asthma. Classically, olfactory dysfunction is not a major complaint for them; however, they also tend to be steroid responsive. Sinonasal symptoms that dominate include congestion, itch, sneeze, and rhinorrhea. Lastly, there are non-type 2 dominant unified airway inflammatory conditions that can also present with similar symptoms; however, these patients also tend to be older (50s to 60s) and nonsteroid responsive. There are also associations between obesity and female gender in this subtype of patients. Lastly, it is important to perform a thorough review of symptoms as secondary subtypes of unified airway diseases such as immunodeficiency, medium vessel vasculitides (granulomatous with polyangiitis [GPA] and eosinophilic granulomatous with polyangiitis [EGPA]), and genetic disorders (cystic fibrosis [CF] and primary ciliary dyskinesia [PCD]) may present with systemic symptoms that can direct further diagnostic testing.[1]

PHYSICAL EXAMINATION

Physical examination may further direct diagnostic testing in efforts to accurately subtype patients. Important features associated with disease subtypes/endotypes include polyp status, presence of purulence/edema, and signs of eosinophil activation (such as allergic mucin). In developed countries, polyps have a strong association with type 2 inflammation; however, in more developing countries such as China, polyps are skewed toward type 1 inflammation.[6] Polyps are associated with various subtypes of CRS including eosinophilic CRS (eCRS), aspirin exacerbated respiratory disease (AERD), CCAD, CF, and EGPA, among others. However, it is evident that patients with these subtypes may present with or without polyps in varying frequencies. Although there has been a shift away from polyp status within some national guidelines, polyp status remains a useful biomarker for type 2 inflammation in appropriate geographic regions.[4] Auscultation of the lungs for signs of lower airway disease (wheeze and ronchi) may further help narrow the differential for disease subtypes as certain primary and secondary CRS subtypes such as ecRS, allergic fungal sinusitis (AFS), AERD, CF, PCD, EGPA, GPA, immunodeficiency, among others are associated with lower airway disease. Although it is important to focus on upper and lower airway examination, a complete physical examination should be performed. Facial dysmorphia can be present in patients with AFS and in patients with expanding mucoceles; therefore, complete facial examination should be performed. Oral cavity examination may elucidate an odontogenic source of CRS. Several secondary types of diffuse CRS may present with systemic findings such as saddle nose, peripheral neuropathies, cardiac disease, pulmonary disease, central nervous system degeneration, susceptibility to infections, weight loss, and failure to thrive.

Diagnostic Tests and Unified Airway

Even though it is routine practice to disengage upper airway inflammation (managed by otorhinolaryngologist or allergist specializing in rhinitis and sinusitis) and lower airway inflammation manifesting as asthma or other inflammatory airways disorders (managed by pulmonologist or allergist with special interest in asthma), a diagnostic approach to characterization of underlying inflammation common to both upper and lower airway provides for a holistic picture. Even though disease may be predominantly in one part of the airway, subtle impacts on the other parts of the respiratory tract may become clinically significant over longer period. Chronic sinusitis will often coexist with lower airway inflammation such as asthma.[6] In a small study of 25 patients, 60% of patients with CRS were shown to have associated lower airway involvement, that is, 24% had asthma and 36% had small airway disease.[7] Conversely, more than 40% of asthmatics have CRS[8] and 15% of patients with AERD are unaware of nonsteroidal anti-inflammatory drug/Acetylsalicylic acid (Aspirin) intolerance and will be diagnosed only after ASA challenge.[9] Accurate diagnostic phenotyping will acquire utilization of more than one modality and diagnostic tests involve in more than 1 part of the airway. For example, diagnosis of chronic sinusitis rests on presence of subjective as well as objective finding showed and a CT scan or rhinolaryngoscopy[4] and

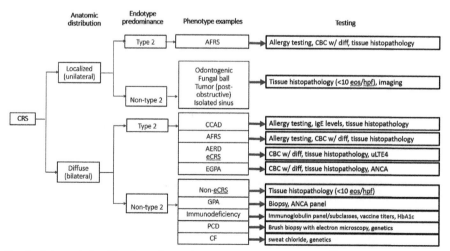

Fig. 2. Adapted classification scheme from Harvey and colleagues[45] and EPOS 2020[4] that highlights potentially clinically useful testing by CRS subtype. AFRS, allergic fungal rhinosinusitis.

quantification of asthma severity requires objective testing such as spirometry and assessment of forced expiratory volume in 1 second (FEV1).[10]

The following diagnostic tests are part of the tool kit that a clinician can use for sub-phenotyping underlying disease in upper and lower airway inflammation.

There has been a shift toward classifying upper and lower airway pathology by incorporating underlying disease endotype. With the development of prognostic and therapeutic biomarkers and a better understanding of disease endotypes, we are likely to see more personalized care pathways for upper and lower airway disease moving forward. **Fig. 2** is an adapted image from EPOS 2020 document on CRS that classifies CRS subtypes by localization of disease and endotype dominance.[4] This adapted figure organizes potentially useful diagnostic testing by CRS subtypes.

IMAGING AND RADIOLOGY

CT scan of the paranasal sinuses. CT scan of the sinuses allows for appreciation of presence of polyps, thereby allowing classification of the sinus disease into CRS with nasal polyps versus that without. CT scans are also a useful adjunct to the diagnosis of AFS.[11] In addition, isolated involvement of the sinuses especially maxillary might point to a local anatomic cause such as odontogenic sinusitis with maxillary sinusitis,[12] and isolated sphenoid sinusitis with fungal sinusitis. Sinus imaging of the paranasal sinuses allows characterization of the sinonasal inflammation and assists in diagnosis.

CT scan of the chest, normal, and expiratory views. CT scan of the chest allows for assessment of pulmonary architecture with regards to comorbid pulmonary conditions that can coexist with inflammatory sinus disease. For example, CT scan of the lungs can show accurate phenomena such as air trapping, bronchiolitis, in severe asthma, and excessive dynamic collapse of the airway, especially in expiratory views in tracheobronchomalacia.[13] Asthma is often associated with eosinophilic or atopic inflammation and can coexist with chronic sinusitis. CT scan of the chest is not used for diagnosis of asthma but can provide important clues that can further delineate the subtype.[14] Additional CT scan findings such as bronchiectasis that can be associated with profound inflammation of the airways as seen with immunodeficiency, and genetic disorders that can present with sinopulmonary syndromes.

Other imaging. CT scan is the standard imaging for the diagnosis of sinusitis; however, in complicated sinusitis with intracranial or orbital involvement MRI frequently is necessary.[15]

ASSESSMENT OF AIRWAY FUNCTION

Spirometry. Airflow limitation is a characteristic of diseases such as asthma (reversible), chronic obstructive pulmonary disease, and bronchiectasis (less than reversible). Spirometry allows for the measurement of several parameters that can not only help diagnose asthma but also assist in quantifying the severity of airflow limitation based on FEV1. In addition, response to bronchodilator can also be documented, with the significant response being 12% or more and more than 200 mL improvement compared with pre-bronchodilator FEV1.[16]

PFT with lung volumes and DLCO (Diffusing capacity for carbon monoxide). PFTs allow for accurate characterization of pulmonary function beyond the spirometry assessment. They allow for the measurement of lung volumes, lung capacities, and diffusion capacity across the alveolar membrane. PFTs are a crucial component of pulmonary assessment in case of lower airway symptoms that often accompany upper airway inflammation. Patients who undergo Functional Endoscopic Sinus Surgery

(FESS) have shown to have a variable improvement in either the pulmonary function assessments or symptom improvement without objective improvement in pulmonary function.[17,18] In any case, the impact of lower airway involvement on their symptoms needs to be assessed and spirometry and PFTs are a crucial component of this unified approach to CRS.

Bronchial provocation tests. Bronchial provocation with methacholine, mannitol, or other measures is useful to show airway hyperresponsiveness that often accompanies lower airway inflammation in diseases such as asthma. Methacholine challenge used as increasing doses of methacholine administered whether respiratory route at the same time monitoring a drop in the pulmonary parameters. A positive methacholine challenge indicates airway hyperresponsiveness.[19] Hypertonic saline and mannitol can also be used to induce bronchial provocation. They are thought to induce bronchoconstriction by release of mediators from bronchial inflammatory cells. Thus, mechanistically this differs from methacholine-induced provocation and is thought to reflect a more accurate mechanism of bronchoconstriction in atopic asthmatics.[20] These are potentially risky tests and patients need to be excluded if they have a low FEV1 of less than 50% baseline, they have a borderline or baseline obstruction to begin with, a history of myocardial infarction or stroke in the past, hypertension (systolic blood pressure greater than 200 or diastolic >100), history of aortic aneurysm, myasthenia gravis (especially with regards to methacholine challenge), current pregnancy or breastfeeding.

Exhaled nitric oxide. Exhaled nitric oxide has been used as a biomarker of eosinophilic lower airway inflammation.[21] This is often elevated in patients who have concomitant comorbid eosinophilic asthma. Characterization of exhaled nitric oxide assists in sub-phenotyping the nature of inflammation at the same time allows for consideration of optimal strategies to control airway inflammation in the tracheobronchial tree.[22] On the contrary, nasal nitric oxide (NO) levels are low in nasal polyposis. This is thought to be due to blockage of flow of paranasal sinus generated NO into the nasal cavity due to the impaired nasal flow anatomy.[23]

BLOOD AND SERUM-BASED TESTS
Measures of Type 2 Inflammation

Blood eosinophil levels. Blood eosinophils are commonly used as a surrogate marker of eosinophilic inflammation in the tissues. Blood eosinophil levels typically tend to correlate well with tissue eosinophilia, and elevation of eosinophils in blood of more than 500 cells per mm cube is an indication of a type 2/eosinophil driven disease. Lower cutoffs (eg, 300 cells/mm^3) have been also shown to be useful in selecting patients for anti-IL-5 therapies.[24] Caution is recommended in interpreting eosinophil count in an isolated manner because therapeutic interventions such as corticosteroids her and new agents such as biologics mepolizumab can reduce blood eosinophilia faster than tissue eosinophil levels.

Total serum IgE. Total serum IgE can assist in sub-phenotyping inflammatory airways disorder as well. Total serum IgE can be elevated from the specific increase in allergen-specific IgE, thereby increasing the total IgE. This is often seen in highly atopic individuals who have a higher burden of allergen-specific IgE. Total IgE is also elevated in patients who have allergic fungal hypersensitivities such as seen with AFS and allergic bronchopulmonary aspergillosis.[25] Total serum IgE can also be elevated often nonspecifically in CRS with nasal polyposis,[26] patients who have AERD,[27] and patients who have intense inflammatory skin disorder such as atopic dermatitis.[28] Caution is recommended in interpreting serum Ig alone without consideration of the underlying clinical presentation.

Allergen-specific IgE. Allergen-specific Ig testing can be used by in-vitro methods such as a RAST (radioallergosorbent assay) or detecting IgE through a sandwich Elisa. The latter methods are more common because they have done away with the need for radioactivity as a laboratory agent. They are accurate and allow for the detection of allergen-specific sensitivities. Atopic sensitization can manifest with allergic rhinitis and allergen-driven atopic asthma, underscoring the unified nature of airway inflammation.

IgG and IgE testing including mold hypersensitivity. Fungal hypersensitivity manifesting as airway inflammation such as AFS in the paranasal sinuses and allergic bronchopulmonary aspergillosis in the lower airways can be clinically suspected if in-vitro tests of mold hypersensitivity are positive. Serum IgE for molds can assist with the diagnosis of fungal sensitization while. In addition, in the case of mold hypersensitivity where the immune response is characterized by presence of IgG antibodies to mold a serum precipitin to Alternaria or Aspergillus is also informative.[29]

Assessment of immune function. These group of tests are important components for the diagnosis of recurrent sinusitis, CRS which has a basis in an underlying immunodeficiency, recurrent pulmonary infections, and sinopulmonary syndromes.

Immunoglobulins including IgG, IgA and IgM. Quantitative immunoglobulin such as IgG, IgA, and IgM allows for the detection of hypogammaglobulinemia and assessment of immune function. Common variable immunodeficiency (CVID) will present commonly with significant reductions in all three immunoglobulin levels.[30] Isolated antibody deficiency such as selective IgA deficiency can also predispose to recurrent sinus infections or lower respiratory tract infections. IgG subclasses usually provide low-yield information because the implication of specific IgG subclass deficiency in the manifestation of the sinonasal disease is not clear. Elevations in IgG 4 are clearly associated with IgG 4-related disease that can present with recurrent sinusitis and inflammatory changes elsewhere in the respiratory tract.[31] IgG subclasses can be measured if there is another antibody deficiency such as IgA deficiency.[32]

Lymphocyte subsets by flow cytometry. Quantification of lymphocytes by flow cytometry is an in dispense able to assess for quantitative deficiencies in the lymphocyte subsets. CD4, CD8 T-cells along with B and NK cell quantification allows to diagnose specific immune deficiencies. For example, in secondary immunodeficiencies such as human immunodeficiency virus, and isolated CD4 lymphopenia CD4 counts are often suppressed relative to other lymphocyte subtypes. B-cell deficiencies can be seen after B-cell ablating therapy such as rituximab and can persist even after therapy has been completed.

Lymphocyte proliferation assay to mitogens, antigens, and anti-CD3. Lymphocyte proliferation assay is part of the immune assessment tools that can be used to assess for immunodeficiency. Stimulation with might agents is especially robust and can detect significant defects in intracellular signaling that leads to immunodeficiency states. Antigen stimulation and anti-CD3 stimulation assays usually help detect more subtle defects as the degree of stimulation is lower order magnitude but specific compared with mitogens.[33]

Antigen-specific immune responses to diphtheria, tetanus, and pneumococcal serotypes and other vaccines. Assessment of the humoral response depends on functional testing of the immune system. Vaccine responses to diphtheria and tetanus look for antigen-specific responses to protein antigens allowing for assessment of immune response with regards to antigen specificity, immune memory, and immune recall. Serotype-specific titers to 23 pneumococcal antigens allow for measurement of humoral response to polysaccharide antigens present on the pneumococcus.

Assessment of Autoimmune Pathology

Antineutrophil Cytoplasmic Antibodies (ANCA) serologies ANCA serologies especially anti-MPO and anti-PR3 are important for the diagnosis of eosinophilic vasculitic syndromes that can present with sinopulmonary conditions. In presence of significant eosinophilia and presence of rheumatologic symptoms, ANCA serologies help diagnosis of EGPA.

Connective tissue autoantibodies and other autoimmune workup. Other autoimmune diseases as well as rarer disorders like sarcoidosis and IgG 4-related disease can present with sinonasal inflammation and pulmonary manifestations. Obtaining a specific rheumatologic workup can often help narrow down the possibilities in presence of an appropriate clinical presentation.

General markers of inflammation C-Reactive Protein (CRP) and Erythrocyte Sedimentation Rate (ESR). General markers of inflammation like CRP and ESR are usually not very helpful for phenotyping airway inflammation but can signify ongoing inflammation or uncontrolled disease.

Skin Tests

Allergen sensitivity including aeroallergens and molds. Skin prick test to aeroallergens including environmental allergens and molds allows for diagnosis of allergen sensitivity. Although the blood tests detect presence of allergen-specific IgE, the skin tests offer a functional assessment of immunoreactivity. Not only to the skin test allow for the demonstration of presence of IgE but the ability of the allergen-specific IgE to bind to the mast cells in the skin, cross-link the receptor and lead to mast cell degranulation. Therefore, skin tests offer it direct evidence of the ability of the allergen to trigger an immune response.

Sweat chloride. Assessment of chloride in the sweat is useful for screening as well as diagnosis of CF as a cause of recurrent sinopulmonary symptoms. In the setting of appropriate clinical history, family history such as a presentation at a young age or presence of extrapulmonary organ involvement obtaining sweat chloride helps consider the differentials of CF.[34]

URINE TESTS

Urine leukotriene E4. Leukotriene E4 metabolites of the Arachidonic acid pathway and are converted sequentially from an AA to leukotriene A metabolite, leukotriene B metabolite, subsequently to cystine leukotrienes. Leukotriene E4 is a stable metabolite of the leukotriene pathway and can be measured in urine. LTE4 measurement has shown clinical utility in diagnosis of aspirin-exacerbated respiratory disorder.[35–37]

TISSUE DIAGNOSIS AND PATHOLOGY

Histopathology. Histopathological examination of the samples obtained from the airway (such as ethmoid tissue obtained during surgery or nasal polyps) can offer an insight into the nature of the inflammation. Perhaps the most frequently useful measure is the degree of eosinophilia that often correlates with the underlying subtype of eosinophilic airway disorder, although other immune cell types can also be noted. Numerous reports have been published investigating the utility of structured histopathology. Most studies define tissue eosinophilia as greater than 10 eosinophils (eos) per high-powered field (hpf). Numerous studies have shown that patients with elevated tissue eosinophilia have worse symptom burden, worse olfactory loss,

Variable	Reported Categories
Degree of inflammation	Mild, moderate, severe
Eosinophil count	≤10 per HPF, >10 per HPF
Neutrophil infiltrate	Absent, present
Inflammatory predominance	Lymphocytic, lymphoplasmacytic, eosinophilic, other
Basement membrane thickening	<7.5 microns, 7.5–15 microns, >15 microns
Subepithelial edema	Absent/mild, moderate, severe
Hyperplastic/papillary change	Absent, present
Mucosal ulceration	Absent, present
Squamous metaplasia	Absent, present
Fibrosis	Absent, present
Fungal elements	Absent, present
Charcot-Leyden crystals	Absent, present
Eosinophil aggregates	Absent, present

HPF = high power field.

Fig. 3. Structured histopathology report used to evaluate sinonasal specimens.

and more frequent relapses.[38] In addition, sinonasal tissue eosinophilia has been associated with worse asthma and bronchial hyperresponsiveness. Soler and colleagues[39] showed that the worst prognostic group after surgery was the cohort with tissue eosinophilia without nasal polyps. However, there is some debate regarding the exact cut-off (eos/hpf) to define tissue eosinophilia. A recent systematic review by McHugh and colleagues[40] showed that a cut-off of greater than 55 eos/hpf best predicted the likelihood of disease recurrence of ECRS. Lymphoplasmacytic/lymphocytic infiltrate is seen in other chronic sinusitis such as IgG 4-related disease and an eosinophil poor infiltrate can be seen in CRS without nasal polyposis. Fungal elements and presence of fungal mucin suggest to AFS/fungal hypersensitivity.[41] Granulomatous inflammation with necrosis may be seen in ANCA-related vasculitides. A recent study by Marino and colleagues[42] showed that fibrosis was associated with less favorable outcomes in SNOT 22 for chronic rhinosinusitis with nasal polyps (CRSwNP) patients at 12 months and may be a prognosticator for poorer long-term outcomes. The variables assessed as part of the structured histopathology report is presented in **Fig. 3**.

SPECIFIC GENETIC TESTS

CF. Genetic testing for CF gene abnormalities can be specifically sent for in patients who have a sinonasal disease. Strong history of familial disease along with the appropriate presentation including chronic sinusitis, bronchiectasis, recurrent pulmonary infections at a engage indicate the possibility of an underlying genetic disorder such as CF.[34] The most common mutation is the delta 508 variant found in the past majority of patients who have CF; however, other mutations are also found in certain ethnic groups.[43]

PCD and other genetic disorders. Specific genetic testing for clinical syndromes is considered when sinopulmonary involvement presents with additional features. Strong family history, and presence of other clinical features such as infertility, GI-related symptoms, history of disease starting at young age etc. are all suggestive of genetic disorders an appropriate testing can be sent for.

SUMMARY

Accurate subtyping of unified airway disease is of growing interest and will continue to evolve. Current research efforts are focusing on targeted therapies, the development of prognostic and therapeutic biomarkers, and understanding disease endotypes. These efforts will lead us to improved personalized care pathways for patients with CRS. Early studies have published improved outcomes using an approach that aims to subtype CRS/Unified airway disease.[44] Even among clinical trials we are seeing a shift away from polyp status and increasing focus on studies that target specific disease subtypes. Accurate subtyping will allow for more personalized management and will aid in optimizing patient outcomes.

CLINICS CARE POINTS

- Clinical history, physical examination (of both upper and lower airways), and imaging are useful in the workup of patients with unified airway disease.

- In appropriate clinical circumstances, further workup to accurately subtype (eg, eosinophilic chronic rhinosinusitis and aspirin exacerbated respiratory disease) unified airway disease may be used. Further testing can include allergy testing, laboratories (eg, autoimmune workup, serum eosinophil levels, urinary leukotriene E4, and immune function testing), pulmonary function testing, genetics, and tissue histopathology.

- A multidisciplinary approach addressing both upper and lower airways may be used to accurately subtype unified airway disease.

- Accurate subtyping will allow for more personalized management and may optimize outcomes.

REFERENCES

1. Kicic A, de Jong E, Ling K-M, et al. Assessing the unified airway hypothesis in children via transcriptional profiling of the airway epithelium. J Allergy Clin Immunol 2020;145(6):1562–73.
2. Kim C, Han J, Wu T, et al. Role of Biologics in Chronic Rhinosinusitis With Nasal Polyposis: State of the Art Review. Otolaryngol Neck Surg Off J Am Acad Otolaryngol Neck Surg 2021;164(1):57–66.
3. Divekar R, Lal D. Recent advances in biologic therapy of asthma and the role in therapy of chronic rhinosinusitis. F1000Research 2018;7:412.
4. Fokkens WJ, Lund VJ, Hopkins C, et al. European Position Paper on Rhinosinusitis and Nasal Polyps 2020. Rhinology 2020;58(Suppl S29):1–464.
5. Grayson JW, Cavada M, Harvey RJ. Clinically relevant phenotypes in chronic rhinosinusitis. J Otolaryngol - Head Neck Surg = Le J D'oto-rhino-laryngologie Chir Cervico-faciale 2019;48(1):23.

6. Chapurin N, Wu J, Labby AB, et al. Current insight into treatment of chronic rhinosinusitis: Phenotypes, endotypes, and implications for targeted therapeutics. J Allergy Clin Immunol 2022;150(1):22–32.

7. Ragab A, Clement P, Vincken W. Objective assessment of lower airway involvement in chronic rhinosinusitis. Am J Rhinol 2004;18(1):15–21.

8. Halawi AM, Smith SS, Chandra RK. Chronic rhinosinusitis: epidemiology and cost. Allergy Asthma Proc 2013;34(4):328–34.

9. Szczeklik A, Nizankowska E, Duplaga M. Natural history of aspirin-induced asthma. AIANE Investigators. European Network on Aspirin-Induced Asthma. Eur Respir J 2000;16(3):432–6.

10. McCracken JL, Veeranki SP, Ameredes BT, et al. Diagnosis and Management of Asthma in Adults: A Review. JAMA 2017;318(3):279–90.

11. Aribandi M, McCoy VA, Bazan C 3rd. Imaging features of invasive and noninvasive fungal sinusitis: a review. Radiogr A Rev Publ Radiol Soc North Am Inc 2007; 27(5):1283–96.

12. Patel NA, Ferguson BJ. Odontogenic sinusitis: an ancient but under-appreciated cause of maxillary sinusitis. Curr Opin Otolaryngol Head Neck Surg 2012; 20(1):24–8.

13. Gilkeson RC, Ciancibello LM, Hejal RB, et al. Tracheobronchomalacia: dynamic airway evaluation with multidetector CT. AJR Am J Roentgenol 2001;176(1):205–10.

14. Gupta S, Siddiqui S, Haldar P, et al. Qualitative analysis of high-resolution CT scans in severe asthma. Chest 2009;136(6):1521–8.

15. Younis RT, Anand VK, Davidson B. The role of computed tomography and magnetic resonance imaging in patients with sinusitis with complications. Laryngoscope 2002;112(2):224–9.

16. Lung function testing: selection of reference values and interpretative strategies. American Thoracic Society. Am Rev Respir Dis 1991;144(5):1202–18.

17. Goldstein MF, Grundfast SK, Dunsky EH, et al. Effect of functional endoscopic sinus surgery on bronchial asthma outcomes. Arch Otolaryngol Head Neck Surg 1999;125(3):314–9.

18. Dhong HJ, Jung YS, Chung SK, et al. Effect of endoscopic sinus surgery on asthmatic patients with chronic rhinosinusitis. Otolaryngol Neck Surg Off J Am Acad Otolaryngol Neck Surg 2001;124(1):99–104.

19. Crapo RO, Casaburi R, Coates AL, et al. Guidelines for methacholine and exercise challenge testing-1999. This official statement of the American Thoracic Society was adopted by the ATS Board of Directors, July 1999. Am J Respir Crit Care Med 2000;161(1):309–29.

20. Anderson SD, Brannan J, Spring J, et al. A new method for bronchial-provocation testing in asthmatic subjects using a dry powder of mannitol. Am J Respir Crit Care Med 1997;156(3 Pt 1):758–65.

21. Kharitonov SA, Barnes PJ. Clinical aspects of exhaled nitric oxide. Eur Respir J 2000;16(4):781–92.

22. Smith AD, Cowan JO, Brassett KP, et al. Use of exhaled nitric oxide measurements to guide treatment in chronic asthma. N Engl J Med 2005;352(21): 2163–73.

23. Colantonio D, Brouillette L, Parikh A, et al. Paradoxical low nasal nitric oxide in nasal polyposis. Clin Exp Allergy J Br Soc Allergy Clin Immunol 2002;32(5): 698–701.

24. Brusselle GG, Koppelman GH. Biologic Therapies for Severe Asthma. N Engl J Med 2022;386(2):157–71.

25. Kurup VP, Banerjee B, Hemmann S, et al. Selected recombinant Aspergillus fumigatus allergens bind specifically to IgE in ABPA. Clin Exp Allergy J Br Soc Allergy Clin Immunol 2000;30(7):988–93.

26. Tripathi A, Conley DB, Grammer LC, et al. Immunoglobulin E to staphylococcal and streptococcal toxins in patients with chronic sinusitis/nasal polyposis. Laryngoscope 2004;114(10):1822–6.

27. Johns CB, Laidlaw TM. Elevated total serum IgE in nonatopic patients with aspirin-exacerbated respiratory disease. Am J Rhinol Allergy 2014;28(4):287–9.

28. Hu Y, Liu S, Liu P, et al. Clinical relevance of eosinophils, basophils, serum total IgE level, allergen-specific IgE, and clinical features in atopic dermatitis. J Clin Lab Anal 2020;34(6):e23214.

29. Vlahakis NE, Aksamit TR. Diagnosis and treatment of allergic bronchopulmonary aspergillosis. Mayo Clin Proc 2001;76(9):930–8.

30. Ameratunga R, Woon S-T, Gillis D, et al. New diagnostic criteria for common variable immune deficiency (CVID), which may assist with decisions to treat with intravenous or subcutaneous immunoglobulin. Clin Exp Immunol 2013;174(2):203–11.

31. Campbell SN, Rubio E, Loschner AL. Clinical review of pulmonary manifestations of IgG4-related disease. Ann Am Thorac Soc 2014;11(9):1466–75.

32. Oxelius VA, Laurell AB, Lindquist B, et al. IgG subclasses in selective IgA deficiency: importance of IgG2-IgA deficiency. N Engl J Med 1981;304(24):1476–7.

33. Stone KD, Feldman HA, Huisman C, et al. Analysis of in vitro lymphocyte proliferation as a screening tool for cellular immunodeficiency. Clin Immunol 2009;131(1):41–9.

34. Farrell PM, Rosenstein BJ, White TB, et al. Guidelines for diagnosis of cystic fibrosis in newborns through older adults: Cystic Fibrosis Foundation consensus report. J Pediatr 2008;153(2):S4–14.

35. Divekar R, Hagan J, Rank M, et al. Diagnostic Utility of Urinary LTE4 in Asthma, Allergic Rhinitis, Chronic Rhinosinusitis, Nasal Polyps, and Aspirin Sensitivity. J Allergy Clin Immunol Pract 2016;4(4):665–70.

36. Bochenek G, Stachura T, Szafraniec K, et al. Diagnostic Accuracy of Urinary LTE4 Measurement to Predict Aspirin-Exacerbated Respiratory Disease in Patients with Asthma. J Allergy Clin Immunol Pract 2018;6(2):528–35.

37. Choby G, Low CM, Levy JM, et al. Urine Leukotriene E4: Implications as a Biomarker in Chronic Rhinosinusitis. Otolaryngol Neck Surg Off J Am Acad Otolaryngol Neck Surg 2022;166(2):224–32.

38. Snidvongs K, Lam M, Sacks R, et al. Structured histopathology profiling of chronic rhinosinusitis in routine practice. Int Forum Allergy Rhinol 2012;2(5):376–85.

39. Soler ZM, Sauer D, Mace J, et al. Impact of mucosal eosinophilia and nasal polyposis on quality-of-life outcomes after sinus surgery. Otolaryngol Neck Surg Off J Am Acad Otolaryngol Neck Surg 2010;142(1):64–71.

40. McHugh T, Snidvongs K, Xie M, et al. High tissue eosinophilia as a marker to predict recurrence for eosinophilic chronic rhinosinusitis: a systematic review and meta-analysis. Int Forum Allergy Rhinol 2018;8(12):1421–9.

41. Schleimer RP. Immunopathogenesis of Chronic Rhinosinusitis and Nasal Polyposis. Annu Rev Pathol 2017;12:331–57.

42. Marino MJ, Garcia JO, Zarka M, et al. A structured histopathology-based analysis of surgical outcomes in chronic rhinosinusitis with and without nasal polyps. Laryngoscope Investig Otolaryngol 2019;4(5):497–503.

43. Cutting GR. Cystic fibrosis genetics: from molecular understanding to clinical application. Nat Rev Genet 2015;16(1):45–56.
44. Miglani A, Divekar RD, Azar A, et al. Revision endoscopic sinus surgery rates by chronic rhinosinusitis subtype. Int Forum Allergy Rhinol 2018;8(9):1047–51.
45. Grayson JW, Hopkins C, Mori E, et al. Contemporary Classification of Chronic Rhinosinusitis Beyond Polyps vs No Polyps: A Review. JAMA Otolaryngol Head Neck Surg 2020;146(9):831–8.

Unified Airway Disease: Genetics and Epigenetics

Tripti Brar, MBBS, MD, Michael J. Marino, MD, Devyani Lal, MD*

KEYWORDS

- Genomics • Epigenetics • Genetics • Unified airway • Sinusitis • Rhinosinusitis
- Chronic rhinosinusitis • Nasal polyps • UAD

KEY POINTS

- Currently identified risk/susceptibility genes for unified airway disease (UAD) participate in cytokine signaling (especially type 2 pathway), tissue remodeling, innate immunity, arachidonic acid metabolism, and other proinflammatory pathways.
- Replicated genome-wide association studies (GWAS) of asthma and allergies have identified key risk alleles and loci that are common across the globe; about 60% to 80% of patients with asthma have allergic rhinitis (AR), whereas 20% to 40% of patients with AR have asthma. Unfortunately, similar quality studies of the key risk alleles for chronic rhinosinusitis (CRS) with asthma or bronchiectasis are lacking.
- Genetic predisposition of common polymorphisms linked with CRS with nasal polyposis (CRSwNP), and the association of CRSwNP with asthma and aspirin-exacerbated respiratory disease (AERD) have been identified.
- Genetics of non-type 2 UAD such as CRS associated with bronchitis/bronchiectasis and CRS without nasal polyps (CRSsNP) have not yet been elucidated satisfactorily.
- Genetic discoveries in UAD can advance patient care through identification of novel therapeutic targets, preventative strategies, prognostication, and personalized medicine.

INTRODUCTION

The coexistence of upper and lower airway diseases (allergic rhinitis [AR]-asthma, AR-chronic rhinosinusitis [CRS]-asthma; CRS-bronchitis/bronchiectasis) is now well recognized.[1] Genetic risk/susceptibility factors that underlie coexistent inflammatory responses in the upper and lower airways merit investigation given that the prevalence of allergies,[2] asthma,[2] and CRS[3] have been noted to increase over the past decades.

Funding Sources: None.
Financial disclosure: D. Lal: Consultant GSK; Consulting Fee; T. Brar: None.
Conflicts of interest: D. Lal: None, T. Brar: None.
Department of Otolaryngology- Head & Neck Surgery, Division of Rhinology, Mayo Clinic in Arizona, 5777 East Mayo Boulevard, Phoenix, AZ 85054, USA
* Corresponding author. Department of Otolaryngology- Head & Neck Surgery, Division of Rhinology, Mayo Clinic in Arizona, 5777 East Mayo Boulevard, Phoenix, AZ 85054.
E-mail address: lal.devyani@mayo.edu

Otolaryngol Clin N Am 56 (2023) 23–38
https://doi.org/10.1016/j.otc.2022.09.002
0030-6665/23/© 2022 Elsevier Inc. All rights reserved.
oto.theclinics.com

Abbreviations	
ABPA	allergic broncho-pulmonary aspergillosis
AERD	aspirin exacerbated respiratory disease
AFRS	allergic fungal rhinosinusitis
AHR	airway hyper-responsiveness
AIA	aspirin-intolerant asthma
AR	allergic rhinitis
ATA	aspirin-tolerant asthma
CF	cystic fibrosis
CFTR	cystic fibrosis transmembrane regulator
CRS	chronic rhinosinusitis
CRSsNP	chronic rhinosinusitis without nasal polyps
CRSwNP	chronic rhinosinusitis with nasal polyps
DNA	deoxyribonucleic acid
EWAS	epigenome wide association studies
GWAS	genome wide association studies
HLA	human leukocyte antigen
IL	Interleukin
mRNA	messenger RNA
NP	nasal polyp
NSAID	non-steroidal anti-inflammatory drug
OR	odds ratio
PBMC	peripheral blood mononuclear cells
RNA	ribonucleic acid
SNP	single nucleotide polymorphisms
UAD	unified airway disease

Genetic studies and predictive biomarkers can provide information on disease susceptibility, prognostication, and therapeutic responsiveness, facilitating earlier and personalized management approaches. This review focuses on genetic studies that investigate unified airway disease (UAD). The reader is referred to contemporary reviews on the genetics of CRS, asthma, and allergy individually because these are outside the scope of the review.

For certain diseases like cystic fibrosis (CF) and primary ciliary dyskinesia, genetic mutations underlying the combined airway pathology are understood. Mutations in the cystic fibrosis transmembrane regulator (CFTR) gene that affects chloride channel opening in epithelial cells can impact the entire airway and other organ systems in CF. The reader is referred to Do-Yeon Cho and colleagues article, "Unified Airway - Cystic Fibrosis," in this issue for detailed information on CF.

Most pathologic conditions of the airway likely do not result from single genetic mutations, and genetic susceptibility may be one of several factors that result in airway disease. Studies support a large genetic contribution to asthma predisposition ("heritability") with estimates of 55% to 74% heritability in adults and almost 90% in children.[4] AR is one of the most common atopic diseases worldwide. The heritability of AR has been estimated to be 33% to 90%.[4,5]

As a chronic disease of the upper airway that is postulated to result from unfavorable environmental interactions in the susceptible host, CRS also likely has a heritable component. However, estimates of the heritability of CRS are currently unavailable. Most common forms of CRS likely have polygenic heritability, with many genetic variants making small contributions to the disease risk. Supporting this premise are prevalence studies among genetically related and unrelated individuals who may or may not share living environments. In Sweden, Bohman and colleagues[6] found that the relative risk of CRS with nasal polyps (CRSwNP) in first-degree relatives was 4.9; the prevalence of CRSwNP in relatives was 13.4% versus a 2.7% in the control population. In a study from Utah, CRS was also reported to have familial clustering.[7] In this large population-based study, subjects included 1638 subjects with CRSwNP and 24,200 subjects with CRS without nasal polyps (CRSsNP) as well as matched random controls. First- and second-degree relatives of subjects with CRSwNP were found to have a 4.1-fold and 3.3-fold elevated risk for CRSwNP, respectively. For subjects with CRSsNP, first- and second-degree relatives had a 2.4- and 1.4-fold risk of developing CRSsNP, respectively. In addition, an interesting finding with respect to spouses of subjects with CRS was also reported. Spouses of subjects with CRSsNP (but not CRSwNP) were also found to be at a 2-fold increased risk of CRSsNP. These findings suggest that both genetic and environmental factors may impact pathogenesis of CRS, with a stronger genetic component for the CRSwNP subtype.[7] These findings offer support to the hypothesis that similar to asthma, in the susceptible host exposed to unfavorable environmental insults, CRS is likely the product of genetic and environmental interactions. It is proposed that among susceptible host, environmental factors such as microbes, smoking exposure, and pollution may induce epithelial barrier disruptions that result in a self-perpetuating inflammatory cascade mediated by innate and adaptive immune responses.[8,9]

In exploring the genetics of the unified airway, the association and overlap of genetic and environmental etiologic factors for AR and asthma has been known for decades.[10] Twin studies have illustrated genetic susceptibility in asthma, atopic dermatitis, and rhinitis, noting significantly higher concordance rates in monozygotic versus dizygotic twins.[11–13] Indeed, asthma may have 50% to 90% concordance in identical twins.[11,14] High-quality GWAS have further advanced the understanding of asthma, AR, and coexistent AR and asthma.[15] These disease phenotypes seem to have common polymorphisms related to type 2 inflammatory pathways. Studies of the genetics of CRS, however, are relatively nascent and composed of small sample sizes. Nevertheless, susceptibility genes involving type 2 inflammatory pathways, especially interleukin (IL)-4, IL-5, IL-13, IL-33, and periostin, have been implicated in CRS with coexistent asthma.[16–19] A GWAS on combined datasets from Iceland and the United Kingdom that included 4366 nasal polyp cases (CRSwNP subjects), 5608 CRS cases (CRSsNP), and more than 700,000 controls found 27 signals linked to nasal polyps (CRSwNP), of which 7 associated with CRS and 13 with asthma.[20]

DISCUSSION

Over the last 2 decades, rapid developments in genetics have aided studies of UAD. Although early studies focused on single nucleotide polymorphisms (SNPs) in candidate genes (candidate gene association studies [CGAS]), genome-wide association studies (GWAS) are now being used for the study of airway diseases.[5,15] These GWAS can examine the entire genome of several individuals simultaneously to identify novel variants and associations with disease or traits.[21] To our knowledge, there are no studies that have investigated the GWAS of CRS in association with AR/asthma.

In addition, the expanding field of epigenetics allows deeper dives into the mechanisms of host-environment interaction on gene expression.[22] Mechanisms through which environmental factors impact gene expression such as DNA methylation, histone modifications, or noncoding RNA expression have been studied in asthma and AR.[14,23] Smaller studies have investigated the epigenetics of CRS, but to our knowledge there are no studies that have investigated the epigenomics of combined CRS and AR/asthma. As epigenetic changes are heritable and occur as a result of the internal or external environmental influence, epigenome-wide association studies (EWAS) may prove invaluable in studying the UAD coexistent with CRS.

Most studies on the genetics and epigenetics of CRS have focused on CRSwNP. Martin and colleagues[24] recently performed a systematic review on the epigenetics and genetics of nasal polyps. After reviewing 80 genetic studies and 24 epigenetic studies, the investigators identified 99 genes and more than 150 SNPs and genetic variants related to nasal polyposis. The investigators then further performed unsupervised cluster analysis of the susceptibility genes (**Tables 1 and 2**). A total of 8 clusters were identified, of which the highest populated cluster was composed of HLA genes that were associated with pathways related to immune responses, cell surface receptor signaling pathway, antigen processing, and presentation. The other clusters were associated with cytokine signaling, immune system processes, stress response, response to chemical stimulus, and signal transcription. Among these 8 clusters, 5 clusters were related to genes associated with increased risk of nasal polyposis; these included COX gene (associated in aerobic electron transport) and cytokine cluster genes. IL-1A and IL-10 were reported to be related to both heightened and lowered risk of nasal polyps depending on the SNP studied. Three clusters of genes associated with a reduced risk for nasal polyposis. HLA gene variants associated with increased risk of nasal polyposis include DQA1*0201 in Hungarian and Mexican patients and HLA-DRB1*03 and HLA-DRB1*04 in Turkish and Mexican patients, whereas HLA-DQB1*0301 reduced risk of nasal polyps in Hungarian and Iranian subjects. Although different allele frequencies exist between subjects with nasal polyp and controls with respect to the CD8 gene, TNF gene, and IL genes, these data are sometimes conflicting or unreplicated.[24] Polymorphisms of IL-1A, IL-1B, IL-4, and IL-10 alleles may be associated with increased or decreased risk of nasal polyps. Taste receptor genes also show different allele frequencies between patients and controls.[25] In a review of 19 TAS receptor genes, 57 SNPs in TAS2R genes and 16 SNPs in TAS1R genes were found. SNPs for TAS2R38 have been further implicated in influencing CRSwNP for risk of polyps and gram-negative infections.[24] MET, SERPINA1, and LAM genes are also associated with increased nasal polyposis risk. Certain alleles of the IRAK4 gene were found to be associated with high serum levels of IgE in patients with NP by Tewfik and colleagues[26] in 206 patients with severe CRS and asthma.

Allergic Rhinitis, Atopic Dermatitis, and Asthma

The association between AR and asthma is relatively well explored. About 60% to 80% of patients with asthma have AR, whereas 20% to 40% of patients with AR have asthma.[27] Genetic association studies have identified common genes that are related to the allergic pathway. Among other pathways, genes involved in the immune barrier and inflammation/homeostasis have been identified.

A 2017 GWAS (n = 360,838) studied the shared genetic origin of asthma, AR, and atopic dermatitis using SNP-based analysis on subjects.[13] The investigators identified 136 independent risk variants located at 99 loci implicating 132 plausible genes.[13] Interestingly, only 6 variants were disease specific, raising the possibility that most gene variants identified were common to the "allergic phenotype." In addition, the investigators also identified 36 genes where CpG methylation influenced transcription, highlighting the impact of environmentally induced epigenetic changes.[13] In a subsequent study, the investigators performed a GWAS using gene-based analysis comparing subjects with asthma, AR, and atopic dermatitis with healthy controls.[28] The investigators reported 30 significant gene-based associations, and 19 novel genes with 11 loci. Most of the newly identified 11 risk variants were shared between asthma, hay fever, and eczema and did not have differential association with the 3

Table 1 Cluster analysis of genes associated with chronic rhinosinusitis with nasal polyps[24]	
Name of Cluster	**List of Genes**
HLA Genes	HLA-A, HLA-B, HLA-C, HLA-DQA1, HLA-DQB1, HLA-DRA, HLA-DRB1, HLA-DRB5, TAPBP, CD8A, CIITA
IL and related genes	IL1A, IL1B, IL1RN, IL1RL1, IRAK4, IL10, IL33
TNF and related genes	TNF, LTA, MTCO2, NOS2
ALOX genes	ALOX5, ALOX5AP, ALOX15, LTC4S
TAS genes	TAS2R13, TAS2R20, TAS2R38, ADORA1
Other genes	FCER1A, FCER1G, MS4A2, CFTR, MET, SERPINA1, LAMA2, LAMB1, PTGDR, MMP2, MMP9, NOS1, NOS1AP, CACNA11, CD14, CCR11, ADRB2, CACNG6, RYBP, HSPA2

individual diseases.[28] In reviewing the top-ranked genes identified individually for asthma and AR, Choi and colleagues[14] reported 25 independent loci related to both diseases. The commonly identified genes are associated with type 2 inflammatory processes, immune signaling, and epithelial barrier regulation.

Chronic Rhinosinusitis and Asthma

Table 3 lists genetic studies and genes that have found to be significant variants commonly between CRS and lower airway diseases.

The concept of allergic inflammatory memory in airway epithelial cells was studied through single-cell RNA sequencing (scRNAseq) in patients with CRS versus controls by Ordovas-Montanes and colleagues.[29] The investigators showed that reduced epithelial diversity in patients with CRSwNP resulted from changes in basal progenitor cells and that epithelial stem cells may serve as repositories for allergic memories.[29] Epithelial barrier dysfunction is imprinted in the basal progenitor cells as a result of exposure to type 2 inflammatory agents, and studies have shown that diseases like CRS and asthma can result from barrier dysfunction.[30] scRNAseq has promising applications for studying CRS and its association with UADs.

Gill and colleagues[31] compared transcriptional profiles of 594 genes associated with innate and adaptive immunity in those with CRS with asthma versus patients with CRS without asthma. The investigators reported that CRSwNP with asthma had an overrepresentation of genes associated with type 2-driven inflammation compared with patients with CRSwNP without asthma. Furthermore, those patients

Table 2 Genes that increase and decrease risk of chronic rhinosinusitis with nasal polyps[24]	
Increase Risk	**Decrease Risk**
IL1A, IL1B, IL1RN, IL4, IL10, IL1RL1, IL33, TNF, FCER1A, FCER1G, MS4A2, LTF, MMP2, MMP9, MT-CO2, MT-CO3, COX4I1, COX5A, COX5B, COX6B1, COX6C, COX7C, CCL11, CFTR, ADRB2, FANCC, FANCF, FANCG, FANCL	IL1A, IL1R1, IL1B, IRAK4, IL10, HLA-B, HLA-C, HLA-DQA1, HLA-DRB5, CD8A, FANCA, FANCC, FANCG, FANCF, FANCL, FANCM, STRA13, ADRB2, C1orf70, C1orf86

Data from Martin MJ, Garcia-Sanchez A, Estravis M, et al. Genetics and epigenetics of nasal polyposis: A systematic review. *J Investig Allergol Clin Immunol.* 2021;31(3):196-211. https://doi.org/10.18176/jiaci.0673.

Table 3
Genetic studies with common variants between chronic rhinosinusitis and lower airway disease

Genes/Loci	Function	Variant	Type of Study	Phenotype	Population	Reference
Variants associated with CRS, asthma, and AIA						
HLA-A	MHC class I	A*24	CGAS	CRSwNP, asthma, AIA	Turkish	Keles et al,[33] 2008
HLA-C	MHC class I	Cw*12	CGAS	CRSwNP, asthma, AIA	Turkish	Keles et al,[33] 2008
HLA-DR	MHC class II	DRB1*04	CGAS	CRSwNP, asthma, AIA	Turkish	Keles et al,[33] 2008
NOS2A	Synthesizes nitric oxide, a biological mediator in several processes, including neurotransmission and antimicrobial and antitumor activity	Promoter VNTR	CGAS	CRSwNP, asthma, AIA	Caucasian	Benito Pescador et al,[58] 2012
Variants associated with CRS and AIA						
IL1R2	Member of IL-1 involved in various immune responses	rs11688145	CGAS	CRSwNP and AIA	Japanese	Sekigawa et al,[59] 2009
IL-10	Immune regulatory cytokine with anti-inflammatory function	rs1800896	CGAS	CRSwNP and AIA	Korean	Kim S-H et al,[60] 2009
IL-13	Interleukin involved in T$_H$2 response	Multiple SNPs	CGAS	CRSwNP and AIA	Korean	Palikhe et al,[61] 2010
INDO/IDO1	Plays a role in antimicrobial and antitumor defense, neuropathology, immunoregulation, and antioxidant activity	rs7820268	CGAS	CRSwNP and AIA	Japanese	Sekigawa et al,[59] 2009

Gene	Description	Variant		Disease	Ethnicity	Reference
MMP9	Matrix metalloproteinase involved in tissue remodeling	rs3918242	CGAS	CRSwNP and AIA	Turkish	Erbek et al,[39] 2007
TGFB1	Cytokine involved in tissue remodeling	rs1800469	CGAS	CRSsNP and AIA	Korean	Kim S-H et al,[62] 2007
Variants associated with CRS and asthma						
HLA	MHC class I	A1/B8	CGAS	CRSwNP and asthma	Caucasian	Moloney et al,[32] 1980
HLA-DR		DRA_rs9268644, rs3129878, rs3129881, rs2239805	CGAS	CRSwNP and asthma	Korean	Kim J-H et al,[34] 2012
IL1A	Member of IL-1 involved in various immune responses	rs17561	CGAS	CRSwNP and asthma	Finnish Caucasian	Karjalainen et al,[38] 2003
LTC4S	Gene involved in arachidonic acid metabolism. Encodes an enzyme that catalyzes the first step in the biosynthesis of cysteinyl leukotrienes	rs730012	CGAS	CRSwNP and asthma	Caucasian	Benito Pescador et al,[58] 2012
EMID2	Chain of collagen type XXVI	rs6945102-rs4729697-rs221-rs1043533 haplotype	CGAS	CRSwNP and asthma	Korean	Pasaje et al,[35] 2012
DCBLD2	Protein related to neurologic process	rs828618	CGAS	CRSwNP and asthma	Korean	Pasaje et al,[36] 2012

(continued on next page)

Table 3
(continued)

Genes/Loci	Function	Variant	Type of Study	Phenotype	Population	Reference
PTGDR2	Encodes prostaglandin D2 receptor involved in arachidonic acid metabolism	Diplotype[a]	CGAS	CRSwNP and asthma	Caucasian	Pescador et al,[58] 2012
HLA-DQA1	MHC class II	rs1391371	GWAS, variants associated with NP	NP, CRS, asthma, blood eosinophil count	European	Kristjansson et al,[20] 2019
IL33	Interleukin involved in T_H2 response	rs1888909	GWAS, variants associated with NP	NP, asthma, blood eosinophil count	European	Kristjansson et al,[20] 2019
TSLP	Cytokine involved in dendritic cell maturation and allergic inflammation	rs1837253	GWAS, variants associated with NP	NP, asthma, blood eosinophil count	European	Kristjansson et al,[20] 2019
ALOX15	Lipoxygenase with inflammation regulatory function	rs34210653	GWAS, variants associated with NP	NP, CRS, blood eosinophil count	European	Kristjansson et al,[20] 2019
10p14	Near GATA3, a master regulator in T_H2 response	rs1444782	GWAS, variants associated with NP	NP, asthma, blood eosinophil count	European	Kristjansson et al,[20] 2019
IL18R1	Cytokine receptor involved in IL-18-mediated interferon-g synthesis in T_H1 cells	rs6543124	GWAS, variants associated with NP	NP, asthma, blood eosinophil count	European	Kristjansson et al,[20] 2019
SLC22A4	Sodium-ion-dependent	rs1050152	GWAS, variants associated with NP	NP, asthma, blood eosinophil count	European	Kristjansson et al,[20] 2019

	carnitine transporter					
IL33	Interleukin involved in T_H2 response	rs78757963	GWAS, eosinophil variants associated with NP	NP, CRS, asthma	European	Kristjansson et al,[20] 2019
		rs146597587	GWAS, eosinophil variants associated with NP	NP, asthma	European	Kristjansson et al,[20] 2019
BACH2	Transcriptional regulator of adaptive immunity	rs62408225	GWAS, eosinophil variants associated with NP	NP, asthma	European	Kristjansson et al,[20] 2019
GATA3	Master regulator in T_H2 response	rs10905284	GWAS, eosinophil variants associated with NP	NP, asthma	European	Kristjansson et al,[20] 2019
12q13	-	rs7302200	GWAS, eosinophil variants associated with NP	NP, asthma	European	Kristjansson et al,[20] 2019
21q22	Near RUNX1, a transcription factor involved in hematopoiesis	rs8129030	GWAS, eosinophil variants associated with NP	NP, asthma	European	Kristjansson et al,[20] 2019
COG6	Subunit of the oligomeric Golgi complex	rs9532434	GWAS, eosinophil variants associated with NP	NP, CRS, asthma	European	Kristjansson et al,[20] 2019
CLEC16 A	Regulator of mitophagy	rs12935413	GWAS, eosinophil variants associated with NP	NP, asthma	European	Kristjansson et al,[20] 2019
5p13	Near IL-7R, which is a receptor of IL-7 and TSLP	rs1961220	GWAS, eosinophil variants associated with NP	NP, asthma	European	Kristjansson et al,[20] 2019

Abbreviations: AIA, aspirin-intolerant asthma; ATA, aspirin-tolerant asthma; CGAS, candidate gene association studies; CRS, chronic rhinosinusitis; CRSsNP, CRS without nasal polyps; CRSwNP, chronic rhinosinusitis with nasal polyps; GWAS, genome wide association studies; HLA, human leukocyte antigen; IL, interleukin; MHC, major histocompatibility complex; NP, nasal polyp; SNP, single nucleotide polymorphism; VNTR, variable number tandem repeat.

a The study investigators constructed a diplotype for PTGDR (prostaglandin D2 receptor) using polymorphisms 2613C>T, rs8004654, rs803010, and rs11157907 (namely, diplotype CCCT/CCCC).

with CRSsNP and asthma had higher expression of these genes compared with those with CRSsNP without asthma. The presence or absence of asthma, irrespective of polyp status, affects gene expression profiles in nasal cells.[31]

Several CGAS have investigated a variety of associations of CRSwNP, asthma, and serum IgE levels. These are listed in **Table 1**. As early as 1980, Moloney and Oliver reported a significantly higher association of HLA A1/B8 and more severe sinus disease in patients who had both nasal polyps and asthma, but not in those patients with nasal polyps without asthma. This study raised the exciting possibility that HLA typing could help identify those at greater risk of developing asthma.[32] The HLA-A*24, HLA-Cw*12, and HLA-DRB1*04 alleles were next determined to be significantly higher in Turkish subjects with CRSwNP, asthma, aspirin sensitive asthma (ASA) triad.[33] Subsequently in 2012, Kim and colleagues[34] postulated that HLA-DRA polymorphisms might contribute to nasal polyposis susceptibility in patients with asthma.

Pasaje and colleagues[35] studied the role of the EMID2 gene in Korean asthmatic patients and found the EMID2_BL1_ht2 variant to be significantly associated with nasal polyposis. The same group of investigators also found polymorphisms in DCBLD2 gene to be significantly correlated in patients with nasal polyp with asthma.[36] COX-2 and MET-2 gene polymorphisms may have a strong association in patients with nasal polyps, and even greater in those who had underlying allergy or asthma.[37] Karjalainen and colleagues[38] found that certain IL-1A polymorphisms were higher in asthmatic patients with nasal polyps versus asthmatic patients without nasal polyps. In a Turkish cohort, Erbek and colleagues[39] found certain genotypes of IL-1A, IL-1B, and TNFA to be higher in patients with nasal polyps; however, no association was found with asthma, aspirin intolerance, or atopy. In an attempt to replicate these findings in a Canadian population, Endam and colleagues found that they could replicate the findings associated with IL-1A, but not IL-1B or TNFA. The Canadian group further found the IL-1A polymorphism to be higher in patients with CRS, but not higher in those with nasal polyps or asthma. The investigators also reported 3 new SNPs associated with IL-1A and CRS.[40]

In a replication study of 53 SNPs previously reported in CRS and nasal polyps, Henmyr and colleagues[41] only found 7 variants to have a significant association with CRS (including TGFB1, NOS1 and NOS1AP gene), but the presence of asthma or AR did not influence the results. Of these 7 genes, TGFB1 gene has been previously associated with chronic obstructive pulmonary disease (COPD) and rhinosinusitis in patients with asthma and the NOS1 gene and NOS1AP gene have been identified in asthma and AR.[41]

Despite a sizable number of studies in this area, replication in large sample sizes across different populations seems necessary before strong conclusions can be inferred.

Aspirin-Exacerbated Respiratory Disease

Aspirin-exacerbated respiratory disease (AERD), also referred to as aspirin-intolerant asthma and nonsteroidal anti-inflammatory drug (NSAID)-associated respiratory disease (NERD), is a well-described triad of CRSwNP, asthma, and aspirin hypersensitivity. The disease is associated with overproduction of cys-leukotrienes (cysLTs), type 2 inflammation, and eosinophilic disease. The HLA DPB1*0301 locus identified in Polish[42] and Korean populations[43] is considered a strong genetic marker for AERD. Most AERD genetic studies have been performed in the Korean population.[44] GWAS have identified several significant SNPs associated with AERD.[45] These polymorphisms are related to CysLTs synthesis, G-coupled CysLT receptors that amplify cysLT activity, and prostanoid receptor genes (PTGER2).[44] Polymorphisms causing increased eosinophil activation include chemokine CCR3 receptor

(CCR3 −520 T>C), chemoattractant receptor molecule expressed in Th2 cells (CRTH2 −466 T>C), and IL5R (−5993 G>A).[44]

Recently, Choi and colleagues[46] reported that the path of physiologic function of TGF-beta 1 in AERD was higher than in patients with aspirin-tolerant asthma. Ex vivo and in vitro experiments showed an association between TGF-beta 1 and cysLT overproduction in AERD pathogenesis and that increased LTE4 levels induced eosinophil degranulation, which further stimulated TGF-beta 1 production.

Stevens and colleagues performed scRNAseq on nasal polyp cells from AERD and non-AERD CRSwNP subjects to compare transcriptional profiles of genes involved in arachidonic acid metabolism via 5-lipoxygenase, COX, and 15-lipoxygenase (15-LO) enzymatic pathways. High ALOX15 was noted in asthma and CRSwNP, even in the absence of aspirin intolerance/AERD phenotype. The levels of the ALOX15 gene encoding for 15-LO were significantly elevated in subjects with AERD versus those with CRSwNP and controls. ALOX15 gene expression was also associated with increasing disease severity in CRSwNP as well as CRSwNP with asthma versus CRSwNP without asthma. ALOX15 gene levels did not vary based on asthma status in CRSsNP tissue.

Experts have reviewed the prevalence of AERD to NSAID exposure, and it is possible that NSAID exposure may lead to AERD pathogenesis through epigenetic mechanisms.[47]

Allergic Bronchopulmonary Aspergillosis and Allergic Fungal Rhinosinusitis

A recent study performed in a murine model investigated the unified airway response to *Aspergillus niger* exposure. Sinonasal and lung tissue were studied for gene expression, flow cytometry, and immunohistochemistry. The investigators found type 2 inflammation at both subsites. In addition to upregulation of JAK-STAT and helper T-cell pathways, pathways governing the spliceosome, osteoclast differentiation, and coagulation were also upregulated at each site.[48]

ROLE OF GENETIC STUDIES IN EARLY DISEASE IDENTIFICATION AND PROGNOSTICATION

The implications of uncovering common shared pathways between diseases of upper and lower airways are significant for prognostication and early therapy. Preschoolers who are not treated for AR have a 3-fold increased risk of asthma in adulthood.[49] Accessible, noninvasive sampling of the nasal passages could provide insights into lower airway disease. Kicic and colleagues[50] looked at similarities in transcriptomic profiles from the upper and lower airways irrespective of airway symptoms (wheeze) or allergy. The investigators discovered that gene expression profiles were conserved between both sites, irrespective of the presence of overt symptoms, suggesting that early insight into lower airway disease could potentially be provided by studying the nasal epithelium.[50] Similarly, DNA methylation patterns of bronchial cells closely represent those of nasal epithelial cells, although DNA methylation in blood is not a good surrogate to study these changes.[51–54] mRNA expression in sputum of patients with AR and asthma was studied by Sohn and colleagues.[55] The investigators subdivided subjects with AR into those with and without airway hyperresponsiveness (AHR) and found that vascular endothelial growth factor and IL-5 mRNA were significantly higher in AR with AHR versus AR without AHR (although levels were lower than those with asthma).[55] AHR is a risk factor for developing asthma, and thus cytokine signatures in sputum may have a predictive role in early diagnosis.

FUTURE DIRECTIONS

- As evident from the earlier discussion, there appear to be mechanisms at the gene level that are common to upper and lower airway pathologic conditions for some disease phenotypes. Although the association between AR and asthma is well known, a small number of studies have explored the association of CRS with asthma, as well as unified airway pathology such as AERD, AFRS, or ABPA. Further studies are warranted to validate these early results. In addition, investigations are necessary across diverse genetic and geographic populations. It is important to conduct these studies in well-characterized phenotypes and cohorts. Uncovering genetic variants common to upper and lower airway disease may aid identification of novel therapeutic agents and strategies. Therapeutic agents that are currently approved for lower airway pathology may have applicability to treating CRS that is coexistent. In addition, the characterization of pathogenetic pathways in CRS that are similar to those in other airway pathologies may also open up the possibility of trials specifically for CRS. For example, biologics targeting IgE- and eosinophil-mediated inflammation that were initially approved for asthma have now been trialed and approved for use in CRSwNP.[56,57] In the future, patients without nasal polyps (CRSsNP) could be potential candidates for trials should they also have pathogenetic mechanisms underlying their disease that similarly respond to these biologics. Significant gaps in research of the combined airway genetics need to be filled, particularly with regard to CRSsNP and non-type 2 diseases such as CRS associated with bronchiectasis/bronchitis.[58–62]

Future directions for investigations in the genetics of UAD include:

- Genetic studies on CRS-associated UAD on very well-characterized phenotype and endotype cohorts
- Unsupervised cluster analysis of UAD in large subject populations replicated across the globe
- Genetics and epigenetics of CRSsNP and CRS characterized by non-type 2 immunopathogenesis
- Characterization of CRS associated with non-type 2 lower airway disease (COPD, bronchiectasis)
- Investigations that concomitantly study tissue or cells from upper and lower airways to identify accessible upper airway biomarkers for lower airway disease

SUMMARY

Studies on asthma, AR, and CRS have illustrated common and shared genetic variants in diseases affecting both upper and lower airway subsites. The most commonly identified genetic variations relate to genes controlling innate and adaptive immunity, cytokine signaling, tissue remodeling, arachidonic acid metabolism, and other proinflammatory mechanisms. Larger replicable studies across different populations need to be undertaken in well-characterized disease cohorts.

CLINICS CARE POINTS

- Genetic studies have begun to reveal genetic variations that are present in coexistent upper and lower airway diseases
- Genetic predisposition is stronger in patients with CRSwNP compared with CRSsNP

- Genetic factors account for 25% to 80% of asthma risk and upto 90% of AR risk but risk contributions are unknown for CRS.
- Specifically in the context of CRS-associated UAD, a limited number of studies have identified genetic polymorphisms associated with asthma coexistent with CRSwNP, as well as asthma and CRS in AERD
- Currently identified genes control innate immunity, cytokine signaling, tissue remodeling, arachidonic acid metabolism, and other proinflammatory mechanisms.

REFERENCES

1. Tiotiu A, Novakova P, Baiardini I, et al. Manifesto on united airways diseases (UAD): an Interasma (global asthma association–GAA) document. J Asthma 2022;59(4):639–54.
2. Pawankar R. Allergic diseases and asthma: A global public health concern and a call to action. World Allergy Organ J 2014;7(1):1–3.
3. Rudmik L, Fleurence R, Fleurence R, et al. Chronic rhinosinusitis: An under-researched epidemic. J Otolaryngol - Head Neck Surg 2015;44(1):1–6.
4. Hernandez-Pacheco N, Pino-Yanes M, Flores C. Genomic predictors of asthma phenotypes and treatment response. Front Pediatr 2019;7(FEB):1–19.
5. Laulajainen-Hongisto A, Lyly A, Hanif T, et al. Genomics of asthma, allergy and chronic rhinosinusitis: novel concepts and relevance in airway mucosa. Clin Transl Allergy 2020;10(1):1–17.
6. Bohman A, Juodakis J, Oscarsson M, et al. A family-based genome-wide association study of chronic rhinosinusitis with nasal polyps implicates several genes in the disease pathogenesis. PLoS One 2017;12(12). https://doi.org/10.1371/JOURNAL.PONE.0185244.
7. Oakley G, Curtin K, Orb Q, et al. Familial risk of chronic rhinosinusitis with and without nasal polyposis: Genetics or environment. Int Forum Allergy Rhinol 2015;5(4):276–82.
8. Kato A, Schleimer RP, Bleier BS. Mechanisms and pathogenesis of chronic rhinosinusitis. J Allergy Clin Immunol 2022;149(5):1491–503.
9. Klingler AI, Stevens WW, Tan BK, et al. Mechanisms and biomarkers of inflammatory endotypes in chronic rhinosinusitis without nasal polyps. J Allergy Clin Immunol 2021;147(4):1306–17.
10. Ober C, Yao TC. The genetics of asthma and allergic disease: A 21st century perspective. Immunol Rev 2011;242(1):10–30.
11. van Beijsterveldt CEM, Boomsma DI. Genetics of parentally reported asthma, eczema and rhinitis in 5-yr-old twins. Eur Respir J 2007;29(3):516–21.
12. Nystad W, Røysamb E, Magnus P, et al. A comparison of genetic and environmental variance structures for asthma, hay fever and eczema with symptoms of the same diseases: a study of Norwegian twins. Int J Epidemiol 2005;34(6):1302–9.
13. Ferreira MA, Vonk JM, Baurecht H, et al. Shared genetic origin of asthma, hay fever and eczema elucidates allergic disease biology. Nat Genet 2017;49(12):1752–7.
14. Choi BY, Han M, Kwak JW, et al. Genetics and Epigenetics in Allergic Rhinitis. Genes (Basel). 2021;12(12). https://doi.org/10.3390/GENES12122004.
15. Schoettler N, Rodríguez E, Weidinger S, et al. Advances in asthma and allergic disease genetics: Is bigger always better? J Allergy Clin Immunol 2019;144(6):1495–506.

16. Alzobaidi N, Rehman S, Naqvi M, et al. Periostin: A Potential Biomarker and Therapeutic Target in Pulmonary Diseases. J Pharm Pharm Sci 2022;25:137–48.

17. Buysschaert ID, Grulois V, Eloy P, et al. Genetic evidence for a role of IL33 in nasal polyposis. Allergy 2010;65(5):616–22.

18. Grotenboer NS, Ketelaar ME, Koppelman GH, et al. Decoding asthma: translating genetic variation in IL33 and IL1RL1 into disease pathophysiology. J Allergy Clin Immunol 2013;131(3). https://doi.org/10.1016/J.JACI.2012.11.028.

19. Milonski J, Zielinska-Blizniewska H, Majsterek I, et al. Expression of POSTN, IL-4, and IL-13 in Chronic Rhinosinusitis with Nasal Polyps. DNA Cell Biol 2015;34(5):342–9.

20. Kristjansson RP, Benonisdottir S, Davidsson OB, et al. A loss-of-function variant in ALOX15 protects against nasal polyps and chronic rhinosinusitis. Nat Genet 2019;51(2):267–76.

21. Bossé Y, Bacot F, Montpetit A, et al. Identification of susceptibility genes for complex diseases using pooling-based genome-wide association scans. Hum Genet 2009;125(3):305–18.

22. Allis CD, Jenuwein T. The molecular hallmarks of epigenetic control. Nat Rev Genet 2016;17(8):487–500.

23. Ntontsi P, Photiades A, Zervas E, et al. Genetics and epigenetics in asthma. Int J Mol Sci 2021;22(5):1–14.

24. Martin MJ, Garcia-Sanchez A, Estravis M, et al. Genetics and epigenetics of nasal polyposis: A systematic review. J Investig Allergol Clin Immunol 2021;31(3):196–211.

25. Mfuna Endam L, Filali-Mouhim A, Boisvert P, et al. Genetic variations in taste receptors are associated with chronic rhinosinusitis: a replication study. Int Forum Allergy Rhinol 2014;4(3):13–5.

26. Tewfik MA, Bossé Y, Lemire M, et al. Polymorphisms in interleukin-1 receptor-associated kinase 4 are associated with total serum IgE. Allergy Eur J Allergy Clin Immunol 2009;64(5):746–53.

27. Bousquet J, Van Cauwenberge P, Khaltaev N, et al. Allergic rhinitis and its impact on asthma. In collaboration with the World Health Organization. Executive summary of the workshop report. 7-10 December 1999, Geneva, Switzerland. Allergy 2002;57(9):841–55.

28. Ferreira MAR, Vonk JM, Baurecht H, et al. Eleven loci with new reproducible genetic associations with allergic disease risk. J Allergy Clin Immunol 2019;143(2):691–9.

29. Ordovas-Montanes J, Dwyer DF, Nyquist SK, et al. Allergic inflammatory memory in human respiratory epithelial progenitor cells. Nature 2018;560(7720):649–54.

30. Ruysseveldt E, Martens K, Steelant B. Airway Basal Cells, Protectors of Epithelial Walls in Health and Respiratory Diseases. Front Allergy 2021;2. https://doi.org/10.3389/FALGY.2021.787128.

31. Gill AS, Pulsipher A, Sumsion JS, et al. Transcriptional Changes in Chronic Rhinosinusitis with Asthma Favor a Type 2 Molecular Endotype Independent of Polyp Status. J Asthma Allergy 2021;14:405–13.

32. Moloney JR, Oliver RT. HLA antigens, nasal polyps and asthma. Clin Otolaryngol Allied Sci 1980;5(3):183–9.

33. Keles B, Cora T, Acar H, et al. Evaluation of HLA-A, -B, -Cw, and -DRB1 alleles frequency in Turkish patients with nasal polyposis. Otolaryngol Neck Surg 2008;139(4):580–5.

34. Kim J-H, Park BL, Cheong HS, et al. HLA-DRA polymorphisms associated with risk of nasal polyposis in asthmatic patients. Am J Rhinol Allergy 2012; 26(1):12–7.
35. Pasaje CFA, Bae JS, Park BL, et al. Possible role of EMID2 on nasal polyps pathogenesis in Korean asthma patients. BMC Med Genet 2012;13. https://doi.org/10.1186/1471-2350-13-2.
36. Pasaje CFA, Bae JS, Park BL, et al. DCBLD2 gene variations correlate with nasal polyposis in Korean asthma patients. Lung 2012;190(2):199–207.
37. Zielinska-Blizniewska H, Sitarek P, Milonski J, et al. Association of the -33C/G OSF-2 and the 140A/G LF gene polymorphisms with the risk of chronic rhinosinusitis with nasal polyps in a Polish population. Mol Biol Rep 2012;39(5):5449–57.
38. Karjalainen J, Joki-Erkkilä VP, Hulkkonen J, et al. The IL1A genotype is associated with nasal polyposis in asthmatic adults. Allergy 2003;58(5):393–6.
39. Erbek SS, Yurtcu E, Erbek S, et al. Proinflammatory cytokine single nucleotide polymorphisms in nasal polyposis. Arch Otolaryngol Head Neck Surg 2007; 133(7):705–9.
40. Mfuna Endam L, Cormier C, Bossé Y, et al. Association of IL1A, IL1B, and TNF gene polymorphisms with chronic rhinosinusitis with and without nasal polyposis: A replication study. Arch Otolaryngol Head Neck Surg 2010;136(2):187–92.
41. Henmyr V, Vandeplas G, Halldén C, et al. Replication study of genetic variants associated with chronic rhinosinusitis and nasal polyposis. J Allergy Clin Immunol 2014;133(1):273–5.
42. Dekker JW, Nizankowska E, Pile K, et al. Aspirin-induced asthma and HLA-DRBI and HLA-DPBI genotypes 1997;27:574–7.
43. Choi JH, Lee KW, Oh HB, et al. HLA association in aspirin-intolerant asthma: DPB1*0301 as a strong marker in a Korean population. J Allergy Clin Immunol 2004;113(3):562–4.
44. Woo SD, Luu QQ, Park HS. NSAID-Exacerbated Respiratory Disease (NERD): From Pathogenesis to Improved Care. Front Pharmacol 2020;11:1–11.
45. Park BL, Kim TH, Kim JH, et al. Genome-wide association study of aspirin-exacerbated respiratory disease in a Korean population. Hum Genet 2013; 132(3):313–21.
46. Choi Y, Sim S, Lee DH, et al. Effect of TGF-β1 on eosinophils to induce cysteinyl leukotriene E4 production in aspirin-exacerbated respiratory disease. PLoS One 2021;16(8 August 2021):1–13.
47. Lee JU, Park JS, Chang HS, et al. Complementary participation of genetics and epigenetics in development of nsaid-exacerbated respiratory disease. Allergy Asthma Immunol Res 2019;11(6):779–94.
48. Sun H, Damania A, Mair ML, et al. STAT6 Blockade Abrogates Aspergillus-Induced Eosinophilic Chronic Rhinosinusitis and Asthma, A Model of Unified Airway Disease. Front Immunol 2022;13. https://doi.org/10.3389/FIMMU.2022.818017.
49. Rochat MK, Illi S, Ege MJ, et al. Allergic rhinitis as a predictor for wheezing onset in school-aged children. J Allergy Clin Immunol 2010;126(6):1170–5.e2.
50. Kicic A, de Jong E, Ling KM, et al. Assessing the unified airway hypothesis in children via transcriptional profiling of the airway epithelium. J Allergy Clin Immunol 2020;145(6):1562–73.
51. Legaki E, Arsenis C, Taka S, et al. DNA methylation biomarkers in asthma and rhinitis: Are we there yet? Clin Transl Allergy 2022;12(3). https://doi.org/10.1002/CLT2.12131.

52. Brugha R, Lowe R, Henderson AJ, et al. DNA methylation profiles between airway epithelium and proxy tissues in children. Acta Paediatr 2017;106(12):2011–6.
53. Sridhar S, Schembri F, Zeskind J, et al. Smoking-induced gene expression changes in the bronchial airway are reflected in nasal and buccal epithelium. BMC Genomics 2008;9. https://doi.org/10.1186/1471-2164-9-259.
54. Baccarelli A, Rusconi F, Bollati V, et al. Nasal cell DNA methylation, inflammation, lung function and wheezing in children with asthma. Epigenomics 2012;4(1): 91–100.
55. Sohn SW, Lee HS, Park HW, et al. Original article: Evaluation of cytokine mRNA in induced sputum from patients with allergic rhinitis: relationship to airway hyper-responsiveness. Allergy 2008;63(3):268–73.
56. Laidlaw TM, Mullol J, Fan C, et al. Dupilumab improves nasal polyp burden and asthma control in patients with CRSwNP and AERD. J Allergy Clin Immunol Pract 2019;7(7):2462–5.e1.
57. Gevaert P, Omachi TA, Corren J, et al. Efficacy and safety of omalizumab in nasal polyposis: 2 randomized phase 3 trials. J Allergy Clin Immunol 2020;1–11. https://doi.org/10.1016/j.jaci.2020.05.032.
58. Benito Pescador D, Isidoro-García M, García-Solaesa V, et al. Genetic association study in nasal polyposis. J Investig Allergol Clin Immunol 2012;22(5):331–40.
59. Sekigawa T, Tajima A, Hasegawa T, et al. Gene-expression profiles in human nasal polyp tissues and identification of genetic susceptibility in aspirin-intolerant asthma. Clin Exp Allergy 2009;39(7):972–81.
60. Kim S-H, Yang E-M, Lee H-N, et al. Combined effect of IL-10 and TGF-beta1 promoter polymorphisms as a risk factor for aspirin-intolerant asthma and rhinosinusitis. Allergy 2009;64(8):1221–5.
61. Palikhe NS, Kim SH, Cho BY, et al. IL-13 Gene Polymorphisms are Associated With Rhinosinusitis and Eosinophilic Inflammation in Aspirin Intolerant Asthma. Allergy Asthma Immunol Res 2010;2(2):134–40.
62. Kim SH, Park HS, Holloway JW, et al. Association between a TGFbeta1 promoter polymorphism and rhinosinusitis in aspirin-intolerant asthmatic patients. Respir Med 2007;101(3):490–5.

Unified Airway Disease
Environmental Factors

Jesse Siegel, MD[a], Navroop Gill, MD[b],
Murugappan Ramanathan Jr, MD[c], Monica Patadia, MD[a],*

KEYWORDS

- Unified airway disease • Environment • Air pollution • Allergy
- Occupational exposure

KEY POINTS

- Allergens, occupational exposures, and ambient air pollutants can have significant impact on incidence of unified airway disease.
- Allergens including house dust mites, household pets, pollens, and mold are strongly associated with the development of upper airway disease, namely allergic rhinitis.
- Occupational exposures are categorized into high and low molecular weight agents, which trigger different allergic pathways and are linked to the development of rhinitis, asthma, and non-asthmatic eosinophilic bronchitis.
- Air pollutants continue to be a concern with progressive urbanization and have been linked with the development of childhood asthma, exacerbation of chronic rhinosinusitis, and altered airway microbiomes.
- There is conflicting evidence regarding environmental exposures and their impact on clinical course and outcome.

ENVIRONMENTAL ALLERGENS

Allergic rhinitis is the most significant environmentally triggered disease of the upper airway, with lifetime prevalence estimated between 10% and 33%.[1] Consistent with the unified airway concept, allergic disease of the upper airway is closely related to that of the lower airway; it is estimated that up to one-third of individuals with allergic rhinitis will go on to develop asthma and more than half of asthmatics also have allergic rhinitis.[2] However, it is not clear whether allergic rhinitis is a predisposing factor for asthma or an earlier manifestation of a single entity. Exposure to allergens in

[a] Department of Otolaryngology, Head and Neck Surgery, Loyola University Medical Center, 2160 South First Avenue, Maguire Center, Room 1870, Maywood, IL 60153, USA; [b] Department of General Surgery, Loyola University Medical Center, 2160 South First Avenue, Bldg. 110, Room 3276, Maywood, IL 60153, USA; [c] Department of Otolaryngology-Head and Neck Surgery, Johns Hopkins Medical Institutions, N. Caroline Street. JHOC 6263, Baltimore, MD 21287, USA
* Corresponding author.
E-mail address: mpatadia@lumc.edu

Otolaryngol Clin N Am 56 (2023) 39–53
https://doi.org/10.1016/j.otc.2022.09.003
0030-6665/23/Published by Elsevier Inc.
oto.theclinics.com

both the upper and lower airways can lead to increased epithelial permeability, IgE sensitization, and eosinophilia, which lead to global airway inflammation. In this section, the authors review some of the most common sources of environmental allergic airway disease and their association with allergic rhinitis, asthma, and chronic rhinosinusitis (CRS) (**Fig. 1**).

House Dust Mites

House dust mites (HDMs) are one of the foremost causes of allergic disease worldwide,[3] producing allergens which stimulate atopic reactions in both the upper and lower airway. HDMs are eight-legged arachnids which are photophobic and depend on ambient water vapor and therefore thrive in dark, humid environments.[4] High concentrations of HDM are particularly found in pillows, mattresses, and carpeted floors.[5] These products easily become airborne when their resting location is disturbed (eg, walking on a carpet or laying on a bed) and then can be inhaled and potentially elicit an allergic response in the airway. Several studies have shown a nonlinear dose-dependent response to HDM allergens; children exposed to the lowest and highest levels of dust mite allergen have shown lower rates of sensitization than those exposed to mid-range levels.[6,7] This suggests that although sufficient exposure is needed for sensitization, there may also be a "high-dose tolerance."

HDMs produce a variety of allergens throughout the course of their lifecycle, including DNA, fragments of shed exoskeleton, and waste pellets.[4] One of the most common dust mites in temperate climates, *Dermatophagoides pteronyssinus* (Der p), produces serine and cysteine proteases which disrupt epithelial tight junctions and expose allergens to underlying antigen-presenting cells,[8] which induces proinflammatory cytokine release and IgE response. These proteases also activate protease-activating receptors which stimulate itching, further cytokine release, and can cause hypertrophy of bronchial smooth muscle in asthmatics.[4,9] In addition, pathogen-associated molecular patterns present in a variety of HDM-produced allergens stimulate the innate immune system and cleave B-cell receptors, thereby skewing a Type 2 versus Type 1 predominant response. Thus, HDM components can not only cause sensitization, but by disrupting epithelial barrier integrity and inducing Th2 polarization, they can predispose hosts to increased atopy and magnified allergic

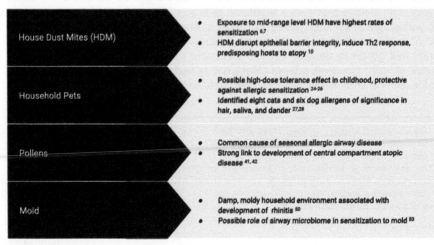

Fig. 1. Summary of environmental allergens.

responses to other pathogens. Given the airborne nature of these particles and their effects on the upper and lower airway, it can be presumed that most exposure occurs due to inhalation; however, there is evidence that the Der p 1 allergen can be found in the human colon where it increases epithelial permeability through cytokine protease activity.[10] It is not clear whether this gastrointestinal exposure can lead to systemic allergy sensitization, but oral exposure to Der p 1 in a mouse model spurred sensitization for asthma, and in humans Der p 10 tropomyosin has strong cross-reactivity with invertebrate tropomyosin and thus can sensitize individuals to ingested seafoods.[11,12]

HDM sensitivity has a well-documented role in disease of the unified airway. One study found that approximately half of patients with allergic rhinitis and two-thirds with CRS were sensitized to HDM. In children with asthma, allergen levels have been shown to correlate with symptom severity,[13] and HDM sensitization has been shown to correlate with bronchial hyperresponsiveness in non-asthmatic children with allergic rhinitis.[14] Although the etiology of CRS is likely multifactorial and variable among individuals, there is evidence that inhaled allergens can be an inciting or exacerbating factor in some.[15] One study found that patients with CRS with nasal polyps and high levels of eosinophilia had increased sensitivity to HDM[16]; another developed a mouse model in which nasal polyps were induced by administering HDM allergen along with *Staphylococcus aureus* endotoxin.[17]

Mitigation strategies for unified airway disease caused by HDM allergy include household interventions such as decreasing humidity, using vacuum cleaners with high efficiency particulate air (HEPA) filtration, and frequently washing bedding (particularly with hot water and bleach).[18,19] In patients with moderate to severe rhinitis or asthma which seem related to allergen exposure and are not well controlled by usual pharmacotherapy, subcutaneous immunotherapy (SCIT), and sublingual immunotherapy (SLIT) have been shown to be effective in reducing symptom severity.[20,21]

Household Pets

Domesticated animals, particularly cats and dogs, carry a high potential for allergic sensitization, and allergy to these animals is a risk factor for development of allergic rhinitis and asthma.[22] Although allergic sensitivity and symptoms of rhinitis and asthma are higher in adults with pets,[23] there are data that suggest that exposure in early childhood is not necessarily a risk for sensitization. Several large studies showed that young children with pets had equal or even lower development of asthma and allergic rhinitis compared with those who did not.[24-26] This suggests that similar to HDM exposure, there may be a high-dose tolerance in early childhood that is protective against allergic sensitization.

There are eight currently identified allergens produced by domestic cats. The major allergen (Fel d 1) is present in cat skin and hair follicles; however, at least four of the allergens are found primarily in cat saliva.[27] Of note, Fel d 4 is a saliva-borne cat allergen which has significant cross-reactivity with dog allergens and may play a role in cosensitization.[28] There are six major dog allergens, which are found most significantly in dog dander but can also be present in dog hair and saliva.[27] Although there is much interest in hypoallergenic pets, it is important to note that some of the allergens for both cats and dogs are proteins such as albumin and immunoglobulins that will be present in all animals even if other allergens are absent. Therefore, there can be no truly nonallergenic cats or dogs, and one study showed that dog allergen levels did not differ in homes with hypoallergenic versus non-hypoallergenic dogs.[29]

The recommended intervention for individuals with significant allergic response to a household pet is removal. However, cat allergens in particular can contaminate an environment for months after removal,[30] and allergic responses can be triggered by contact with others who have pets at home (and allergens adherent to their clothing), making avoidance of exposure difficult for individuals with pet allergies even after removal of their own.[31] Although data are still limited on SCIT and SLIT for cat and dog allergies, there is emerging evidence that these treatment modalities can alleviate symptoms in pet-induced allergic rhinitis and asthma.[32,33] To date, there are no data on SLIT and extremely limited data on SCIT for treatment of CRS, particularly with respect to pet allergy.[34,35]

Pollens

One of the most common causes of seasonal allergic airway disease is pollen grains. The causative pollens differ geographically and seasonally; in North America, the contribution is generally greatest from tree pollen in the spring, grass pollen in the summer, and weed pollen in the late summer and autumn.[36] Within the weed pollen category, ragweed (*Ambrosia* spp.) is the most significant contributor to allergic airway disease; with studies finding rates of skin test responsiveness ranging from 10 to greater than 33% of individuals.[37,38] Ragweed-responsive patients have increased rates of rhinitis symptoms and bronchial hyperresponsiveness, which may be a predisposing feature for the development of asthma.[39,40] Data on the role of pollen allergy in CRS are conflicting, but there are certain subtypes that have been strongly associated with perennial allergy. For example, central compartment atopic disease (CCAD), a variant of CRS characterized by polypoid changes of the middle turbinate and in more severe cases the superior turbinates and posterosuperior nasal septum, seems to have a strong link with environmental aeroallergen sensitivity.[41,42]

The prevalence of ragweed allergy has increased in recent years in both North America and Europe.[43,44] Of note, the length of the ragweed pollen season has also significantly increased in the last 20 years. This can be geographically correlated with the increasing effect of anthropogenic climate change and may be related not only to number of frost-free days but also environmental CO_2 level, which increases ragweed pollen production.[36,45]

Compared with the indoor allergens described earlier, prevention via removal or avoidance is less feasible for outdoor airborne allergens such as pollens. Standard pharmacotherapy including nasal corticosteroids and oral or nasal antihistamines can control symptoms but are insufficient for many patients and do not have sustained benefit after cessation of use.[46] For patients with seasonal allergic airway disease refractory to pharmacotherapy, immunotherapy is an option which can be targeted to multiple allergens including grass, tree, and ragweed pollens and can be administered via subcutaneous or sublingual routes. SCIT and SLIT have been shown in multiple randomized controlled trials to decrease symptom burden and improve quality of life.[47] Furthermore, there is emerging evidence that specific immunotherapy in children with allergic rhinitis can decrease the risk for the future development of asthma.[48,49] Evidence for efficacy of immunotherapy in CRS is mixed[35]; however, this has yet to be tested in specific endotypes such as CCAD which seem to have a stronger allergic component.

Mold

The evidence for mold's contribution to allergic disease of the unified airway remains mixed; however, there is a body of data suggesting that damp and moldy conditions in the household are associated with rhinitis.[50] The evidence for the role of mold in asthma is also equivocal. Although some studies have reported correlation with mold exposure to asthma development or severity, others have failed to measure such an association.[51,52] One possible reason for this heterogeneity is the wide variability in environmental and patient factors that affect sensitization to mold, including potentially the gut or airway microbiomes. There is some evidence that alterations in the microbiome early in life may play an important role in allergic sensitization to mold. One study found that mold exposure and antibiotic use in infancy (which would alter the microbiome at a young age) have additive effects on the risk of developing allergic rhinitis.[53] In this sense, it has been argued that the internal microbiome can be conceptualized as a separate, internal type of environment that individuals are exposed to which modulates their reactions to potential allergens.[54]

OCCUPATIONAL EXPOSURES

Occupational rhinitis (OR) is defined as rhinitis that develops from workplace exposure to an inciting agent in a previously asymptomatic individual.[55,56] OR develops before occupational asthma (OA), with 10% to 40% of OR patients developing OA over time, consistent with the concept of united airway disease.[57,58] Ambient air pollution continues to be a matter of public health concern owing to increasing urbanization, energy consumption, and transportation emissions.[15,59] Air pollutants have been linked to the development and exacerbation of both upper and lower airway disease.[15,59–62]

The inciting occupational agents are classified as either high molecular weight (HMW) or low molecular weight (LMW), capable of eliciting different types of allergic responses.[55] HMW agents are typically biological substances and enzymes that trigger specific IgE-mediated sensitization and induce a Th2 response.[55,63,64] HMW agents, specifically, act in a dose-dependent manner where higher level of exposure is correlated with a significant impact on the development of sensitization and OR.[55,63] LMW agents are haptens that bind to carrier proteins, becoming immunogenic in a mechanism that is yet unknown.[55,64] Regardless of the molecular weight of the agent, both are characterized by the presence of eosinophils as demonstrated in nasal lavage fluid or nasal secretions after specific inhalation challenge testing.[63,65–68]

The incidence of OR is highest among laboratory animal workers (10%–42%) and bakers (23%–50%), with other high-risk occupations including farming, food processing, boat building, and textile workers.[55,69] A study of textile workers revealed that increasing nasal obstruction and overall impairment was positively correlated with time spent at work with the aggravating agent.[70] OR and OA often remain underdiagnosed due to the lack of association with environmental work agents, and many workers with severe impairments leave their positions, leading to a remaining population of healthy workers, known as the healthy worker effect.[55] Closely related to OA is non-asthmatic eosinophilic bronchitis (NAEB), which is characterized by chronic cough and eosinophils in the sputum without airflow obstruction or airway hyperresponsiveness. The etiology of NAEB is thought to be exposure to an environmental allergen or occupational sensitizer, welding fumes, formaldehyde exposure, and baking flour have been reported as inciting agents.[71–73] Although patients may have repeated episodes associated with persistent sputum eosinophilia, especially when presenting with rhinitis, studies have shown that unlike OA, there is little to no risk of long-term chronic airway obstruction.[74]

Combat experience as a form of occupational exposure results in a large population of veteran soldiers with post-deployment pathology of their aerodigestive systems.[75] Respiratory diseases, including sinusitis, allergic rhinitis, and asthma are documented as the leading nonpsychiatric diagnoses among Iraq and Afghanistan veterans. The proposed risk factors of combat-related airway disease include outdoor living conditions, close living quarters, and inhalation of ambient particulate matter including several combustive materials, including burn pits.[75] Similarly, protective service occupations such as firefighters have reported rates of occupational-related asthma at a rate of 300/1,000,000 due to exposure to high levels of combustive materials and smoke.[76]

Construction workers and insulators define another population with occupational exposures that have been linked to various health conditions. Specifically, asbestos is well established with its role in the development of pulmonary fibrosis, pleural abnormalities, mesothelioma, and other pulmonary malignancies; however, its role in benign airway disease is still relatively unknown.[77,78] Asbestos is banned by most western countries, however, the production of asbestos and mineral forms of asbestos, including actinolite, anthophyllite, and tremolite, continued as recently as 2018 in some western countries and still continues in China, making its impact on respiratory health an important consideration.[77,78] One study seeking to understand the benign manifestations of asbestos exposures looked at a group of 1043 insulators in Alberta, Canada, from 2011 to 2017 and found that asbestos had no impact on the development of asthma, but was the only insulate material with a marginally increased risk for chronic obstructive pulmonary disorder (COPD).[77] The pathophysiology of asbestos-associated disease is largely attributed to its induction of pulmonary fibrosis; however, studies of patients with confirmed asbestosis have found that asbestos exposure results in duration-dependent small airway obstructive defects.[78] Newer insulation materials such as aerogels have been reported in a small study to cause irritation of the nose and throat including epistaxis and nasal congestion.[79] The investigators were unable to point to aerogel as the cause for the respiratory symptoms, however given that aerogel is a new product, its impact on upper respiratory disease cannot be excluded and warrants further exploration.

AMBIENT AIR POLLUTION

The US Environmental Protection Agency has defined six criteria air pollutants which include ozone, particulate matter (PM), carbon monoxide, lead, sulfur dioxide (SO_2), and nitrogen dioxide (NO_2)[80] (**Fig. 2**). Epidemiologic evidence has documented the detrimental acute and chronic effects of these pollutants on morbidity and mortality including exacerbations of cardiovascular and pulmonary diseases.[15,61] Traffic-related air pollutants (TRAP), cigarette smoke, and PM have been shown to exacerbate chronic inflammatory airway disorders.[15] Both in vivo and in vitro studies have demonstrated that regardless of the kind of pollutant, air pollutants upregulate reactive

		Production of Pollutant	Impact on Unified Airway
1	Ozone	Greenhouse gas generated by atmospheric reactions between NO_2, hydrocarbons, and ultraviolet light.[59,60]	• Strong smell leading to airway discomfort, increased sputum, and emphysema [59,60,108] • Time and dose dependent production of ROS that damage epithelial barrier function [108]
2	Particulate Matter	Generated as TRAP, combustion or from soil/sand with varying sizes, shape, surface area, and chemical composition [96]	• PM2.5 able to penetrate entire airway, reaching alveoli [60,81,97] • Correlated with incidence of CRS, microbiome alteration, and childhood asthma [86,88-90,92,95,100]
3	Sulfur Dioxide (SO_2)	Formed by combustion of fossil fuels and smoke stacks [106,107]	• Correlated with exacerbation of COPD[106] • Possible synergistic effect on asthma development when combined with NO_2[107]
4	Nitrogen Based Pollutants (NOx)	From combustion of fossil fuels which generate photochemical smog [59,60]	• Correlated with incidence/prevalence of CRS, and developing childhood asthma [89-90,97,95,100-102] • Conflicting evidence on exacerbation of asthma and AR symptoms [15,69,103-105]

Fig. 2. Summary of environmental air pollutants.

oxygen species (ROS) leading to oxidative stress and inflammation, and this mechanism is thought to drive exacerbations of airway diseases.[59,60,62]

Urbanization

Epidemiologic studies of airway disease have investigated the comparative risk of disease development across different locations and environments. Analysis from rapidly developing cities such as Shanghai and Bengaluru have shown increased incidence and prevalence of asthma among children from the early 1990s to 2010s.[81,82] It is theorized that this trend is a result of increased urbanization and environmental pollution from personal products, household appliances, and building materials.[82] Residence in urban and inner-city areas is hypothesized to be a risk factor for the development of airway disease secondary to increased ambient air pollution, pest allergens, and HDM; however, after adjusting for race/ethnicity, region, and sex, there is no significant difference in the prevalence of asthma between inner-city and non-inner city residents. In adjusted models, Black race, Puerto Rican ethnicity, and lower socioeconomic status increased risk for the development of asthma and asthma-related morbidity.[83] Looking at global trends, a World Health Survey of adults found that the highest prevalence of patients with clinical asthma were Australia, Sweden, United Kingdom, Netherlands, and Brazil. As these represent highly developed countries, this was thought to be due to increased urbanization, including energy consumption, and higher levels of air pollution.[84]

Particulate Matter and Traffic-Related Air Pollution

Another category of environmental airway pollution is TRAPs which include nitrogen oxides, NO_2, diesel exhaust particles, black carbon, SO_2, and PM less than 10 μm in size (PM10).[85–95] PM may be composed of solid and liquid particles of various sizes, shapes, surface areas, and chemical compositions.[96] The size and composition of the PM determine its site of deposition in the respiratory tract where particles 2.5 μm (PM2.5) or smaller are able to penetrate the entire airway, carrying condensed toxic air pollutants all the way to the alveoli.[60,81,97] Animal studies analyzing the effect of PM2.5 exposure on airway inflammation have found Type 2 sinonasal inflammation, epithelial barrier dysfunction, and increased expression of proinflammatory mediators.[98] Nitrogen pollutants (NOx) are most significantly produced from the combustion of fossil fuels by automobiles, generating photochemical smog that has acute toxic effects on the human airway.[59,60] Several cohort studies have found a positive correlation between PM (both PM2.5 and PM10) and NOx and incidence/prevalence of CRS.[88–90,92,94] It was also found that pollutants have varied effects on subtypes of disease. When looking at CRS with nasal polyposis (CRSwNP) versus CRS without nasal polyposis (CRSsNP), it was found that CRSwNP had higher PM2.5 exposure, however, CRSsNP had worsened disease severity with increasing PM2.5 exposure.[99] There is also evidence that TRAPs can cause disturbances in the airway microbiome; one study found that increasing levels of neighborhood PM2.5 was associated with decreased relative abundance of *Corynebacterium* in the nasal cavities.[86] This suggests that TRAPs' mechanism of airway inflammation may be multifactorial, involving both production of ROS as well as induction of microbiome changes.

Studies have also focused on the impact of NOx and PM on the development of childhood airway disease, namely asthma, finding that closer proximity to roadways and increased exposure to TRAPs increases the risk for development of asthma.[95,100–102] Studies in adults, however, have found conflicting evidence. A cohort study of US women with asthma found that NO_2 and PM2.5 were both significantly associated with increased wheezing, whereas a large Canadian cohort study failed to find any association between long-term exposure to ultrafine particulates and the incidence of respiratory disease.[69,103] In patients with allergic rhinitis, researchers found a positive correlation between disease severity and increasing automobile air pollution, whereas a different cohort study found no correlation between TRAPs and risk of allergic rhinitis.[15,104,105] Although the growing consensus supports a correlation between TRAPs and risk/exacerbation of united airway disease, further research is needed to define this relationship.

SO_2 as a TRAP and its specific impact on the airway receives significantly less attention. Briefly, it is formed from the combustion of fossil fuels and burning of smokestacks. SO_2 is found to be associated with respiratory symptoms including shortness of breath, wheezing, and increased risk of obstructive airway disease.[106,107] SO_2 exposure is correlated significantly with increased exacerbations of COPD and has questionable impact on asthma.[106] Together with NO_2, areas high in SO_2 have been found to increase risk for development of asthma over areas only high in NO_2 or with moderate SO_2.[107] It warrants further research to understand the individual role of SO_2 on airway disease and its possible synergistic role with other ambient air pollutants.

Ozone

Ozone as a greenhouse gas is considered to be one of the most toxic photochemical air pollutants, generated at the ground level through atmospheric reactions between NO_2, hydrocarbons, and ultraviolet light.[59,60] Ozone is associated with an extremely strong smell that is irritating to the respiratory system and may lead to swelling of the throat, discomfort in the chest, coughing, increased sputum production, and even emphysema.[59,60,108] Ozone is extremely reactive, inducing the production of ROS within the fluid-lined compartment of the lung, leading to activation of intracellular signaling pathways within the cells lining the airway and thus increased inflammation and remodeling of tissues.[109] Studies have also shown that ROS cause dysfunction of epithelial cell tight junctions by disrupting claudin expression.[109] The effect of ozone on the airways is shown to be dependent on concentration, duration of exposure, and level of exertion.[59] Animal studies have indicated that acute ozone exposure is enough to cause respiratory epithelial cell disruption with bronchoalveolar lavage fluids showing strong neutrophil recruitment, protein leak, and airway hyperresponsiveness.[108] When exposure to ozone was increased in concentration and time, the effect was amplified as demonstrated through collagen deposition, reduced epithelial barrier height, distended bronchioles, and evidence of alveolar damage indicative of emphysema.[108] Patel and colleagues continued to find a concentration-dependent effect of ozone on upper airway disease with increasing inflammation and the presence of Charcot–Leyden crystals in patients with CRSwNP with increasing ozone exposure.[87] However, other studies failed to find any impact of ozone on development or outcomes in patients with upper airway disease.[88,89] As ambient greenhouse gas emissions continue to increase, ozone's impact on the incidence and exacerbations of airway diseases remains an important area of concern.

SUMMARY

In this section, the authors reviewed several common environmental factors impacting the development of united airway disease. Although innovative research has advanced the understanding of inciting environmental agents and their specific role in the pathogenesis of airway disease, we continue to learn about how race, gender, and socioeconomic factors further influence environmentally induced respiratory disease. With increased understanding of the profound impact that environmental factors play in development of unified airway disease, it is crucial to address these to improve morbidity and mortality globally. Changes in housing regulations, occupational safety procedures, and environmental protection measures to decrease emissions may have significant impacts on outcomes for patients suffering from airway disease.

CLINICS CARE POINTS

- High concentrations of house dust mites (HDMs) are found in pillows, mattresses, and carpeted floors. Children exposed to mid-range level concentrations have higher rates of sensitization than low or high concentrations, termed "high-dose tolerance." Treatment strategies for HDM-induced airway disease include decreasing household humidity, use of HEPA filtration, frequent washing of bedding, pharmacologic agents, and immunotherapies.

- Household pets as allergens follow a high-dose tolerance pattern of sensitization, and studies have shown that there is no difference in allergen levels between hypoallergenic and non-hypoallergenic dogs. Interventions for those with pet allergies include pet removal; however, allergens may linger in the environment for months making this challenging.

- Pollen contribution is most significantly from tree pollen, grass pollen, and weed pollen throughout spring, summer, and autumn, respectively. Allergy prevalence is increasing, particularly for ragweed, and correlates with increasing pollen season length which may be due in part to anthropogenic climate change. Treatment includes nasal corticosteroids, antihistamines, and for refractory symptoms, immunotherapy.

- Occupational exposures are underdiagnosed due to the lack of association with environmental work agents. Patients will often leave their positions, leading to a remaining population of health workers, the healthy worker effect. Treatment involves removal of the inciting agent from the environment or enhanced protective equipment.

- Air pollutants continue to increase secondary to increased urbanization and energy consumption. Proximity to roadways and increased exposure to air pollutants have been associated with development and exacerbation of airway diseases. Strategies for mitigation include global measures to decrease air pollutants and energy consumption.

DISCLOSURE

The authors declare no relevant conflicts of interest.

REFERENCES

1. Wise SK, Lin SY, Toskala E, et al. International Consensus Statement on Allergy and Rhinology: Allergic Rhinitis. Int Forum Allergy Rhinol 2018;8(2):108–352.
2. Compalati E, Ridolo E, Passalacqua G, et al. The link between allergic rhinitis and asthma: the united airways disease. Expert Rev Clin Immunol 2010;6(3): 413–23.
3. Sánchez-Borges M, Fernandez-Caldas E, Thomas WR, et al. International consensus (ICON) on: clinical consequences of mite hypersensitivity, a global problem. World Allergy Organ J 2017;10(1):14.
4. Miller JD. The Role of Dust Mites in Allergy. Clin Rev Allergy Immunol 2019; 57(3):312–29.
5. Sidenius KE, Hallas TE, Brygge T, et al. House dust mites and their allergens at selected locations in the homes of house dust mite-allergic patients. Clin Exp Allergy 2002;32(9):1299–304.

6. Tovey ER, Almqvist C, Li Q, et al. Nonlinear relationship of mite allergen exposure to mite sensitization and asthma in a birth cohort. J Allergy Clin Immunol 2008;122(1):114–8.

7. Schram-Bijkerk D, Doekes G, Boeve M, et al. Nonlinear relations between house dust mite allergen levels and mite sensitization in farm and nonfarm children. Allergy 2006;61(5):640–7.

8. Wan H, Winton HL, Soeller C, et al. Der p 1 facilitates transepithelial allergen delivery by disruption of tight junctions. J Clin Invest 1999;104(1):123–33.

9. Trian T, Allard B, Dupin I, et al. House dust mites induce proliferation of severe asthmatic smooth muscle cells via an epithelium-dependent pathway. Am J Respir Crit Care Med 2015;191(5):538–46.

10. Tulic MK, Vivinus-Nébot M, Rekima A, et al. Presence of commensal house dust mite allergen in human gastrointestinal tract: a potential contributor to intestinal barrier dysfunction. Gut 2016;65(5):757–66.

11. Macchiaverni P, Rekima A, Turfkruyer M, et al. Respiratory allergen from house dust mite is present in human milk and primes for allergic sensitization in a mouse model of asthma. Allergy 2014;69(3):395–8.

12. Popescu FD. Cross-reactivity between aeroallergens and food allergens. World J Methodol 2015;5(2):31–50.

13. Chan-Yeung M, Manfreda J, Dimich-Ward H, et al. Mite and cat allergen levels in homes and severity of asthma. Am J Respir Crit Care Med 1995;152(6): 1805–11.

14. Kim HB, Hong SJ, Lee SY. House dust mite sensitization is associated with bronchial hyperresponsiveness in children with allergic rhinitis. J Allergy Clin Immunol 2020;145(2):AB39.

15. London NR, Lina I, Ramanathan M. Aeroallergens, air pollutants, and chronic rhinitis and rhinosinusitis. World J Otorhinolaryngology- Head Neck Surg 2018;04(03):209–15.

16. Xu M, Ye X, Zhao F, et al. Allergogenic profile in patients with different subtypes of chronic rhinosinusitis with nasal polyps. ORL J Otorhinolaryngol Relat Spec 2015;77(1):10–6.

17. Khalmuratova R, Lee M, Kim DW, et al. Induction of nasal polyps using house dust mite and Staphylococcal enterotoxin B in C57BL/6 mice. Allergologia et Immunopathologia 2016;44(1):66–75.

18. Portnoy J, Miller JD, Williams PB, et al. Environmental assessment and exposure control of dust mites: a practice parameter. Ann Allergy Asthma Immunol 2013; 111(6):465–507.

19. Sarwar M. House Dust Mites: Ecology, Biology, Prevalence, Epidemiology and Elimination. IntechOpen 2020. https://doi.org/10.5772/intechopen.91891.

20. Tang RB. House dust mite-specific immunotherapy alters the natural course of atopic march. J Chin Med Assoc 2020;83(2):109–12.

21. Virchow JC, Backer V, Kuna P, et al. Efficacy of a House Dust Mite Sublingual Allergen Immunotherapy Tablet in Adults With Allergic Asthma: A Randomized Clinical Trial. JAMA 2016;315(16):1715–25.

22. Konradsen JR, Fujisawa T, van Hage M, et al. Allergy to furry animals: New insights, diagnostic approaches, and challenges. J Allergy Clin Immunol 2015; 135(3):616–25.

23. Bener A, Mobayed H, Sattar HA, et al. Pet ownership: its effect on allergy and respiratory symptoms. Eur Ann Allergy Clin Immunol 2004;36(8):306–10.

24. Hesselmar B, Aberg N, Aberg B, et al. Does early exposure to cat or dog protect against later allergy development? Clin Exp Allergy 1999;29(5):611–7.

25. Carlsen KCL, Roll S, Carlsen KH, et al. Does Pet Ownership in Infancy Lead to Asthma or Allergy at School Age? Pooled Analysis of Individual Participant Data from 11 European Birth Cohorts. PLoS One 2012;7(8):e43214.
26. Sandin A, Björkstén B, Bråbäck L. Development of atopy and wheezing symptoms in relation to heredity and early pet keeping in a Swedish birth cohort. Pediatr Allergy Immunol 2004;15(4):316–22.
27. Portnoy JM, Kennedy K, Sublett JL, et al. Environmental assessment and exposure control: a practice parameter–furry animals. Ann Allergy Asthma Immunol 2012;108(4):223.
28. Spitzauer S, Pandjaitan B, Mühl S, et al. Major cat and dog allergens share IgE epitopes. J Allergy Clin Immunol 1997;99(1 Pt 1):100–6.
29. Nicholas CE, Wegienka GR, Havstad SL, et al. Dog allergen levels in homes with hypoallergenic compared with nonhypoallergenic dogs. Am J Rhinol Allergy 2011;25(4):252–6.
30. Wood RA, Chapman MD, Adkinson NF, et al. The effect of cat removal on allergen content in household-dust samples. J Allergy Clin Immunol 1989; 83(4):730–4.
31. Wang DY. Risk factors of allergic rhinitis: genetic or environmental? Ther Clin Risk Manag 2005;1(2):115–23.
32. Virtanen T. Immunotherapy for pet allergies. Hum Vaccin Immunother 2017; 14(4):807–14.
33. Uriarte SA, Sastre J. Subcutaneous Immunotherapy With High-Dose Cat and Dog Extracts: A Real-life Study. J Investig Allergol Clin Immunol 2020;30(3): 169–74.
34. Borish L, Baroody FM, Kim MS, et al. Yardstick for the medical management of chronic rhinosinusitis. Ann Allergy Asthma Immunol 2022;128(2):118–28.
35. DeYoung K, Wentzel JL, Schlosser RJ, et al. Systematic review of immunotherapy for chronic rhinosinusitis. Am J Rhinol Allergy 2014;28(2):145–50.
36. Ziska L, Knowlton K, Rogers C, et al. Recent warming by latitude associated with increased length of ragweed pollen season in central North America. Proc Natl Acad Sci 2011;108(10):4248–51.
37. Gergen PJ, Turkeltaub PC, Kovar MG. The prevalence of allergic skin test reactivity to eight common aeroallergens in the U.S. population: results from the second National Health and Nutrition Examination Survey. J Allergy Clin Immunol 1987;80(5):669–79.
38. Chapman JA. Aeroallergens of southeastern missouri, usa. Grana 1986;25(3): 235–46.
39. Braman SS, Barrows AA, DeCotiis BA, et al. Airway hyperresponsiveness in allergic rhinitis. A risk factor for asthma. Chest 1987;91(5):671–4.
40. Townley RG, Ryo UY, Kolotkin BM, et al. Bronchial sensitivity to methacholine in current and former asthmatic and allergic rhinitis patients and control subjects. J Allergy Clin Immunol 1975;56(6):429–42.
41. White LJ, Rotella MR, DelGaudio JM. Polypoid changes of the middle turbinate as an indicator of atopic disease. Int Forum Allergy Rhinology. 2014;4(5): 376–80.
42. DelGaudio JM, Loftus PA, Hamizan AW, et al. Central Compartment Atopic Disease. Am J Rhinol Allergy 2017;31(4):228–34.
43. Oswalt ML, Marshall GD. Ragweed as an Example of Worldwide Allergen Expansion. Allergy Asthma Clin Immunol 2008;4(3):130–5.
44. Lake IR, Jones NR, Agnew M, et al. Climate Change and Future Pollen Allergy in Europe. Environ Health Perspect 2017;125(3):385–91.

45. Rogers CA, Wayne PM, Macklin EA, et al. Interaction of the onset of spring and elevated atmospheric CO2 on ragweed (Ambrosia artemisiifolia L.) pollen production. Environ Health Perspect 2006;114(6):865–9.

46. White P, Smith H, Baker N, et al. Symptom control in patients with hay fever in UK general practice: how well are we doing and is there a need for allergen immunotherapy. Clin Exp Allergy 1998;28(3):266–70.

47. Dretzke J, Meadows A, Novielli N, et al. Subcutaneous and sublingual immunotherapy for seasonal allergic rhinitis: A systematic review and indirect comparison. J Allergy Clin Immunol 2013;131(5):1361–6.

48. Fiocchi A, Fox AT. Preventing progression of allergic rhinitis: the role of specific immunotherapy. Arch Dis Child - Education Pract 2011;96(3):91–100.

49. Alviani C, Roberts G, Mitchell F, et al. Primary prevention of asthma in high-risk children using HDM SLIT; assessment at age 6 years. J Allergy Clin Immunol 2020;145(6):1711–3.

50. Jaakkola MS, Quansah R, Hugg TT, et al. Association of indoor dampness and molds with rhinitis risk: A systematic review and meta-analysis. J Allergy Clin Immunol 2013;132(5):1099–110.e18.

51. Oluwole O, Kirychuk SP, Lawson JA, et al. Indoor mold levels and current asthma among school-aged children in Saskatchewan, Canada. Indoor Air 2017;27(2):311–9.

52. Vincent M, Corazza F, Chasseur C, et al. Relationship between mold exposure, specific IgE sensitization, and clinical asthma: A case-control study. Ann Allergy Asthma Immunol 2018;121(3):333–9.

53. Yang SI, Lee E, Jung YH, et al. Effect of antibiotic use and mold exposure in infancy on allergic rhinitis in susceptible adolescents. Ann Allergy Asthma Immunol 2014;113(2):160–5.e1.

54. Sbihi H, Boutin RCT, Cutler C, et al. Thinking bigger: How early-life environmental exposures shape the gut microbiome and influence the development of asthma and allergic disease. Allergy 2019;74(11):2103–15.

55. Shao Z, Bernstein JA. Occupational Rhinitis: Classification, Diagnosis, and Therapeutics. Curr Allergy Asthma Rep 2019;19(12):54.

56. Lau A, Tarlo SM. Update on the management of occupational asthma and work-exacerbated asthma. Allergy Asthma Immunol Res 2019;11(2):188–200.

57. Kurt OK, Basaran N. Occupational Exposure to Metals and Solvents: Allergy and Airway Diseases. Curr Allergy Asthma Rep 2020;20:38.

58. Balogun RA, Siracusa A, Shusterman D. Occupational rhinitis and occupational asthma: association or progression? Am J Ind Med 2018;61(4):293–307.

59. Kelly FJ, Fussell JC. Air pollution and airway disease. Clin Exp Allergy 2011;41(8):1059–71. PMID: 21623970.

60. Lee YG, Lee PH, Choi SM, et al. Effects of Air Pollutants on Airway Diseases. Int J Environ Res Public Health 2021;18(18):9905.

61. Pope CA, Lefler JS, Ezzati M, et al. Mortality Risk and Fine Particulate Air Pollution in a Large. Representative Cohort U.S Adults." Environ Health Perspect 2019;127(7):77007.

62. Ghio AJ, Carraway MS, Madden MC. Composition of air pollution particles and oxidative stress in cells, tissues, and living systems. J Toxicol Environ Health B Crit Rev 2012;15(1):1-21.

63. Quirce S, Lemière C, Walusiak-Skorupa J, et al. Occupational Rhinitis. In: Asthma in the workplace. Taylor and Francis: CRC Press; 2021. p. 273–8.

64. Dufour MH, Lemière C, Prince P, et al. Comparative airway response to high-versus low-molecular weight agents in occupational asthma. Eur Respir J 2009;33(4):734–9. Epub 2009 Jan 7. PMID: 19129274.
65. Palczynski C, Walusiak J, Ruta U, et al. Nasal provocation test in the diagnosis of natural rubber latex allergy. Allergy 2000;55(1):34–41.
66. Pałczyński C, Walusiak J, Krakowiak A, et al. Nasal lavage fluid examination in diagnostics of occupational allergy to chloramine. Int J Occup Med Environ Health 2003;16(3):231–40. Erratum in: Int J Occup Med Environ Health. 2003;16(4):328. Szymczak Wojciech [corrected to Szymczak Wies¿aw]. PMID: 14587536.
67. Krakowiak A, Ruta U, Górski P, et al. Nasal lavage fluid examination and rhino-manometry in the diagnostics of occupational airway allergy to laboratory animals. Int J Occup Med Environ Health 2003;16:125–32.
68. Walusiak J, Wiszniewska M, Krawczyk-Adamus P, et al. Occupational allergy to wheat flour. Nasal response to specific inhalative challenge in asthma and rhinitis vs. isolated rhinitis: a comparative study. Int J Occup Med Environ Health 2004;17(4):433–40. PMID: 15852757.
69. Young MT, Sandler DP, DeRoo LA, et al. Ambient air pollution exposure and incident adult asthma in a nationwide cohort of U.S. women. Am J Respir Crit Care Med 2014;190:914–21.
70. Maoua M, Maalel OE, Kacem I, et al. Quality of life and work productivity impairment of patients with allergic occupational rhinitis. Tanaffos 2019;18:58–65.
71. Di Stefano F, Di Giampaolo L, Verna N, et al. Occupational eosinophilic bronchitis in a foundry worker exposed to isocyanate and a baker exposed to flour. Thorax 2007;62(4):368–70.
72. Pala G, Pignatti P, Gentile E, et al. La bronchite eosinofila professionale: considerazioni e nuovi strumenti diagnostici a margine di un caso clinico [Professional eosinophilic bronchitis: considerations and new diagnostic methods in a clinical case]. G Ital Med Lav Ergon 2010;32(2):145–8. Italian. PMID: 20684434.
73. Côté A, Russell RJ, Boulet LP, et al, CHEST Expert Cough Panel. Managing Chronic Cough Due to Asthma and NAEB in Adults and Adolescents: CHEST Guideline and Expert Panel Report. Chest 2020;158(1):68–96. Epub 2020 Jan 20. PMID: 31972181.
74. Lai K, Liu B, Xu D, et al. Will nonasthmatic eosinophilic bronchitis develop into chronic airway obstruction?: a prospective, observational study. Chest 2015; 148(4):887–94. PMID: 25905627.
75. Parsel SM, Riley CA, McCoul ED. Combat zone exposure and respiratory tract disease. Int Forum Allergy Rhinol 2018;00:1–6.
76. Arif AA, Delclos GL, Whitehead LW, et al. Occupational exposures associated with work-related asthma and work-related wheezing among U.S. workers. Am J Ind Med 2003;44(4):368–76.
77. Moitra S, Farshchi Tabrizi A, Idrissi Machichi K, et al. Non-Malignant Respiratory Illnesses in Association with Occupational Exposure to Asbestos and Other Insulating Materials: Findings from the Alberta Insulator Cohort. Int J Environ Res Public Health 2020;17(19):7085.
78. Yang X, Yan Y, Xue C, et al. Association between increased small airway obstruction and asbestos exposure in patients with asbestosis. Clin Respir J 2018;12(4):1676–84. Epub 2017 Nov 23. PMID: 29087047.
79. NIOSH [2015]. Health hazard evaluation report: evaluation of aerogel insulation particulate at a union training facility. By Feldmann K, Musolin K, Methner M. Cincinnati, OH: U.S. Department of Health and Human Services, Centers for

Disease Control and Prevention, National Institute for Occupational Safety and Health, NIOSH HHE Report No. 2014-0026-3230.

80. Criteria Air Pollutants." EPA, Environmental Protection Agency, https://www.epa.gov/criteria-air-pollutants.

81. Paramesh H. Air Pollution and Allergic Airway Diseases: Social Determinants and Sustainability in the Control and Prevention. Indian J Pediatr 2018;85:284–94.

82. Huang C, Liu W, Hu Y, et al. Updated prevalences of asthma, allergy, and airway symptoms, and a systematic review of trends over time for childhood asthma in Shanghai, China. PLoS One 2015;10(4):e0121577. PMID: 25875829; PMCID: PMC4395352.

83. Keet CA, McCormack MC, Pollack CE, et al. Neighborhood poverty, urban residence, race/ethnicity, and asthma: Rethinking the inner-city asthma epidemic. J Allergy Clin Immunol 2015;135(3):655–62. Epub 2015 Jan 20. PMID: 25617226; PMCID: PMC4391373.

84. Enilari O, Sinha S. The Global Impact of Asthma in Adult Populations. Ann Glob Health 2019;85(1):2. PMID: 30741503; PMCID: PMC7052341.

85. Leland EM, Vohra V, Seal SM, et al. Environmental air pollution and chronic rhinosinusitis: A systematic review. Laryngoscope Investig Otolaryngol 2022;7(2):349–60.

86. Padhye LV, Kish JL, Batra PS, et al. The impact of levels of particulate matter with an aerodynamic diameter smaller than 2.5 μm on the nasal microbiota in chronic rhinosinusitis and healthy individuals. Ann Allergy Asthma Immunol 2021;126(2):195–7.

87. Patel TR, Tajudeen BA, Brown H, et al. Association of air pollutant exposure and sinonasal histopathology findings in chronic rhinosinusitis. Am J Rhinol Allergy 2021;35(6):761–7.

88. Zhang Z, Kamil RJ, London NR, et al. Long-term exposure to particulate matter air pollution and chronic rhinosinusitis in non-allergic patients. Am J Respir Crit Care Med 2021;204(7):859–62.

89. Lu M, Ding S, Wang J, et al. Acute effect of ambient air pollution on hospital outpatient cases of chronic sinusitis in Xinxiang, China. Ecotoxicol Environ Saf 2020;202:110923.

90. Velasquez N, Moore JA, Boudreau RM, et al. Association of air pollutants, airborne occupational exposures, and chronic rhinosinusitis disease severity. Int Forum Allergy Rhinol 2020;10(2):175–82.

91. Park M, Lee JS, Park MK. The effects of air pollutants on the prevalence of common ear, nose, and throat diseases in South Korea: a national population-based study. Clin Exp Otorhinolaryngol 2019;12(3):294–300.

92. Mady LJ, Schwarzbach HL, Moore JA, et al. The association of air pollutants and allergic and nonallergic rhinitis in chronic rhinosinusitis. Int Forum Allergy Rhinol 2018;8(3):369–76.

93. Sommar JN, Ek A, Middelveld R, et al. Quality of life in relation to the traffic pollution indicators NO2 and NOx: results from the Swedish GA(2)LEN survey. BMJ Open Respir Res 2014;1(1):e000039.

94. Wolf C. Urban air pollution and health: an ecological study of chronic rhinosinusitis in Cologne, Germany. Health Place 2002;8(2):129–39.

95. McConnell R, Islam T, Shankardass K, et al. Childhood incident asthma and traffic-related air pollution at home and school. Environ Health Perspect 2010;118:1021–6.

96. Gehring U, Beelen R, Eeftens M, et al. Particulate matter composition and respiratory health: the PIAMA birth cohort study. Epidemiology 2015;26:300–9.

97. Dong J, Shang Y, Tian L, et al. Ultrafine particle deposition in a realistic human airway at multiple inhalation scenarios. Int J Numer Method Biomed Eng 2019; 35(7):e3215. Epub 2019 May 29. PMID: 31077567.

98. Ramanathan M Jr, London NR Jr, Tharakan A, et al. Airborne particulate matter induces nonallergic eosinophilic sinonasal inflammation in mice. Am J Respir Cell Mol Biol 2017;57:59–65.

99. Mady LJ, Schwarzbach HL, Moore JA, et al. Air pollutants may be environmental risk factors in chronic rhinosinusitis disease progression. Int Forum Allergy Rhinol 2018;8(3):377–84.

100. Thurston GD, Balmes JR, Garcia E, et al. Outdoor Air Pollution and New-Onset Airway Disease. An Official American Thoracic Society Workshop Report. Ann Am Thorac Soc 2020;17(4):387–98.

101. Garcia E, Berhane KT, Islam T, et al. Association of changes in air quality with incident asthma in children in California, 1993–2014. JAMA 2019;321:1906–15.

102. Khreis H, Nieuwenhuijsen MJ. Traffic-Related Air Pollution and Childhood Asthma: Recent Advances and Remaining Gaps in the Exposure Assessment Methods. Int J Environ Res Public Health 2017;14(3):312.

103. Weichenthal S, Bai L, Hatzopoulou M, et al. Long-term exposure to ambient ultrafine particles and respiratory disease incidence in in Toronto, Canada: a cohort study. Environ Health 2017;16(1):64.

104. Nicolussi FH, Santos AP, André SC, et al. Air pollution and respiratory allergic diseases in schoolchildren. Rev Saude Publica 2014;48:326–30.

105. Yi SJ, Shon C, Min KD, et al. Association between exposure to traffic-related air pollution and prevalence of allergic diseases in children, Seoul, Korea. Biomed Res Int 2017;2017:421610.

106. Saygın M, Gonca T, Öztürk Ö, et al. To Investigate the Effects of Air Pollution (PM10 and SO2) on the Respiratory Diseases Asthma and Chronic Obstructive Pulmonary Disease. Turk Thorac J 2017;18(2):33–9.

107. Greenberg N, Carel RS, Derazne E, et al. Different effects of long-term exposures to SO2 and NO2 air pollutants on asthma severity in young adults. J Toxicol Environ Health A 2016;79(8):342–51. PMID: 27092440.

108. Michaudel C, Fauconnier L, Jule Y, et al. Functional and morphological differences of the lung upon acute and chronic ozone exposure in mice. Sci Rep 2018;8:10611.

109. Mumby S, Chung KF, Adcock IM. Transcriptional Effects of Ozone and Impact on Airway Inflammation. Front Immunol 2019;10:1610.

Sex Differences in Airway Diseases

Mackenzie Latour, MD[a], Devyani Lal, MD[b], Michael T. Yim, MD[a],*

KEYWORDS

- Sex disparity • Gender gap • Unified airway • Unified airway disease
- Respiratory disease

KEY POINTS

- Patient sex impacts epidemiology, disease progression, and treatment outcomes for diseases of the unified airway.
- Sex-related disparities have been described for many diseases affecting the unified airway, including chronic rhinosinusitis, asthma, chronic obstructive pulmonary disease, and cystic fibrosis.
- The mechanisms responsible for these male-female differences have not been fully elucidated and are likely multifactorial.

INTRODUCTION

Sex- and gender-related differences in health and disease have gained significant attention in recent years, and increasing emphasis is being placed on understanding the differences between women and men as a crucial step in improving outcomes.[1] Sex (a biological and physiological construct) and gender (a societal and cultural construct) both function as known modifiers for a variety of diseases, including those affecting the upper and lower airway.

Patient sex influences epidemiology,[2–5] symptoms,[6–8] disease progression,[3,9–11] and treatment outcomes[3,8,12–14] in men and women suffering from diseases of the unified airway. Sex-related disparities have been described for many diseases affecting the unified airway, including chronic rhinosinusitis (CRS),[5] asthma,[3] chronic obstructive pulmonary disease,[15] and cystic fibrosis.[10,16] Sex hormones, genetic predisposition, and environmental factors are among many components thought to be related to sexual dimorphism of disease, although the exact mechanisms responsible for sex-related differences in unified airway disease are likely multifactorial and have not yet been fully elucidated.[9,10,17,18]

---

[a] Department of Otolaryngology – Head and Neck Surgery, Louisiana State University Health, 1501 Kings Hwy, Shreveport, LA 71103, USA; [b] Department of Otolaryngology – Head and Neck Surgery, Mayo Clinic, 5777 E Mayo Blvd, Phoenix, AZ 85054, USA
* Corresponding author.
E-mail address: Michael.yim@lsuhs.edu

Otolaryngol Clin N Am 56 (2023) 55–63
https://doi.org/10.1016/j.otc.2022.09.004
oto.theclinics.com
0030-6665/23/© 2022 Elsevier Inc. All rights reserved.

DISCUSSION
Differences in Individual Airway Diseases

Chronic rhinosinusitis
The National Center for Health Statistics in the United States reports a higher prevalence of sinusitis in female individuals than in male individuals from 2015 to 2018, with a prevalence ranging from 13.8% to 15.7% in female individuals compared with 8.0% to 9.2% in male individuals over that timeframe.[19] In 2018, females accounted for 58% of total sinusitis diagnoses. These data were claims based, and otolaryngologist-confirmed diagnosis was not required; therefore, sensitivity and specificity can be considered generally low with the potential to skew reported prevalence in this case. Studies are conflicting on CRS phenotype prevalence by sex, with studies from North America and England reporting higher rates of Chronic Rhinosinusitis with Nasal Polyposis (CRSwNP) in men and higher rates of Chronic Rhinosinusitis without Nasal Polyposis (CRSsNP) in women whereas other studies from Europe and Asia show no difference.[5]

In addition to population-level prevalence variation, male-female differences account for variation in the patient's individual perception of CRS symptoms. One prospective study evaluating sex-related differences in CRS patients undergoing endoscopic sinus surgery (ESS) found that despite similar objective measures of disease (CT and endoscopic scoring), patient-reported quality of life (QOL) was lower on rhinosinusitis disability index (RSDI) and chronic sinusitis survey for female individuals compared with male individuals in both the preoperative and postoperative setting. This effect was negated on multivariate analysis, which revealed that QOL differences reflected the confounding effect of comorbid aspirin intolerance or depression, which were both associated with female sex in their study. The authors concluded that sex, independent of other comorbid illness, was not predictive of CRS-related QOL outcomes following ESS.[13]

Another similar study found that, compared with males, females reported higher total 22-item sino-nasal outcome test (SNOT-22) scores despite lower Lund–Mackay computed tomography (CT) scores.[7] In this study, there were no differences in comorbid illness between sexes and they concluded that despite the higher symptom burden reported by women in the preoperative and early postoperative period, subjective and objective outcomes were comparable between women and men at 1-year following ESS.[20] A third study retrospectively utilizing the total polyp score (TPS) and the German adapted version of the SNOT-20 to compare QOL outcomes between men and women suffering from either CRSwNP or aspirin exacerbated respiratory disease (AERD) also failed to find any significant differences between the two groups.[6]

In contrast to the described outcomes following surgical treatment, the impact of gender dimorphism on response to medical therapy in CRS has not been well characterized. There is evidence that differential absorption and metabolism of oral antibiotics may impact responsiveness to therapeutics in females versus males.[21] Additionally, it has been suggested that corticosteroid responsiveness may be lower in females. Duma and colleagues evaluated glucocorticoid regulation of gene expression in male and female rat liver model and found that glucocorticoid administration broadened the expression of sexually dimorphic genes. They describe 84 additional glucocorticoid-responsive genes in the male, suggesting that the anti-inflammatory actions of glucocorticoids may be more effective in male rats.[22] This has not been reproduced outside of animal studies, and so the presence and significance of these additional genes in humans remains unknown. Even still, this hypothesis has potential clinical implications and could help to explain heightened symptoms among women and their propensity to elect for surgical management under lower objective disease burden compared with men. This understudied topic also has relevance in many other inflammatory disorders affecting the unified airway and needs attention in future studies.

The mechanisms driving sexual dimorphism in CRS subtype prevalence and relative symptom perception are multifactorial. Subtype prevalence discrepancies may be due to variations in study methodology, disease definitions, or perhaps due to global differences in sex-specific prevalence of CRS.[5] Several mechanisms have been postulated to account for the observed differences in symptom perception between men and women with CRS. Relevant comorbid illness (including migraine, allergic rhinitis, and depression) is more common among women and has been cited as a potential confounding contributor to CRS symptoms.[13] It is important to note however, that SNOT-22 subdomain scores are not consistently lower in the psychological subdomain category for women, and that more severe symptom burden was perceived in several studies in which there were no differences in relevant comorbid illness.[8,20,23] Current literature has yet to convincingly demonstrate that these sex-related differences affect subjective or objective outcomes, and ultimately conclude that CRS treatment improves outcomes regardless of patient sex. Still, there is a paucity of literature evaluating mechanisms driving these sex- and gender-specific differences in CRS and as such it is certainly an area ripe for additional research and investigation.

Lower airway. A plethora of literature has been published on the sex and gender differences in disease primarily affecting the lower airways (asthma, chronic obstructive pulmonary disease, bronchiectasis, etc). Although a comprehensive review in this area is beyond the scope of this article, several key differences will be highlighted here.

Asthma. Sex disparities affecting asthma patients have been well-described and account for differences in prevalence and progression of the disease in men and women throughout various stages of life. During childhood, boys have a higher prevalence of asthma with increased hospitalizations for exacerbations compared with girls. The prevalence of asthma between the two sexes normalizes in adolescence and eventually develops a female predominance during the reproductive years.[9] In adulthood, females experience a higher number of associated exacerbations, hospitalizations, and asthma-related deaths compared with males.[3,9] Furthermore, according to the Centers for Disease Control (CDC) asthma data from 2019, adult women also have approximately a 50% greater mortality rate compared with adult males.[24]

Airway anatomy develops differently based on sex, with ever-present changes occurring in infancy and throughout adolescence, resulting in morphometric differences between the male and female airway. These differences begin in the neonatal period and initially benefit female airways, but increasingly become more disease protective for males (and less so for females) as they approach maturity in adolescence. Female neonates experience earlier lung maturity, surfactant production, and fetal breathing sooner than male neonates.[17] After birth, upper airway growth lags behind lung parenchymal growth for boys, but not for girls. The parallel and synchronous growth of the upper and lower airway in girls allows for their higher baseline respiratory capacity (higher FEV1 to FVC ratio) compared to boys of the same height.[25] During puberty, this phenomenon reverses, when the growth ratio of thoracic height to standing height is relatively higher in men, resulting in a reported 25% increased lung function compared to women of the same height.[26] This anatomic dichotomy has well-described implications in respiratory diseases, and likely explains (to some degree) why young men suffer from many respiratory diseases more than women and why this reverses after puberty.[17]

Sex hormones are also thought to play an important role in the inflammatory pathways involved in asthma, as it is well known that sex disparities evolve alongside major hormonal fluctuations throughout life. Although the exact mechanisms have not yet been fully elucidated, numerous animal studies have revealed that estrogen increases, and testosterone decreases, Th2-mediated airway inflammation during puberty, with these differences becoming more pronounced with increasing age.[9]

There is also evidence of some genetic predisposition in asthma, namely the association of the *17q12-q21* gene with childhood onset of disease. There is now evidence that these known genetic risk factors may also be modified over time, potentially contributing to the observed changes occurring between men and women. One study described sex-driven differences in DNA methylation of the *17q12-q21* promoter gene, which they also associated with differences in age.[18]

Despite known anatomic, hormonal, and genetic mechanisms contributing to sex-related differences in asthma, the literature has not consistently shown a difference in treatment response to inhaled beta-agonists, anticholinergics, or corticosteroids between men and women.[17] As in CRS, there are some smaller studies that suggest a decreased efficacy of inhaled corticosteroids in women compared to men. A study by Dijkstra and colleagues[27] found that treatment with inhaled corticosteroids in adults with moderate to severe asthma was associated with dose-dependent reduction in the decline of FEV1 in men but not in women. One randomized control trial showed that inhaled corticosteroid use was significantly associated with a decrease in airway responsiveness in healthy participants, an effect that was significantly greater in male patients on multivariate regression.[28] There is also some evidence that women, compared with men, are less likely to attend pulmonary rehabilitation and less commonly use the correct inhaler technique.[29,30] This places patient engagement, education, and counseling at the forefront of actionable steps that providers can take to bridge the gender gap in asthma.

Chronic obstructive pulmonary disease

Chronic obstructive pulmonary disease (COPD) has also recently shifted from a historically male-dominant disease to one with an increasingly higher prevalence infemales. Although COPD was classically considered a male-predominant disease, the number of women dying from COPD now surpasses that of men.[31] As smoking is the number one risk factor for development of COPD, this trend is thought to be in large part due to the increases in female smoking. Interestingly, a study evaluating the sex differences in susceptibility to the effects of cigarette smoking found that female sex was associated with reduced lung function and increased severity of disease in patients with either low smoking exposure or early disease onset.[32] Female smokers also experience a greater average decrease in life expectancy than male smokers and have poorer response to smoking cessation attempts.[14,15]

Pathophysiologic variation in response to smoking does not account for the entirety of COPD differences between men and women, as evidenced by the persistence of this male-female disparity among nonsmokers with COPD. For moderate-to-severe cases of COPD lacking any associated smoking history, more than two-thirds of disease is disproportionately over-represented by women compared with men.[4]

The mechanisms driving sex-specific differences in COPD and in pathophysiologic response to smoking and smoking cessation have not been fully elucidated and are likely multifactorial. A hormonal interaction has been described, whereby estrogen promotes increased metabolism of nicotine and an increased expression of lung-carcinogen metabolizing enzyme (CYP1A1).[33,34] These differences in CYP1A1 as well as in nicotine metabolism rates between men and women may account for some sex-related aspects of smoking and disease. Importantly, one meta-analysis of placebo-controlled trials for nicotine patch therapy found that the odds of long-term abstinence from smoking using nicotine patch (versus placebo patch) was lower in women compared with men.[14] There is also some evidence that smoking cessation success varies with cyclic changes in the menstrual cycle, although other psychosocial factors have also been implicated here.[35] Interestingly, one study found that smoking abstinence in women was better at 1 year for those who had concomitant cognitive behavior therapy targeted at reducing weight concerns.[36]

Comorbidities associated with female sex have also been suggested to contribute to disparity in COPD outcomes. For instance, low body mass index and malnutrition, which are more common in females, have been shown to be predictive of mortality in COPD.[37] One prospective study also showed that anxiety and depression was associated with the increased dyspnea and poorer quality of life reported by women compared to men with similar lung function in COPD.[38] Physician bias has also been named as a contributing factor for late and missed diagnosis in women and represents an area of immediate actionable change for individual practitioners.[17]

Cystic fibrosis

The incidence of cystic fibrosis (CF) is near-equal in male and female individuals, although a gender gap in CF outcomes has been well known for decades. An epidemiological study published in 1997 found that females with CF had a 60% higher mortality rate compared with males with CF.[16] Although the life expectancy has more than doubled since then with the advent of cystic fibrosis transmembrane regulator (CFTR) modulator therapies, the survival rate for men is consistently a few percentage points higher than in women as seen in numerous international CF registry databases.[10] One retrospective large database analysis found that median life expectancy in CF was shorter for female compared with male individuals (36.0 vs. 38.7 years) and that female sex alone conferred a significant risk of death compared with males on multivariate analysis, even after controlling for morphometric and comorbid male-female differences.[12] This may be in part due to the increased susceptibility of females with CF to infection by various respiratory pathogens, notably *Pseudomonas aeruginosa* and *Staphylococcus aureus*. Compared with males, females acquire infection earlier in life and experience more rapid decline in pulmonary function thereafter, necessitating more intense therapy and prolonged hospitalizations. Even still, in the setting of these respiratory infections, life expectancy decreases more in women than in men.[10,12] Like in asthma, CF gender discrepancies tend to become more noticeable following puberty and progress throughout adulthood.[17]

There are many multifactorial mechanisms that contribute to the sex differences observed for CF patients. A hormonal basis has been well described as estrogen directly modulates the expression of CFTR and epithelial sodium channel while also inhibiting calcium-mediated chloride channels. This decreases airway cell surface liquid layer, thereby increasing mucous viscosity and decreasing mucociliary clearance.[10,12] Estrogen also promotes microbial virulence and induces an immune hyporesponsive state, further disadvantaging women with CF. High estrogenic states have been associated with the conversion of *P aeruginosa* to a mucoid subtype, which has heightened virulence and more stubborn resistance patterns portending to the increased mortality among those affected.[39]

As CF is a lifespan-shortening disease, the effect of hormonal fluctuations across the lifetime are less well studied in this population. One CF-related infection that has been well correlated with hormonal changes is nontuberculous mycobacterium, which has a predilection for postmenopausal women in CF.[40] Although this further supports the importance of hormonal components of microbiological susceptibility, a genetic predisposition has also been hypothesized here. One prospective study evaluated patients with non-CF, nontuberculous mycobacterial infections and found that 95% of those enrolled were women and that 36% had at least one CFTR mutation, corroborating a genetic basis for this sex-driven disparity.[41]

Hormonal influences on mucociliary clearance, microbiological susceptibility, and immunocompetence, likely account for much, but not the entirely of sex disparity in CF.[12] Genetic variability, morphometric anatomic differences, and decreased nutritional status in women have also been implicated.[10] Although incompletely understood, there is enough evidence to suggest that these mechanisms are related to poorer outcomes for women and indicate the importance of understanding sex differences in managing this disease.[17]

SUMMARY

Sex differences influence health and disease in the unified airway and represent an understudied topic requiring the attention of health care providers who desire improved outcomes for all patients. There is growing evidence exposing the male-female differences in clinical presentation, disease progression, and overall outcomes for diseases of the unified airway. Epidemiology of unified airway disease is clearly affected by patient gender, as evidenced by the sex-specific differences in the prevalence of CRS, COPD, and asthma.[2,3,5] Importantly, disease progression is also affected as seen in asthma, COPD, and cystic fibrosis, in which adult women experience increased morbidity compared with men.[17] Symptom burden is elevated for women compared with men (despite similar objective evidence of disease burden) in CRS and COPD.[8,13,20,42] In CRS, women and men benefit similarly from surgical treatment.[13,20] There is some support for differential treatment response to corticosteroids between sexes although data are generally lacking on this topic.[17,21,22,27] Mortality is higher for adult women compared with men in both CF and in asthma.[3,12] Physician understanding of the male-female differences in unified airway disease is an essential step toward improved outcomes for all patients.

CLINICS CARE POINTS

- Biological sex impacts prevalence and outcomes for airway pathologic conditions such as rhinitis, sinusitis, asthma etc.

- Although women may experience more significant preoperative symptom burden than men with chronic rhinosinusitis (CRS), functional endoscopic sinus surgery improves symptoms by similar magnitudes in both sexes.

- The prevalence of comorbid migraines, depression, anxiety, and currently unknown factors may contribute to increased symptom burden in women with CRS; clinicians should proactively screen for these conditions and manage/refer accordingly.

- Importantly, suspicion or diagnosis of comorbid anxiety or depression should not bias diagnosis or treatment strategy in CRS.

- Male children are at a higher risk for development of asthma and (for increased associated morbidity) compared with female children. This trend reverses during puberty when women garner increased risk of asthma-related morbidity and mortality.

- Improving patient engagement, education, and counseling are paramount in improving outcomes in asthma, especially in adult women, who may be less adherent and who also suffer significantly worse outcomes.

- Chronic obstructive pulmonary disease (COPD), although classically thought of as a male-predominant disease, has become an increasingly important women's health issue.
- Provider conscientiousness of the evolving gender dichotomy in COPD is essential to eliminate physician bias and to ensure timely diagnosis for all patients.
- Alternative strategies addressing patient-specific motivations (including cognitive behavioral therapy) may improve smoking cessation success in women.
- Despite having a near-equal incidence between the sexes, women with cystic fibrosis (CF) have reduced life expectancy compared with men.
- Current literature suggests turning clinical attention to supporting the nutritional status, mucociliary clearance interventions, and early prevention of infection to improve parity between men and women with CF.

DISCLOSURE

M.T. Yim is a consultant for Acclarent and Chitogel.

REFERENCES

1. Mauvais-Jarvis F, Bairey Merz N, Barnes PJ, et al. Sex and gender: modifiers of health, disease, and medicine. Lancet 2020;396(10250):565–82.
2. Akinbami LJ, Liu X. Chronic obstructive pulmonary disease among adults aged 18 and over in the United States, 1998-2009. NCHS Data Brief 2011;(63):1–8.
3. Akinbami LJ, Moorman JE, Bailey C, et al. Trends in asthma prevalence, health care use, and mortality in the United States, 2001-2010. NCHS Data Brief 2012;(94):1–8.
4. Salvi SS, Barnes PJ. Chronic obstructive pulmonary disease in non-smokers. Lancet 2009;374(9691):733–43.
5. Ference EH, Tan BK, Hulse KE, et al. Commentary on gender differences in prevalence, treatment, and quality of life of patients with chronic rhinosinusitis. Allergy Rhinol (Providence) 2015;6(2):82–8.
6. Bartosik TJ, Liu DT, Campion NJ, et al. Differences in men and women suffering from CRSwNP and AERD in quality of life. Eur Arch Otorhinolaryngol 2021;278(5): 1419–27.
7. Lal D, Rounds AB, Divekar R. Gender-specific differences in chronic rhinosinusitis patients electing endoscopic sinus surgery. Int Forum Allergy Rhinol 2016; 6(3):278–86.
8. Ramos L, Massey CJ, Asokan A, et al. Examination of sex differences in a chronic rhinosinusitis surgical cohort. Otolaryngol Head Neck Surg 2022. https://doi.org/ 10.1177/01945998221076468. 1945998221076468.
9. Fuseini H, Newcomb DC. Mechanisms driving gender differences in asthma. Curr Allergy Asthma Rep 2017;17(3):19.
10. Lam GY, Goodwin J, Wilcox PG, et al. Sex disparities in cystic fibrosis: review on the effect of female sex hormones on lung pathophysiology and outcomes. ERJ Open Res 2021;7(1). https://doi.org/10.1183/23120541.00475-2020.
11. Becklake MR, Kauffmann F. Gender differences in airway behaviour over the human life span. Thorax 1999;54(12):1119–38.
12. Harness-Brumley CL, Elliott AC, Rosenbluth DB, et al. Gender differences in outcomes of patients with cystic fibrosis. J Womens Health (Larchmt) 2014;23(12): 1012–20.

13. Mendolia-Loffredo S, Laud PW, Sparapani R, et al. Sex differences in outcomes of sinus surgery. Laryngoscope 2006;116(7):1199–203.
14. Perkins KA, Scott J. Sex differences in long-term smoking cessation rates due to nicotine patch. Nicotine Tob Res 2008;10(7):1245–50. https://doi.org/10.1080/14622200802097506.
15. Aryal S, Diaz-Guzman E, Mannino DM. COPD and gender differences: an update. Transl Res 2013;162(4):208–18.
16. Rosenfeld M, Davis R, FitzSimmons S, et al. Gender gap in cystic fibrosis mortality. Am J Epidemiol 1997;145(9):794–803.
17. Raghavan D, Jain R. Increasing awareness of sex differences in airway diseases. Respirology 2016;21(3):449–59.
18. Naumova AK, Al Tuwaijri A, Morin A, et al. Sex- and age-dependent DNA methylation at the 17q12-q21 locus associated with childhood asthma. Hum Genet 2013;132(7):811–22.
19. National Center for Health Statistics. Crude percentages of sinusitis for adults aged 18 and over, United States, 2015-2018. National Health Interview Survey. Available at: https://www.cdc.gov/nchs/nhis/ADULTS/www/index.htm. Accessed May 19 2022.
20. Lal D, Golisch KB, Elwell ZA, et al. Gender-specific analysis of outcomes from endoscopic sinus surgery for chronic rhinosinusitis. Int Forum Allergy Rhinol 2016;6(9):896–905.
21. Whitley H, Lindsey W. Sex-based differences in drug activity. Am Fam Physician 2009;80(11):1254–8.
22. Duma D, Collins JB, Chou JW, et al. Sexually dimorphic actions of glucocorticoids provide a link to inflammatory diseases with gender differences in prevalence. Sci Signal 2010;3(143):ra74.
23. Bhattacharyya N, Wasan A. Do anxiety and depression confound symptom reporting and diagnostic accuracy in chronic rhinosinusitis? Ann Otol Rhinol Laryngol 2008;117(1):18–23.
24. Centers for Disease Control. Most recent national asthma data. Available at. https://www.cdc.gov/asthma/most_recent_national_asthma_data.htm. Accessed May 22, 2022.
25. Mead J. Dysanapsis in normal lungs assessed by the relationship between maximal flow, static recoil, and vital capacity. Am Rev Respir Dis 1980;121(2): 339–42.
26. DeGroodt E, van Pelt W, Borsboom G, et al. Growth of lung and thorax dimensions during the pubertal growth spurt. Eur Respir J 1988;1(2):102–8.
27. Dijkstra A, Vonk JM, Jongepier H, et al. Lung function decline in asthma: association with inhaled corticosteroids, smoking and sex. Thorax 2006;61(2):105–10.
28. Convery RP, Leitch DN, Bromly C, et al. Effect of inhaled fluticasone propionate on airway responsiveness in treatment-naive individuals–a lesser benefit in females. Eur Respir J 2000;15(1):19–24.
29. Goodman DE, Israel E, Rosenberg M, et al. The influence of age, diagnosis, and gender on proper use of metered-dose inhalers. Am J Respir Crit Care Med 1994; 150(5 Pt 1):1256–61.
30. Hayton C, Clark A, Olive S, et al. Barriers to pulmonary rehabilitation: characteristics that predict patient attendance and adherence. Respir Med 2013;107(3): 401–7.
31. Mannino DM, Homa DM, Akinbami LJ, et al. Chronic obstructive pulmonary disease surveillance–United States, 1971-2000. MMWR Surveill Summ 2002; 51(6):1–16.

32. Sorheim IC, Johannessen A, Gulsvik A, et al. Gender differences in COPD: are women more susceptible to smoking effects than men? Thorax 2010;65(6):480–5.

33. Son D-S, Roby KF, Rozman KK, et al. Estradiol enhances and estriol inhibits the expression of CYP1A1 induced by 2,3,7,8-tetrachlorodibenzo-p-dioxin in a mouse ovarian cancer cell line. Toxicology 2002;176(3):229–43.

34. Dempsey D, Jacob P 3rd, Benowitz NL. Accelerated metabolism of nicotine and cotinine in pregnant smokers. J Pharmacol Exp Ther 2002;301(2):594–8.

35. Allen SS, Bade T, Center B, et al. Menstrual phase effects on smoking relapse. Addiction 2008;103(5):809–21.

36. Perkins KA, Marcus MD, Levine MD, et al. Cognitive-behavioral therapy to reduce weight concerns improves smoking cessation outcome in weight-concerned women. J Consult Clin Psychol 2001;69(4):604–13.

37. Celli BR, Cote CG, Marin JM, et al. The body-mass index, airflow obstruction, dyspnea, and exercise capacity index in chronic obstructive pulmonary disease. N Engl J Med 2004;350(10):1005–12.

38. Di Marco F, Verga M, Reggente M, et al. Anxiety and depression in COPD patients: The roles of gender and disease severity. Respir Med 2006;100(10): 1767–74.

39. Chotirmall SH, Greene CM, Oglesby IK, et al. 17Beta-estradiol inhibits IL-8 in cystic fibrosis by up-regulating secretory leucoprotease inhibitor. Am J Respir Crit Care Med 2010;182(1):62–72.

40. Mirsaeidi M, Machado RF, Garcia JG, et al. Nontuberculous mycobacterial disease mortality in the United States, 1999-2010: a population-based comparative study. PLoS One 2014;9(3):e91879.

41. Kim RD, Greenberg DE, Ehrmantraut ME, et al. Pulmonary nontuberculous mycobacterial disease: prospective study of a distinct preexisting syndrome. Am J Respir Crit Care Med 2008;178(10):1066–74.

42. Han MK, Postma D, Mannino DM, et al. Gender and chronic obstructive pulmonary disease: why it matters. Am J Respir Crit Care Med 2007;176(12):1179–84.

Unified Airway Disease

Examining Prevalence and Treatment of Upper Airway Eosinophilic Disease with Comorbid Asthma

Mitesh P. Mehta, MD, Sarah K. Wise, MD, MSCR*

KEYWORDS

- Unified airway • Rhinitis • Rhinosinusitis • Asthma • Eosinophilia
- Type 2 inflammation • Nasal polyp

KEY POINTS

- The "unified airway" concept highlights that inflammation affects the upper and lower airways by similar mechanisms.
- There are multiple subtypes of upper airway eosinophilic pathology, each with characteristic symptoms, histology, and imaging findings.
- These upper airway conditions often coexist with lower airway eosinophilic conditions with varying levels of comorbid prevalence.
- Treatment guided by considering upper and lower airway pathology together generally leads to improved overall outcomes across the entire airway.

INTRODUCTION

The concept of unified airway disease has been prevalent in the literature for decades with multiple reports establishing the fact that coinciding inflammation affects the upper and lower airways by similar mechanisms.[1–4] Unified airway pathophysiology often manifests as rhinitis, rhinosinusitis, and/or nasal polyposis in the upper airway with associated asthma or bronchial inflammation in the lower airways.[1] Eosinophilia and airway remodeling may be seen in chronic rhinosinusitis with and without nasal polyposis (CRSwNP and CRSsNP, respectively), as well as in asthma. These similar histologic hallmarks in the upper and lower airways have been suggested to represent the same pathologic disease process, further supporting the unified airway concept.[5]

This report specifically highlights the clinical relationships between eosinophilic diseases in the upper and lower airways by examining their prevalence and recommended treatment regimens (**Tables 1** and **2**). The following upper airway eosinophilic

Department of Otolaryngology–Head and Neck Surgery, Emory University School of Medicine, 550 Peachtree Street, Northeast, Atlanta, GA 30308, USA
* Corresponding author.
E-mail address: skmille@emory.edu

Otolaryngol Clin N Am 56 (2023) 65–81
https://doi.org/10.1016/j.otc.2022.09.005
0030-6665/23/

diseases are reviewed: allergic rhinitis (AR), non-allergic rhinitis with eosinophilia syndrome (NARES), chronic rhinosinusitis with nasal polyps (CRSwNP), aspirin-exacerbated respiratory disease (AERD), allergic fungal rhinosinusitis (AFRS), central compartment atopic disease (CCAD), and eosinophilic mucin rhinosinusitis (EMRS). Recognizing the interrelatedness of type 2 inflammatory diseases of the upper and lower airways will better help clinicians assess and manage patients accurately and holistically.

It should be noted that various other disease processes may also affect the upper and lower airways by similar pathophysiologic mechanisms. Examples include sarcoidosis, granulomatosis with polyangiitis (formerly Wegner granulomatosis), infectious causes such as acute sinusitis accompanied by bronchitis or pneumonia, and others. This review, however, strictly addresses eosinophilic disease processes.

DISCUSSION
Allergic Rhinitis

Multiple epidemiologic studies report that AR and asthma frequently coexist.[2,6,7] The prevalence of asthma in patients with AR is 15% to 38%, whereas the prevalence of AR in patients with asthma is between 80% and 100%.[6,8,9] Internationally, studies have shown that AR is associated with, and serves as a significant risk factor for, the onset of asthma with a positive correlation between severity of AR symptoms and severity of asthma symptoms.[10–13] There is significant overlap in the causative agents inducing asthma and AR exacerbations, including dust mites, animal dander, and pollen.[14] AR is also associated with increased risk for bronchial hyperresponsiveness and methacholine challenge positivity.[15,16] Although the temporal relationship of onset can be variable, the diagnosis of AR often precedes that of asthma.[17] According to Bousquet and colleagues,[18] in an average patient, the onset of rhinitis typically occurs 2 years before the presenting symptoms of asthma. Globally, multiple studies have shown that patients with AR and comorbid asthma suffer from increased use of health care resources, emergency department visits, rates of hospitalization, and greater lengths of hospital stay.[12,19,20] Given the association of asthma with AR, along with the substantial additional use of health care resources in asthmatic patients, the potential for comorbid asthma in the patient with AR should be considered.

For patients with AR and associated asthma, it has been shown that treating one condition may alleviate symptoms of the other. A 2013 systematic review showed improvements in asthma outcomes with intranasal corticosteroids (INCS) for patients with AR with concomitant asthma.[21] Studies have shown that only 2% of intranasally administered corticosteroid reaches the lungs, suggesting this effect on the lower airway may be related to its intranasal effects.[22] Using an oral H_1 antihistamine is a mainstay treatment of AR. In patients with asthma and comorbid AR, oral antihistamines can improve nonspecific bronchial hyperresponsiveness and persistent asthma symptoms, especially for those with intermittent AR.[23–25] One study showed that combining oral H_1 antihistamines and decongestants for rhinitis was more effective in treating asthma symptoms than using an antihistamine alone.[26] Leukotriene receptor agonists (LTRAs) (eg, montelukast) target cysteinyl leukotrienes, inflammatory mediators in AR and asthma, and evidence suggests this class of medications reduces AR symptoms to a similar level as antihistamines and oral decongestants; LTRAs may additionally improve lung function in patients with asthma.[26] The International Consensus Statement on Allergy and Rhinology: Allergic Rhinitis recommends LTRAs not to be used as monotherapy for AR but can be considered as part of the treatment of comorbid asthma and AR.[22]

Table 1
Prevalence of comorbid asthma and eosinophilic upper airway disease subtypes

Upper Airway Disease	Prevalence of Asthma in Patients with Disease	Prevalence of Disease in Patients with Asthma
AR	15%–38%[8,9]	80%–100%[6,9]
NARES	23%–28%[37,38]	unk
CRSwNP	20%–60%[44]	15%–26%[44]
AERD	100%[67]	7%, 14% (severe asthma)[68]
AFRS	19%–73%[66,84,85]	unk
CCAD	9.8%–17.1% (isolated CCAD), 30.8% (sinonasal + CC polyps),[66,94,95] 16.1% (peds)[97]	unk
EMRS	73%–100%[100–102]	unk

Abbreviations: AERD, aspirin exacerbated respiratory disease; AFRS, allergic fungal rhinosinusitis; AR, allergic rhinitis; CC, central compartment; CCAD, central compartment atopic disease; EMRS, eosinophilic mucin rhinosinusitis; NARES, nonallergic rhinitis with eosinophilia syndrome; peds, pediatric population; unk, unknown.

Oral corticosteroids (OCSs) have been shown to be beneficial in treating refractory AR and asthma exacerbations; however, the side effect profile of these medications must be carefully considered.[27,28] Marogna and colleagues[29] found that sublingual immunotherapy (SLIT) has a durable effect on AR with persistent benefits for 8 years following an optimal 4-year course of SLIT, and SLIT reduces the risk of moderate or severe allergic asthma exacerbations.[30] Allergen immunotherapy (AIT) generally has demonstrated benefit in concomitant AR and asthma, leading to decreased symptoms, bronchial hyperresponsiveness, and rescue medication usage along with reduced development of asthma in patients with AR only.[22] Omalizumab, an anti-IgE monoclonal antibody, has also been shown to be effective in patients with both intermittent and persistent AR and moderate-to-severe allergic asthma, improving symptoms, enhancing quality of life (QOL), and reducing asthma exacerbations.[31–33] However, it should be noted that omalizumab is not approved by the United States Food and Drug Administration (FDA) for the treatment of AR alone.

Non-Allergic Rhinitis with Eosinophilia Syndrome

NARES is a clinical syndrome that was first described in 1981 and is considered a subtype of rhinitis, representing approximately 15% to 33% of adults with nonallergic rhinitis.[34,35] Patients with NARES have symptoms consistent with AR but lack allergen sensitivity on skin testing; in these patients, nasal cytology analysis demonstrates more than 20% eosinophils. The pathophysiology of NARES is poorly understood, but a key component involves a self-perpetuating, chronic eosinophilic nasal inflammation with development of nasal micropolyposis.[36] Meng and colleagues[37] describe NARES as a disease likely associated with the upper and lower airway in that it may be a precursor for CRSwNP, asthma, and AERD. The investigators enrolled a small sample of patients with NARES and showed that 23% of patients had concomitant asthma.[37] Another study examining patients with NARES found that 28% of enrolled patients also had asthma.[38] Some studies report that concomitant asthma is uncommon, whereas others show that NARES is associated with developing late-onset asthma.[36,39] Overall, there remains a paucity of epidemiologic literature currently regarding the correlation between NARES and asthma.

Table 2
Treatment effects on comorbid asthma in eosinophilic upper airway disease subtypes

Upper Airway Disease	Treatments	Effect on Asthma
AR	AIT	Reduces BH, asthma exacerbations, asthma symptoms. Decreases risk of developing asthma in patients with AR only[22,30]
	Antihistamine	Improves nonspecific BH and persistent asthma symptoms[23–25]
	INCS	Improvements in asthma outcomes[21]
	LTRAs	Improves lung function[22,26]
	Biologics	Improves asthma symptoms, enhances QOL, reduces asthma exacerbations[31–33]
	OCS	Beneficial in asthma exacerbations[27,28]
NARES	LTRAs	Improved FEV$_1$, asthma symptom scores[38]
CRSwNP	LTRAs	Improved objective and subjective pulmonary symptoms, lung function.[51] Decreased inflammatory mediators, eosinophils[52]
	Biologics	Improved pulmonary symptom scores[53]
	FESS	Improves QOL scores, FEV$_1$, asthma control, asthma attack frequency/hospitalizations, use of OCS/ICS.[56–59] Reduces incidence of new asthma diagnoses[60]
	Erythromycin	Improved pulmonary symptoms in patients refractory to INCS, nasal saline irrigation[51]
AERD	LTRAs	Increased FEV$_1$, improved asthma QOL scores, decreased asthma exacerbations[69,70]
	Biologics	Improved lung function[71,72]
	FESS	Subjective improvement in asthma 1 y postoperatively.[73] Improved asthma symptoms, FEV$_1$, use of OCS/ICS, frequency of asthma attacks, frequency of physician visits for asthma-related concerns, and hospitalizations for asthma exacerbations[58,59]
	Aspirin desensitization	Improved QOL, ACQ scores, respiratory symptoms[53,75]
AFRS	Biologics	Improved FEV$_1$, symptom scores, QOL, rate of revision procedures; decreased OCS use, serum eosinophil levels[89,91,92]

CCAD and EMRS not included because there are no treatment effects on asthma described in the literature currently for these subtypes.

Abbreviations: ACQ, asthma control questionnaire; AERD, aspirin exacerbated respiratory disease; AFRS, allergic fungal rhinosinusitis; AIT, allergen immunotherapy; AR, allergic rhinitis; BH, bronchial hyperresponsiveness; CCAD, central compartment atopic disease; EMRS, eosinophilic mucin rhinosinusitis; FEV$_1$, forced expiratory volume in 1 second; ICS, inhaled corticosteroids; INCS, intranasal corticosteroids; NARES, nonallergic rhinitis with eosinophilia syndrome; OCS, oral corticosteroids; QOL, quality of life.

Formal study of the various treatments for NARES and any subsequent variation in treatment due to the presence of concomitant asthma is limited. NARES is primarily treated with INCS with multiple studies showing clinical evidence of symptom improvement, although patients may eventually require surgery.[40,41] One study showed benefit with the addition of an antihistamine with symptom improvement and decrease in nasal secretion eosinophil count.[42] For refractory symptoms, systemic steroid therapy can be used while weighing the side effect profile.[43] A study of LTRA use in patients with NARES found improved symptom scores, decreased nasal eosinophil infiltration, and higher probability of response to treatment specifically in patients with concomitant asthma.[38]

Chronic Rhinosinusitis with Nasal Polyps

Langdon and Mullol[44] report that 20% to 60% of patients with CRSwNP have comorbid asthma at the time of diagnosis, and up to 45% of patients with CRSwNP will develop asthma. Conversely, only 7% of asthmatic patients have nasal polyps.[45] Patients with concomitant CRSwNP and asthma report more severe symptoms and impaired QOL. Bilodeau and colleagues[46] report that patients with CRSwNP have more poorly controlled asthma, increased airway obstruction, and more marked lower airway inflammation than those with CRSsNP and asthma.[47] Environmental triggers for CRSwNP overlap significantly with those of asthma, including smoking, pollution, pollen, and dander.[1] The temporal relationship between developing asthma and CRSwNP is variable.[48] CRSwNP describes a disease phenotype without specification of the underlying endotype or cause. Prevalence of associated asthma may differ by specific disease endotype as noted in subsequent subsections on AERD, AFRS, and CCAD.

Researchers have concluded that treating CRSwNP either medically or surgically has a beneficial effect on concomitant asthma symptoms.[49,50] The most frequently used medical treatments for CRSwNP and comorbid asthma are LTRAs, monoclonal antibodies, or macrolide antibiotics in addition to INCS and nasal saline irrigations.

Ragab and colleagues[51] examined the use of montelukast as add-on therapy to INCS in patients with CRSwNP with concomitant asthma, demonstrating subjective and objective improvement in pulmonary and nasal symptoms, independent of AERD status. Schaper and colleagues[52] also examined the use of montelukast and found improvements in symptom and nasal endoscopy scores, nasal airflow, inflammatory mediators and eosinophils, and lung function. Patients who failed INCS and nasal saline irrigations who then added erythromycin for 12 weeks also experienced improvement in nasal and pulmonary symptoms.[51]

Until 2019, monoclonal antibody (biologic) therapy could only be prescribed for patients with CRSwNP with comorbid severe asthma. The FDA has since approved the use of dupilumab, omalizumab, and mepolizumab for patients with refractory CRSwNP. Per the European Position Paper on Rhinosinusitis and Nasal Polyps 2020 (EPOS2020), monoclonal antibody therapies including anti-interleukin (IL)-4/13 and anti-IL-5 agents have shown symptomatic improvements in type 2 inflammatory diseases and, once widely approved, will be a paradigm shift in treating CRSwNP and comorbid asthma in the appropriate subset of patients.[53] It will be important to consider specific disease endotypes before treating patients with biologics to make their use most cost-effective. The International Consensus Statement on Allergy and Rhinology: Rhinosinusitis 2021 recommends considering dupilumab for severe CRSwNP refractory to medical and surgical management.[5] Larger trials of anti-IL-5 drugs will be critical because high IL-5 CRS endotypes have the strongest association with nasal polyps and asthma.[53] In patients with CRSwNP, omalizumab reduced periostin, a protein that promotes tissue remodeling and possibly indicates airway allergic inflammation exacerbations.[54] Another study showed that asthmatic patients with high serum periostin react more favorably to omalizumab.[55]

When considering surgical management, functional endoscopic sinus surgery (FESS) has been shown to ameliorate sinus and asthma symptoms in patients with CRSwNP with comorbid asthma, improving QOL scores, forced expiratory volume in 1 second (FEV_1), nasal endoscopy scores, asthma control, asthma attack frequency and hospitalizations, and the use of OCS and inhaled corticosteroids (ICS).[56–59] It has also been shown to reduce the incidence of new asthma diagnoses following surgery.[60] Leung and colleagues[61] simulated an evidence-based risk analysis for patients with CRSwNP and concomitant asthma noting that the threshold at which the risks of repeated courses of OCS exceeded the risks of surgery was a course of steroids more frequently than every 2 years. A 2015 systematic review showed that pulmonary and nasal outcomes did not significantly differ between FESS and medical management with montelukast, omalizumab, or erythromycin for patients with CRSwNP and comorbid asthma.[62]

Aspirin-Exacerbated Respiratory Disease

AERD is a complex syndrome characterized by underlying respiratory tract inflammation in which patients experience the triad of eosinophilic CRSwNP, adult-onset asthma, and acute upper and lower respiratory tract reactions induced by aspirin and other nonsteroidal anti-inflammatory drugs (NSAIDs) that inhibit the cyclooxygenase-1 enzyme.[63] Classically, symptoms develop within 30 to 180 minutes of NSAID exposure and typically include nasal congestion, rhinorrhea, sneezing, coughing, wheezing, and decrease in lung function.[64] Identification of the disease is challenging but critical because patients with AERD experience greater morbidity characterized by more emergency department visits, hospitalizations, and corticosteroid bursts than patients with aspirin-tolerant asthma.[65] Typical computed tomographic (CT) findings can be seen in **Fig. 1**. The prevalence of comorbid asthma in patients with AERD is 100% as would be expected based on the disease's diagnostic criteria.[66] The prevalence of concomitant AERD is approximately 7% among patients with asthma, although that figure increases to 14% in patients with severe asthma.[67]

Management of AERD begins with educating patients to avoid NSAID ingestion to prevent life-threatening reactions; however, it is important to note that because NSAIDs themselves are not the underlying cause of the disease, patients typically continue to experience symptoms even in the setting of NSAID avoidance.[68] For this reason, the mainstays of AERD therapy involve treatment of patients' asthma and CRS.

Basic medical management starts with standard asthma care, INCS, antihistamines, and nasal saline irrigations.[1] In particular, randomized controlled trials of LTRAs in patients with AERD have shown efficacy in increasing FEV_1, improving asthma QOL scores, and reducing asthma exacerbations by as much as 54%.[69,70] Several biologic agents have recently shown promise in alleviating symptoms of both asthma and nasal symptoms as well. Randomized controlled trials of dupilumab in patients with AERD have demonstrated efficacy in reducing nasal congestion and obstruction, reducing scores on the 22-item sinonasal outcome test (SNOT)-22, reducing nasal polyp burden, and improving lung function in patients with AERD.[71,72] FESS has been reported to have durable outcomes in patients with AERD with 94% of patients noting subjective improvement in asthma 1 year postoperatively,[73] and studies show that FESS in patients with AERD leads to improvements in sinus and asthma symptoms, nasal endoscopy scores, FEV_1, use of OCS and ICS, frequency of asthma attacks, frequency of physician visits for asthma-related concerns, and hospitalizations for asthma exacerbations.[58,59]

Aspirin desensitization therapy provides long-lasting clinical benefits, although its reduction of CRS symptoms typically exceeds those of asthma.[74] The protocol is built around physician-supervised administration of increasing dosages of aspirin until symptoms occur. Symptoms are treated, escalating dosages are readministered, and the cycle continues with progressively decreasing symptom response until patients are able to tolerate at least 325 mg and are thus considered "desensitized."[74]

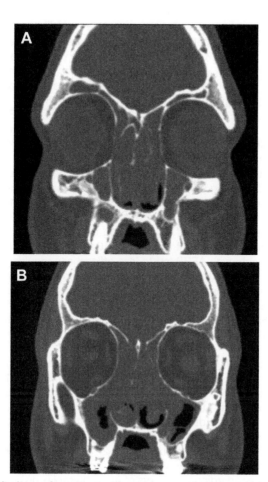

Fig. 1. Typical CT findings of a patient with aspirin-exacerbated respiratory disease preparing to undergo revision surgery. Coronal CT scan in bone window algorithm. (*A*) Anterior section demonstrating extensive opacification of the nasal cavities consistent with nasal polyposis, along with complete opacification of the visualized portions of the bilateral maxillary sinuses and frontal recesses. (*B*) Section through the ethmoid region demonstrating complete ethmoid opacification and lateralization of the middle turbinate remnant on the left.

Following the desensitization procedure, daily high-dose aspirin therapy has been shown by recent studies to improve QOL by SNOT-22 score, Asthma Control Questionnaire scores, and respiratory symptoms[53,75]; benefits of this therapy have been shown as early as 6 months following desensitization and lasting as long as 5 years after the protocol.[76] Importantly, patients must be counseled on daily medication adherence in perpetuity because loss of desensitization has been shown to ensue in as little as 48 hours following discontinuation of therapy.[77]

Allergic Fungal Rhinosinusitis

AFRS is a disorder characterized by a Th2-mediated inflammatory reaction to colonizing, noninvasive fungus in a patient's mucus.[78] Patients with AFRS are typically young and immunocompetent with a history of atopy.[66,79] Allergic or eosinophilic mucin, a thick secretion sometimes compared with peanut butter, is a hallmark of the disease.[53] The Bent and Kuhn criteria are commonly used to diagnose AFRS. Major criteria include type I hypersensitivity, nasal polyposis, eosinophilic mucin without fungal invasion into the surrounding tissue, positive fungal stain, and characteristic CT findings of unilateral sinus involvement, central hyperattenuated areas, and bony erosion (Fig. 2). The minor criteria include a history of asthma.[80,81] Early reports found that approximately 50% of patients with AFRS also suffered from asthma.[82,83] More contemporary studies have found a wider variance with 19% to 73% of patients diagnosed with concomitant AFRS and asthma.[66,84,85]

AFRS is initially treated surgically via FESS with the goal of widely opening the sinuses, removing obstructing polyps and stagnant eosinophilic mucin, and minimizing bony and soft tissue destruction.[86] Surgery alone has been shown to have a high rate of recurrence, and so oral (short-term) and topical (long-term) corticosteroid therapy, along with the possible addition of AIT, are used to improve symptoms and prolong time between surgery for recurrent disease.[53,87] Bassichis and colleagues[88] showed that AIT use in patients with AFRS led to less office visits requiring intervention and less revision surgery. Although systemic antifungal treatments have been shown to reduce nasal symptoms, dependence on OCS, and disease recurrence in AFRS, their potential benefit must be weighed against the harms of chronic antifungal use.[89] The use of LTRAs in AFRS has not been rigorously studied, although Schubert[90] published a case report of a patient having significant symptom improvement following LTRA therapy.

Omalizumab was studied in patients with AFRS with concomitant moderate-to-severe asthma post-FESS, finding a mean SNOT-22 difference of 16.3 points, mean FEV_1 improvement of 9.4%, and 87% of patients reporting improved symptoms and QOL. Most patients were able to reduce their use of corticosteroids, and none required revision procedures during the mean 9.7 month follow-up period.[91] Similarly, mepolizumab, an IL-5 antagonist, given as monthly injections, was found to improve endoscopic inflammation scores, reduce SNOT-22 scores by 13 points, and decrease serum eosinophil levels in patients with recalcitrant AFRS and comorbid asthma.[92] The body of literature regarding the effects of AFRS therapies on concomitant asthma is still developing and will lend important additional findings in the future.

Central Compartment Atopic Disease

CCAD is a recently recognized variant of CRSwNP, characterized by a local inhalant allergy process affecting the central nasal structures of ethmoid origin.[93] The lateral aspects of the sinuses are classically spared (Fig. 3). Studies from the United States and East Asia have shown that the prevalence of concomitant asthma in patients with isolated CCAD was relatively low between 9.8% and 17.1% and that it was 30.8% in patients with both sinonasal and central compartment polyps.[66,94,95] However, patients with CCAD were found to have a high prevalence of comorbid allergy (100%).[96] Marcus and colleagues[66] hypothesized that the low rate of asthma in this CCAD cohort could be due to sampling bias because adult-onset asthma is typically nonallergic or could be attributed to the central compartment's ability to filter inhalant allergens to minimize access to the lower airway. Lee and colleagues[97] found the prevalence of concomitant asthma with CCAD in the pediatric population to be 16.1%, which is concordant with that in the adult population. Because CCAD is a relatively newly described entity, data on the prevalence of concomitant asthma will need to be validated and studied further in the United States and other geographic regions.

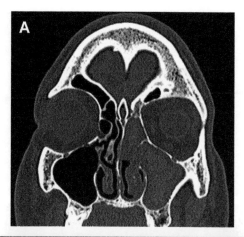

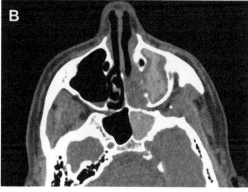

Fig. 2. Typical CT findings of a patient with allergic fungal rhinosinusitis. (*A*) Coronal CT in bone window algorithm demonstrating left maxillary and ethmoid opacification. (*B*) Axial CT in soft tissue algorithm highlights heterogeneous intrasinus densities in the maxillary and sphenoid sinuses.

Literature regarding specific effects of CCAD treatment on concomitant asthma is sparse currently. DelGaudio and colleagues[93] highlight that allergy management is a critical component of CCAD treatment along with nasal steroid irrigations.[98] Sinonasal surgery often plays a role in CCAD disease management. Specifically, surgery involves removing central compartment polyps and addressing concomitantly obstructed sinuses in a relatively limited manner, allowing delivery of topical steroids via nasal irrigations, controlling inhalant allergies, and preserving the protective capabilities of central compartment structures. Steehler and colleagues[98] found that, following FESS, polyp recurrence (8%) and rates of revision surgery (5%) were significantly lower in CCAD than other subtypes of CRSwNP. AIT has also been posited as a potential treatment of CCAD based on the disease pathophysiology, but this has yet to be studied.[66] Further study of the relationship between asthma and CCAD is needed.

Eosinophilic Mucin Rhinosinusitis

EMRS represents a heterogeneous group of pathophysiological mechanisms characterized by systemic dysregulation associated with upper and lower airway eosinophilia. Histopathological findings in EMRS are identical to those of AFRS except that there is

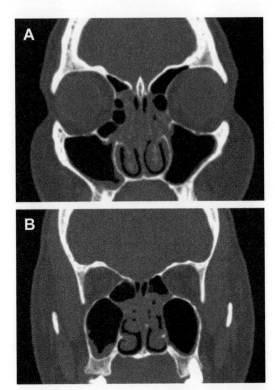

Fig. 3. Typical CT findings of a patient with central compartment atopic disease. Coronal CT scan in bone window algorithm. (*A*) Section through the anterior ethmoid and middle turbinate region demonstrating opacification of the central nasal cavities between the middle turbinates and nasal septum. There is also opacification of the medial aspects of the ethmoid and maxillary sinuses. (*B*) Section through the posterior ethmoid region, which similarly demonstrates posterior-superior nasal cavity opacification and mucosal thickening of the medial aspects of the posterior ethmoid sinuses. In both views, one can appreciate that the lateral aspects of the sinuses, including the lamina papyracea and ethmoid skull base remains relatively free of disease.

absence of fungi, and EMRS eosinophilia is instead proposed to be driven by nonallergic mechanisms.[99] Studies show that 73% to 100% of patients with EMRS have comorbid asthma, which is most commonly adult-onset moderate-to-severe asthma.[99–101]

Unfortunately, although EMRS and asthma are strongly associated, there is a paucity of literature regarding treatment effects on comorbid asthma. Compared with other subtypes of CRS, EMRS is typically more resistant to treatment with a higher relapse rate, and treatment depends on oral corticosteroid (OCS) therapy.[102] FESS is considered a mandatory component of treatment as well.[103] One small study showed that 53% of patients with EMRS found AIT helpful in diminishing symptoms. Antifungal agents, in contrast, were found to be ineffective.[99] Future study of EMRS treatment and its effects on comorbid asthma is necessary.

SUMMARY

It is critical to recognize that upper and lower airway diseases are intricately intertwined under the unified airway paradigm. In patients with upper airway eosinophilic diseases, concomitant asthma is relatively common. Thus, clinicians should evaluate patients for these diseases in conjunction. Across multiple upper airway disease sub-types, the literature supports that treating upper airway disease can improve coexisting lower airway pathology, significantly reducing morbidity, improving QOL, and optimizing health care system utilization. In addition to typical medical management for rhinosinusitis and asthma, which includes standard asthma treatment, topical corticosteroids, antihistamines, and nasal saline irrigations, this report highlights treatments that have been shown to have a synergistic effect in managing both nasal and pulmonary symptoms. In particular, LTRAs, immunotherapies, biologics, FESS, and aspirin desensitization (specifically in patients with AERD) were commonly cited options that improved patients' upper and lower airway symptoms. Opportunities for further study exist with respect to some subtypes of rhinitis and rhinosinusitis, and there is much on the horizon regarding biologic agents. Practices and guidelines must continue to evolve with new treatments, and providers should seek to treat patients' airways holistically, considering treatment effects on both the upper and lower regions to ensure that patients are treated effectively.

CLINICS CARE POINTS

- Patients with upper airway eosinophilic disease should be assessed for comorbid asthma because these diseases frequently occur in conjunction
- Basic medical management for patients with upper and lower airway eosinophilic diseases starts with standard asthma care, nasal saline irrigations, and topical corticosteroids/INCS.
- FESS, leukotriene receptor antagonists, AIT, and biologics show promising benefits for both upper and lower airway symptoms in certain combined airway eosinophilic diseases.
- Further study of the crossover between upper and lower airway eosinophilic diseases is crucial to optimizing treatment of these often comorbid conditions.

DISCLOSURE

Sarah K. Wise (Consultant: NeurENT, Chitogel; Advisory Board: OptiNose).

REFERENCES

1. Ramakrishnan JB, Kingdom TT, Ramakrishnan VR. Allergic rhinitis and chronic rhinosinusitis: their impact on lower airways. Immunol Allergy Clin N Am 2013; 33(1):45–60.
2. Bachert C, Vignola AM, Gevaert P, et al. Allergic rhinitis, rhinosinusitis, and asthma: one airway disease. Immunol Allergy Clin N Am 2004;24(1):19–43.
3. Grossman J. One airway, one disease. Chest 1997;111(2 Suppl):11S–6S.
4. Krouse JH. The unified airway. Facial Plast Surg Clin North Am 2012;20(1): 55–60.
5. Orlandi RR, Kingdom TT, Smith TL, et al. International consensus statement on allergy and rhinology: rhinosinusitis 2021. Int Forum Allergy Rhinol 2021;11(3): 213–739.
6. Leynaert B, Neukirch F, Demoly P, et al. Epidemiologic evidence for asthma and rhinitis comorbidity. J Allergy Clin Immunol 2000;106(5 Suppl):S201–5.
7. Thomas M. Allergic rhinitis: evidence for impact on asthma. BMC Pulm Med 2006;6(Suppl 1):S4.

8. Brozek JL, Bousquet J, Agache I, et al. Allergic Rhinitis and its Impact on Asthma (ARIA) guidelines-2016 revision. J Allergy Clin Immunol 2017;140(4): 950–8.

9. Linneberg A, Henrik Nielsen N, Frolund L, et al. The link between allergic rhinitis and allergic asthma: a prospective population-based study. The Copenhagen Allergy Study. Allergy. 2002;57(11):1048–52.

10. Guerra S, Sherrill DL, Martinez FD, et al. Rhinitis as an independent risk factor for adult-onset asthma. J Allergy Clin Immunol 2002;109(3):419–25.

11. Plaschke PP, Janson C, Norrman E, et al. Onset and remission of allergic rhinitis and asthma and the relationship with atopic sensitization and smoking. Am J Respir Crit Care Med 2000;162(3 Pt 1):920–4.

12. Sazonov Kocevar V, Thomas J 3rd, Jonsson L, et al. Association between allergic rhinitis and hospital resource use among asthmatic children in Norway. Allergy 2005;60(3):338–42.

13. Leger D, Annesi-Maesano I, Carat F, et al. Allergic rhinitis and its consequences on quality of sleep: An unexplored area. Arch Intern Med 2006;166(16):1744–8.

14. Izuhara Y, Matsumoto H, Nagasaki T, et al. Mouth breathing, another risk factor for asthma: the Nagahama Study. Allergy 2016;71(7):1031–6.

15. Boulet LP. Asymptomatic airway hyperresponsiveness: a curiosity or an opportunity to prevent asthma? Am J Respir Crit Care Med 2003;167(3):371–8.

16. Braman SS, Barrows AA, DeCotiis BA, et al. Airway hyperresponsiveness in allergic rhinitis. A risk factor for asthma. Chest 1987;91(5):671–4.

17. Greisner WA 3rd, Settipane RJ, Settipane GA. Co-existence of asthma and allergic rhinitis: a 23-year follow-up study of college students. Allergy Asthma Proc 1998;19(4):185–8.

18. Bousquet J, Van Cauwenberge P, Khaltaev N, et al. Allergic rhinitis and its impact on asthma. J Allergy Clin Immunol 2001;108(5 Suppl):S147–334.

19. Bousquet J, Gaugris S, Kocevar VS, et al. Increased risk of asthma attacks and emergency visits among asthma patients with allergic rhinitis: a subgroup analysis of the investigation of montelukast as a partner agent for complementary therapy [corrected]. Clin Exp Allergy 2005;35(6):723–7.

20. Bjermer L, Bisgaard H, Bousquet J, et al. Montelukast and fluticasone compared with salmeterol and fluticasone in protecting against asthma exacerbation in adults: one year, double blind, randomised, comparative trial. BMJ 2003;327(7420):891.

21. Lohia S, Schlosser RJ, Soler ZM. Impact of intranasal corticosteroids on asthma outcomes in allergic rhinitis: a meta-analysis. Allergy 2013;68(5):569–79.

22. Wise SK, Lin SY, Toskala E, et al. International Consensus Statement on Allergy and Rhinology: Allergic Rhinitis. Int Forum Allergy Rhinol 2018;8(2):108–352.

23. Aaronson DW. Evaluation of cetirizine in patients with allergic rhinitis and perennial asthma. Ann Allergy Asthma Immunol 1996;76(5):440–6.

24. Aubier M, Neukirch C, Peiffer C, et al. Effect of cetirizine on bronchial hyperresponsiveness in patients with seasonal allergic rhinitis and asthma. Allergy 2001; 56(1):35–42.

25. Grant JA, Nicodemus CF, Findlay SR, et al. Cetirizine in patients with seasonal rhinitis and concomitant asthma: prospective, randomized, placebo-controlled trial. J Allergy Clin Immunol 1995;95(5 Pt 1):923–32.

26. Kim H, Bouchard J, Renzi PM. The link between allergic rhinitis and asthma: a role for antileukotrienes? Can Respir J 2008;15(2):91–8.

27. Hox V, Lourijsen E, Jordens A, et al. Benefits and harm of systemic steroids for short- and long-term use in rhinitis and rhinosinusitis: an EAACI position paper. Clin Transl Allergy 2020;10:1.
28. Normansell R, Kew KM, Mansour G. Different oral corticosteroid regimens for acute asthma. Cochrane Database Syst Rev 2016;5:CD011801.
29. Marogna M, Spadolini I, Massolo A, et al. Long-lasting effects of sublingual immunotherapy according to its duration: a 15-year prospective study. J Allergy Clin Immunol 2010;126(5):969–75.
30. Edwards TS, Wise SK. Clinical Applications of Sublingual Immunotherapy. Otolaryngol Clin North Am 2017;50(6):1121–34.
31. Corren J, Casale T, Deniz Y, et al. Omalizumab, a recombinant humanized anti-IgE antibody, reduces asthma-related emergency room visits and hospitalizations in patients with allergic asthma. J Allergy Clin Immunol 2003;111(1):87–90.
32. Holgate ST, Djukanovic R, Casale T, et al. Anti-immunoglobulin E treatment with omalizumab in allergic diseases: an update on anti-inflammatory activity and clinical efficacy. Clin Exp Allergy 2005;35(4):408–16.
33. Vignola AM, Humbert M, Bousquet J, et al. Efficacy and tolerability of anti-immunoglobulin E therapy with omalizumab in patients with concomitant allergic asthma and persistent allergic rhinitis: SOLAR. Allergy 2004;59(7):709–17.
34. Settipane GA, Klein DE. Non allergic rhinitis: demography of eosinophils in nasal smear, blood total eosinophil counts and IgE levels. N Engl Reg Allergy Proc 1985;6(4):363–6.
35. Moneret-Vautrin DA, Hsieh V, Wayoff M, et al. Nonallergic rhinitis with eosinophilia syndrome a precursor of the triad: nasal polyposis, intrinsic asthma, and intolerance to aspirin. Ann Allergy 1990;64(6):513–8.
36. Ellis AK, Keith PK. Nonallergic rhinitis with eosinophilia syndrome. Curr Allergy Asthma Rep 2006;6(3):215–20.
37. Meng Y, Yan B, Wang Y, et al. Diagnosis and management of nonallergic rhinitis with eosinophilia syndrome using cystatin SN together with symptoms. World Allergy Organ J 2020;13(7):100134.
38. De Corso E, Anzivino R, Galli J, et al. Antileukotrienes improve naso-ocular symptoms and biomarkers in patients with NARES and asthma. Laryngoscope 2019;129(3):551–7.
39. Bousquet J, Khaltaev N, Cruz AA, et al. Allergic Rhinitis and its Impact on Asthma (ARIA) 2008 update (in collaboration with the World Health Organization, GA(2)LEN and AllerGen). Allergy 2008;63(Suppl 86):8–160.
40. De Corso E, Seccia V, Ottaviano G, et al. Clinical Evidence of Type 2 Inflammation in Non-allergic Rhinitis with Eosinophilia Syndrome: a Systematic Review. Curr Allergy Asthma Rep 2022;22(4):29–42.
41. Crisci CD, Ardusso LRF. A Precision Medicine Approach to Rhinitis Evaluation and Management. Curr Treat Options Allergy 2020;7(1):93–109.
42. Purello-D'Ambrosio F, Isola S, Ricciardi L, et al. A controlled study on the effectiveness of loratadine in combination with flunisolide in the treatment of nonallergic rhinitis with eosinophilia (NARES). Clin Exp Allergy 1999;29(8):1143–7.
43. Mygind N. Effects of corticosteroid therapy in non-allergic rhinosinusitis. Acta Otolaryngol 1996;116(2):164–6.
44. Langdon C, Mullol J. Nasal polyps in patients with asthma: prevalence, impact, and management challenges. J Asthma Allergy 2016;9:45–53.
45. Tint D, Kubala S, Toskala E. Risk Factors and Comorbidities in Chronic Rhinosinusitis. Curr Allergy Asthma Rep 2016;16(2):16.

46. Bilodeau L, Boulay ME, Prince P, et al. Comparative clinical and airway inflammatory features of asthmatics with or without polyps. Rhinology 2010;48(4): 420–5.
47. Lehrer E, Mullol J, Agredo F, et al. Management of chronic rhinosinusitis in asthma patients: is there still a debate? Curr Allergy Asthma Rep 2014; 14(6):440.
48. Yoshimura K, Kawata R, Haruna S, et al. Clinical epidemiological study of 553 patients with chronic rhinosinusitis in Japan. Allergol Int 2011;60(4):491–6.
49. Lund VJ. The effect of sinonasal surgery on asthma. Allergy 1999;54(Suppl 57): 141–5.
50. Scadding G. The effect of medical treatment of sinusitis upon concomitant asthma. Allergy 1999;54(Suppl 57):136–40.
51. Ragab SM, Lund VJ, Scadding G. Evaluation of the medical and surgical treatment of chronic rhinosinusitis: a prospective, randomised, controlled trial. Laryngoscope 2004;114(5):923–30.
52. Schaper C, Noga O, Koch B, et al. Anti-inflammatory properties of montelukast, a leukotriene receptor antagonist in patients with asthma and nasal polyposis. J Investig Allergol Clin Immunol 2011;21(1):51–8.
53. Fokkens WJ, Lund VJ, Hopkins C, et al. European Position Paper on Rhinosinusitis and Nasal Polyps 2020. Rhinology 2020;58(Suppl S29):1–464.
54. De Schryver E, Derycke L, Calus L, et al. The effect of systemic treatments on periostin expression reflects their interference with the eosinophilic inflammation in chronic rhinosinusitis with nasal polyps. Rhinology 2017;55(2):152–60.
55. Izuhara K, Ohta S, Ono J. Using Periostin as a Biomarker in the Treatment of Asthma. Allergy Asthma Immunol Res 2016;8(6):491–8.
56. Smith TL, Mendolia-Loffredo S, Loehrl TA, et al. Predictive factors and outcomes in endoscopic sinus surgery for chronic rhinosinusitis. Laryngoscope 2005; 115(12):2199–205.
57. Uri N, Cohen-Kerem R, Barzilai G, et al. Functional endoscopic sinus surgery in the treatment of massive polyposis in asthmatic patients. J Laryngol Otol 2002; 116(3):185–9.
58. Awad OG, Fasano MB, Lee JH, et al. Asthma outcomes after endoscopic sinus surgery in aspirin-tolerant versus aspirin-induced asthmatic patients. Am J Rhinol 2008;22(2):197–203.
59. Awad OG, Lee JH, Fasano MB, et al. Sinonasal outcomes after endoscopic sinus surgery in asthmatic patients with nasal polyps: a difference between aspirin-tolerant and aspirin-induced asthma? Laryngoscope 2008;118(7): 1282–6.
60. Benninger MS, Sindwani R, Holy CE, et al. Impact of medically recalcitrant chronic rhinosinusitis on incidence of asthma. Int Forum Allergy Rhinol 2016; 6(2):124–9.
61. Leung TN, Lam PM, Ng PC, et al. Repeated courses of antenatal corticosteroids: is it justified? Acta Obstet Gynecol Scand 2003;82(7):589–96.
62. Rix I, Hakansson K, Larsen CG, et al. Management of chronic rhinosinusitis with nasal polyps and coexisting asthma: A systematic review. Am J Rhinol Allergy 2015;29(3):193–201.
63. Samter M, Beers RF Jr. Intolerance to aspirin. Clinical studies and consideration of its pathogenesis. Ann Intern Med 1968;68(5):975–83.
64. Laidlaw TM. Pathogenesis of NSAID-induced reactions in aspirin-exacerbated respiratory disease. World J Otorhinolaryngol Head Neck Surg 2018;4(3):162–8.

65. Mascia K, Haselkorn T, Deniz YM, et al. Aspirin sensitivity and severity of asthma: evidence for irreversible airway obstruction in patients with severe or difficult-to-treat asthma. J Allergy Clin Immunol 2005;116(5):970–5.

66. Marcus S, Schertzer J, Roland LT, et al. Central compartment atopic disease: prevalence of allergy and asthma compared with other subtypes of chronic rhinosinusitis with nasal polyps. Int Forum Allergy Rhinol 2020;10(2):183–9.

67. Rajan JP, Wineinger NE, Stevenson DD, et al. Prevalence of aspirin-exacerbated respiratory disease among asthmatic patients: A meta-analysis of the literature. J Allergy Clin Immunol 2015;135(3):676–681 e671.

68. Fahrenholz JM. Natural history and clinical features of aspirin-exacerbated respiratory disease. Clin Rev Allergy Immunol 2003;24(2):113–24.

69. Dahlen SE, Malmstrom K, Nizankowska E, et al. Improvement of aspirin-intolerant asthma by montelukast, a leukotriene antagonist: a randomized, double-blind, placebo-controlled trial. Am J Respir Crit Care Med 2002; 165(1):9–14.

70. Dahlen B, Nizankowska E, Szczeklik A, et al. Benefits from adding the 5-lipoxygenase inhibitor zileuton to conventional therapy in aspirin-intolerant asthmatics. Am J Respir Crit Care Med 1998;157(4 Pt 1):1187–94.

71. Bachert C, Han JK, Desrosiers M, et al. Efficacy and safety of dupilumab in patients with severe chronic rhinosinusitis with nasal polyps (LIBERTY NP SINUS-24 and LIBERTY NP SINUS-52): results from two multicentre, randomised, double-blind, placebo-controlled, parallel-group phase 3 trials. Lancet 2019; 394(10209):1638–50.

72. Laidlaw TM, Bachert C, Amin N, et al. Dupilumab improves upper and lower airway disease control in chronic rhinosinusitis with nasal polyps and asthma. Ann Allergy Asthma Immunol 2021;126(5):584–592 e581.

73. Loehrl TA, Ferre RM, Toohill RJ, et al. Long-term asthma outcomes after endoscopic sinus surgery in aspirin triad patients. Am J Otol 2006;27(3):154–60.

74. DeGregorio GA, Singer J, Cahill KN, et al. A 1-Day, 90-Minute Aspirin Challenge and Desensitization Protocol in Aspirin-Exacerbated Respiratory Disease. J Allergy Clin Immunol Pract 2019;7(4):1174–80.

75. Chaaban MR, Moffatt D, Wright AE, et al. Meta-analysis Exploring Sinopulmonary Outcomes of Aspirin Desensitization in Aspirin-Exacerbated Respiratory Disease. Otolaryngol Head Neck Surg 2021;164(1):11–8.

76. Stevens WW, Jerschow E, Baptist AP, et al. The role of aspirin desensitization followed by oral aspirin therapy in managing patients with aspirin-exacerbated respiratory disease: A Work Group Report from the Rhinitis, Rhinosinusitis and Ocular Allergy Committee of the American Academy of Allergy, Asthma & Immunology. J Allergy Clin Immunol 2021;147(3):827–44.

77. Fruth K, Pogorzelski B, Schmidtmann I, et al. Low-dose aspirin desensitization in individuals with aspirin-exacerbated respiratory disease. Allergy 2013;68(5): 659–65.

78. Cho SH, Hamilos DL, Han DH, et al. Phenotypes of Chronic Rhinosinusitis. J Allergy Clin Immunol Pract 2020;8(5):1505–11.

79. Ma C, Mehta NK, Nguyen SA, et al. Demographic Variation in Chronic Rhinosinusitis by Subtype and Region: A Systematic Review. Am J Rhinol Allergy 2022; 36(3):367–77.

80. Bent JP 3rd, Kuhn FA. Diagnosis of allergic fungal sinusitis. Otolaryngol Head Neck Surg 1994;111(5):580–8.

81. Ryan MW, Clark CM. Allergic Fungal Rhinosinusitis and the Unified Airway: the Role of Antifungal Therapy in AFRS. Curr Allergy Asthma Rep 2015;15(12):75.

82. Cody DT 2nd, Neel HB 3rd, Ferreiro JA, et al. Allergic fungal sinusitis: the Mayo Clinic experience. Laryngoscope 1994;104(9):1074–9.

83. Manning SC, Holman M. Further evidence for allergic pathophysiology in allergic fungal sinusitis. Laryngoscope 1998;108(10):1485–96.

84. Philpott CM, Erskine S, Hopkins C, et al. Prevalence of asthma, aspirin sensitivity and allergy in chronic rhinosinusitis: data from the UK National Chronic Rhinosinusitis Epidemiology Study. Respir Res 2018;19(1):129.

85. Barac A, Stevanovic G, Pekmezovic M, et al. Study toward resolving the controversy over the definition of allergic fungal rhinosinusitis. Med Mycol 2018;56(2):162–71.

86. Glass D, Amedee RG. Allergic fungal rhinosinusitis: a review. Ochsner J 2011;11(3):271–5.

87. Rupa V, Jacob M, Mathews MS, et al. A prospective, randomised, placebo-controlled trial of postoperative oral steroid in allergic fungal sinusitis. Eur Arch Otorhinolaryngol 2010;267(2):233–8.

88. Bassichis BA, Marple BF, Mabry RL, et al. Use of immunotherapy in previously treated patients with allergic fungal sinusitis. Otolaryngol Head Neck Surg 2001;125(5):487–90.

89. Gan EC, Thamboo A, Rudmik L, et al. Medical management of allergic fungal rhinosinusitis following endoscopic sinus surgery: an evidence-based review and recommendations. Int Forum Allergy Rhinol 2014;4(9):702–15.

90. Schubert MS. Antileukotriene therapy for allergic fungal sinusitis. J Allergy Clin Immunol 2001;108(3):466–7.

91. Gan EC, Habib AR, Rajwani A, et al. Omalizumab therapy for refractory allergic fungal rhinosinusitis patients with moderate or severe asthma. Am J Otolaryngol 2015;36(5):672–7.

92. Karp J, Dhillon I, Panchmatia R, et al. Subcutaneous Mepolizumab Injection: An Adjunctive Treatment for Recalcitrant Allergic Fungal Rhinosinusitis Patients With Asthma. Am J Rhinol Allergy 2021;35(2):256–63.

93. DelGaudio JM, Loftus PA, Hamizan AW, et al. Central compartment atopic disease. Am J Rhinol Allergy 2017;31(4):228–34.

94. Kong W, Wu Q, Chen Y, et al. Chinese Central Compartment Atopic Disease: The Clinical Characteristics and Cellular Endotypes Based on Whole-Slide Imaging. J Asthma Allergy 2022;15:341–52.

95. Shih LC, Hsieh BH, Ma JH, et al. A comparison of central compartment atopic disease and lateral dominant nasal polyps. Int Forum Allergy Rhinol 2022. https://doi.org/10.1002/alr.22996.

96. DelGaudio JM. Central compartment atopic disease: the missing link in the allergy and chronic rhinosinusitis with nasal polyps saga. Int Forum Allergy Rhinol 2020;10(10):1191–2.

97. Lee K, Kim TH, Lee SH, et al. Predictive Value of Radiologic Central Compartment Atopic Disease for Identifying Allergy and Asthma in Pediatric Patients. Ear Nose Throat J 2021. https://doi.org/10.1177/0145561321997546. 145561321997546.

98. Steehler AJ, Vuncannon JR, Wise SK, et al. Central compartment atopic disease: outcomes compared with other subtypes of chronic rhinosinusitis with nasal polyps. Int Forum Allergy Rhinol 2021;11(11):1549–56.

99. Ferguson BJ. Eosinophilic mucin rhinosinusitis: a distinct clinicopathological entity. Laryngoscope 2000;110(5 Pt 1):799–813.

100. Uri N, Ronen O, Marshak T, et al. Allergic fungal sinusitis and eosinophilic mucin rhinosinusitis: diagnostic criteria. J Laryngol Otol 2013;127(9):867–71.

101. Ramadan HH, Quraishi HA. Allergic mucin sinusitis without fungus. Am J Rhinol 1997;11(2):145–7.
102. Ghorbani J, Hosseini Vajari A, Pourdowlat G, et al. Eosinophilic Mucin Rhinosinusitis in Iranian Patients Undergoing Endoscopic Sinus Surgery. Iran J Otorhinolaryngol 2018;30(101):347–53.
103. Park SK, Park KW, Mo JH, et al. Clinicopathological and Radiological Features of Chronic Rhinosinusitis with Eosinophilic Mucin in Chungcheong Province of Korea. Mycopathologia 2019;184(3):423–31.

Non-Eosinophilic Granulomatous Disease and the Unified Airway

Joanne Rimmer, MBBS, MA, FRCS(ORL-HNS), FRACS[a,b,c,*],
Valerie J. Lund, MBBS, MS, FRCS, FRCSEd, DMHon, FACSHon, CBE[d,e]

KEYWORDS

- Vasculitis • Granuloma • Granulomatosis with polyangiitis • Sarcoidosis • Sinusitis
- Rhinosinusitis

KEY POINTS

- Granulomatous and vasculitic diseases can affect the upper airway in isolation or as part of a more widespread condition involving both the upper and lower airways as well as other organ systems.
- Granulomatous and vasculitis diseases can present with vague symptoms that mimic common conditions such as chronic rhinosinusitis and may present to ear, nose, and throat surgeons initially.
- A high threshold of clinical suspicion is required to consider and make the diagnosis.

INTRODUCTION

Granulomas, an organized collection of macrophages fused to form multinucleated giant cells, can be seen in various inflammatory, neoplastic, and vasculitic diseases of the upper and lower airways. The classification of vasculitis remains mainly based on vessel size according to the revised International Chapel Hill Consensus Conference Nomenclature of Vasculitides,[1] although there are a variety of other classification systems in use. Here, the authors discuss two non-eosinophilic granulomatous conditions that commonly affect the nose and sinuses, either in isolation or as part of a systemic process: granulomatosis with polyangiitis (GPA, formerly Wegener's granulomatosis) and sarcoidosis, a systemic granulomatous condition of unknown etiology. Both can

[a] Department of Surgery, Monash University, Monash Medical Centre Level 5, Block E, 246 Clayton Road, Clayton, 3168 VIC, Australia; [b] Department of Otolaryngology Head & Neck Surgery, Monash Health, ENT Building, Moorabbin Hospital, 823-865 Centre Road, Bentleigh East, VIC 3165, Australia; [c] Department of Otolaryngology Head & Neck Surgery, St Vincent's Hospital, 41 Victoria Parade, Fitzroy, VIC 3065, Australia; [d] Royal National Ear, Nose and Throat and Eastman Dental Hospitals, 47-49 Huntley St, London WC1E 6DG, UK; [e] University College London Ear Institute, 332 Grays Inn Rd, London WC1X 8EE, UK
* Corresponding author. Department of Otolaryngology Head & Neck Surgery, ENT Building, Moorabbin Hospital, 823-865 Centre Road, Bentleigh East, Victoria 3165, Australia.
E-mail address: rimmer.joanne@gmail.com

Otolaryngol Clin N Am 56 (2023) 83–95
https://doi.org/10.1016/j.otc.2022.09.006
0030-6665/23/Crown Copyright © 2022 Published by Elsevier Inc. All rights reserved.

mimic upper airway conditions such as chronic rhinosinusitis (CRS). Eosinophilic GPA (EGPA, formerly Churg Strauss syndrome) is beyond the remit of this article but should not be forgotten in patients with adult-onset asthma, nasal polyps, systemic symptoms, and serum eosinophilia.

GRANULOMATOSIS WITH POLYANGIITIS

GPA is an idiopathic vasculitis typically associated with necrotizing granulomatous inflammation of the upper and lower respiratory tracts and kidneys but can affect any organ system (**Table 1**). Localized or limited disease may progress to become generalized or severe.[2] "Limited" disease is now most commonly accepted to mean GPA without life- or organ-threatening manifestations and without gastrointestinal, ocular, or central nervous system involvement, in contrast to "severe" disease.[3] It is an antineutrophil cytoplasmic antibody (ANCA)-associated vasculitis but ANCA may be negative. Diagnosis can, therefore, be a challenge and the 1990 American College of Rheumatology (ACR) classification of GPA[4] has recently been revised and validated by the ACR and the European Alliance of Associations for Rheumatology.[5]

Epidemiology

The diagnostic difficulty means that the incidence of GPA is probably underestimated but is reported as 2 to 30 cases per million population per year with an overall prevalence of 25 to 250 cases per million.[2] Diagnosis is most common in the fourth and fifth decades, although it can occur at any age. Men and women are equally affected and it is predominantly a disease of Caucasians (93%).[6]

Clinical Manifestations

Ear, nose, and throat (ENT) symptoms are seen in approximately two-thirds of patients at presentation: 40% have rhinological manifestations, 15% have ear symptoms, and 6% complain of laryngopharyngeal problems.[7] During the course of their disease, 95% of patients with GPA will have head and neck involvement, with over 80% complaining of sinonasal symptoms including crusting (75%), discharge (70%), obstruction (65%), bleeding (59%), olfactory loss (52%), and facial pain (33%).[7,8] Up to 25% develop the typical saddle nose deformity (**Fig. 1**), and a septal perforation is seen in approximately 30% of cases.[6] There may be destruction of the lateral nasal wall architecture and the formation of a single sinonasal cavity. In active disease, the mucosa may be inflamed, friable, and granular with significant crusting (**Fig. 2**).

One-third of patients develop otitis media with effusion and associated conductive hearing loss, whereas sensorineural hearing loss occurs in 35%. Patients may complain of dizziness or tinnitus, and 8% to 10% develop a facial nerve palsy. Oral manifestations are rare, but "strawberry" gingival hyperplasia is said to be pathognomonic. Patients may complain of hoarseness, wheeze, or stridor, and subglottic stenosis occurs in up to 16% of patients.

Systemic symptoms can also occur, and malaise that seems out of proportion to the clinical findings should raise the suspicion of an underlying vasculitic or granulomatous disease. The ENT symptoms can mimic more common diseases such as CRS and it is perhaps because of this that the diagnosis is often delayed for several months in such cases.[7] Despite this frequent delay in diagnosis, a retrospective cohort study found that patients who presented with ENT symptoms had a significantly higher 5-year survival rate than those without (98% vs 78%, $P = .049$).[9] The ENT involvement at presentation was also an independent predictor of better long-term outcomes (OR 0.37, 95% CI 0.2–0.8, $P = .019$).

Table 1
Symptoms and signs seen with different system involvement in granulomatosis with polyangiitis and sarcoidosis

	GPA	Sarcoid
Ear	Otalgia, otorrhea, chronic otitis media, otitis externaConductive and sensorineural hearing loss, vestibular dysfunction	Conductive and sensorineural hearing loss, dizziness, tinnitusFacial nerve paralysis
Nose	Nasal obstruction, crusting, bleeding, discharge, facial pain, anosmia, rhinosinusitisAdhesions, septal perforation, external "saddle" deformity	Nasal obstruction, crusting, blood-stained discharge, facial pain, anosmiaAdhesions, septal perforation, "strawberry skin" nasal mucosal nodules, nasal bones rarefaction, soft tissue infiltration, lupus pernio
Mouth	Oral ulceration, gingivitis, fistula	Fistula
Larynx	Hoarseness, stridor, vocal fold palsy, subglottic and tracheal stenosis	Hoarseness, stridor, vocal fold palsy, supraglottic granulomas and stenosis
Lower respiratory tract	Dyspnea, pleuritic pain, hemoptysisPulmonary infiltrates, nodules, abscesses, or hemorrhage	Dyspnea, cough, chest pain, wheeze, hemoptysisPulmonary infiltratesHilar lymphadenopathy (+ fever and polyarthralgia = Lofgren syndrome, mainly Scandinavians)
Eye	Proptosis, pain, visual loss, epiphoraScleritis, episcleritis, retinitisRetro-orbital granuloma	Epiphora, pain, red eye, photophobia, dry eye, visual lossAnterior and posterior uveitis, iridocyclitis, keratoconjunctivitis, scleral plaquesLacrimal gland enlargement
Cardiac	Arrhythmias, pericardial effusion, infarction, myocarditis	Cardiac failure and ventricular arrhythmia—heart block, sudden death
Renal	Glomerulonephritis, renal impairment, renal failure	
Gastrointestinal	Diarrhea, bleeding	
Peripheral nervous system	Sensory or motor polyneuropathy, mononeuritis	Polyneuritis, peripheral mononeuritis, myelopathy
Central nervous system	CNS lesions, meningitis, meningeal vasculitisCranial neuropathies	Lymphocytic meningitisCranial neuropathiesHypothalamic/pituitary dysfunction (rare)
Skin	Purpura, subcutaneous nodules, nonhealing ulceration	Violaceous rash, erythema nodosum, lupus pernioMaculopapular plaques (rare)
Musculoskeletal	Arthralgia, myalgia	Arthralgia, myalgia, dactylitis
General/other	Fever, weight loss, fatigue, nocturnal sweats	Fever, weight loss, fatiguePeripheral lymphadenopathyParotitis (Heerfordt's syndrome) Hepatosplenomegaly

From Fokkens WJ, Lund VJ, Hopkins C, et al. European position paper on rhinosinusitis and nasal polyps 2020. Rhinology 2020 Suppl. 29:1–464.

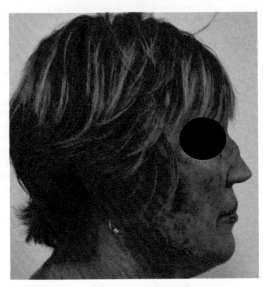

Fig. 1. Typical external saddle nose deformity seen in GPA.

Investigations

Antineutrophil cytoplasmic antibody

Symptoms and signs suggestive of GPA should prompt investigation with a positive ANCA being highly specific.

ANCA has traditionally been classified as either cytoplasmic (c)-ANCA or perinuclear (p)-ANCA based on indirect immunofluorescence, GPA being more commonly associated with c-ANCA and EGPA with p-ANCA.[6] However, enzyme-linked immunosorbent assay testing for antibodies against proteinase 3 (PR3) and myeloperoxidase (MPO) is now much more readily available and is becoming the first-line screening test.[2] A positive PR3-ANCA is found in approximately 90% of patients with severe

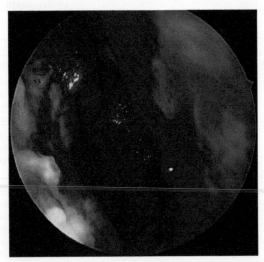

Fig. 2. Endoscopic view of left nasal cavity after de-crusting, showing typical inflamed friable mucosa of active GPA. Biopsy was diagnostic in this case of localized disease.

GPA but may be negative in localized or limited disease or after systemic steroid treatment.[3] MPO-ANCA will be positive in approximately 5%.[6] Patients may become ANCA-positive if their disease progresses to become more severe, and ANCA can, therefore, be a useful tool for monitoring disease activity.[2] The French Vasculitis Study Group recently reviewed over 700 patients and found that ANCA-negative patients were more likely to have limited disease, but their relapse-free survival (RFS) and overall survival rates were similar to ANCA-positive patients.[10] PR3-ANCA-positive patients had lower RFS than the other two groups.

Cocaine abuse must not be forgotten as a differential diagnosis of sinonasal GPA, as similar midline nasal septal inflammation, crusting, and destruction can also be seen with preceding nasal obstruction and epistaxis. PR3-ANCA can be positive in such cases, which further complicates the diagnosis and requires specialist testing for human neutrophil elastase.[11] Other midline destructive processes include NK-T cell lymphoma (formerly midline lethal granuloma) and acute fulminant fungal infection, which require biopsy to exclude if clinical suspicion warrants.

Complementary investigations include renal function, complete blood count erythrocyte sedimentation rate, C-reactive protein, and urinalysis.

Imaging

Imaging of both the chest and sinuses can be helpful in diagnosing this disease which often involves both the upper and lower airways. In the absence of previous sinonasal surgery, the combination of simultaneous bony destruction and neo-osteogenesis on computed tomography (CT) is almost pathognomic of GPA (**Fig. 3**),[12] although nonspecific mucosal thickening is common (87.7%), especially in early and/or limited disease.[13] "Tramlining," a fat signal from the sclerotic sinus wall on MR imaging T1-weighted sequences, is also very suggestive of GPA and is most commonly seen in the maxillary sinuses.[12] Chest CT may show widespread infiltrates, nodules, or progressive cavitation if pulmonary disease is present.[6]

Histology

Histologic diagnosis, with features of necrosis, granulomatous inflammation, and vasculitis, can be difficult to confirm but should be sought where possible, especially

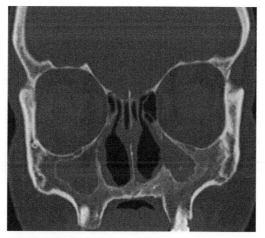

Fig. 3. Coronal CT scan showing both bony destruction and neo-osteogenesis in GPA, with loss of the lateral nasal wall architecture.

if the diagnosis is uncertain.[14] Sinonasal biopsies, even when taken from clinically abnormal mucosa, have low sensitivity (20%–50%).[2] Endobronchial biopsies are only diagnostic in 10% of cases, while open lung biopsies have the highest sensitivity (80%–90%) but are obviously more invasive.[15] Percutaneous ultrasound-guided renal biopsy is an alternative.[16]

Management

Management of vasculitic diseases should be undertaken by a specialist multidisciplinary team.

Systemic Treatment

GPA, and indeed any vasculitis, should be managed by a multidisciplinary team. Untreated systemic GPA has a mean survival time of 5 months.[6] This has improved dramatically since the introduction of immunosuppressant drugs. The current treatment protocols have two phases: remission induction and then maintenance therapy.[2] For severe GPA, remission is generally induced using systemic corticosteroids and either cyclophosphamide or rituximab for 3 to 6 months.[16] The Rituximab in ANCA-associated vasculitis (RAVE) trial and Rituximab versus cyclophosphamide in ANCA-associated vasculitis (RITUXVAS) trial showed that remission can be induced in over 80% of patients with these drugs.[17,18] Recently, the C5a receptor inhibitor avacopan was compared with prednisolone, with either cyclophosphamide or rituximab, in the randomized controlled ADVOCATE trial.[19] Avacopan was non-inferior to prednisolone at inducing remission at 26 weeks (72.3% vs 70.1%, respectively), and superior to prednisolone at 52 weeks (65.7% vs 54.9%, respectively, $P<.001$), and may become the new standard of care.

For more limited disease, steroids and either methotrexate or mycophenolate mofetil are recommended to induce remission.[16] The ABROGATE trial is currently studying abatacept (CTLA4-Ig) for the treatment of relapsing, non-severe GPA (ABROGATE; ClinicalTrials.gov Identifier: NCT02108860).

Once remission has been achieved, it should be maintained with a combination of low-dose corticosteroids and either azathioprine, rituximab, methotrexate, or mycophenolate mofetil for at least 2 years after a period of sustained remission.[16] Rituximab is the most commonly used maintenance therapy, with both the MAINRITSAN and RITAZAREM trials showing superiority of rituximab over azathioprine in preventing relapse.[20,21]

Treatment of Sinonasal Symptoms

Sinonasal symptoms in GPA are rarely helped by surgery, and endoscopic sinus surgery should be avoided unless to treat complications as it can lead to adhesions and additional scarring.[22] The mainstay of treatment for nasal crusting and congestion is with topical rinses, lubricants, and intranasal steroid sprays.[23] Reconstructive septorhinoplasty to correct the saddle nose deformity can be undertaken if remission has been maintained for at least a year, with an overall success rate of 84.1% reported in a systematic review of 44 patients.[24] Similarly, dacryocystorhinostomy can be performed in selected cases.[22] Septal perforation repair is unlikely to be successful and is rarely possible; a septal button may be inserted.[23]

Subglottic stenosis is now most commonly managed by regular balloon dilatations and intralesional steroid injections, and tracheostomy can usually be avoided.[25]

Middle ear ventilation tubes should be avoided due to the risk of chronic discharge.[26]

SARCOIDOSIS

Sarcoidosis is a systemic inflammatory disease of unknown etiology associated with noncaseating granulomas.[6] It most commonly affects the lungs as well as hilar lymph nodes, skin, and eyes, but can affect any organ system including the upper airway.[27] The large European multicenter GenPhenRea epidemiologic study of over 2000 patients described five distinct phenotypes according to the organs involved: (1) abdominal; (2) ocular–cardiac–cutaneous–central nervous system; (3) musculoskeletal–cutaneous; (4) pulmonary and intrathoracic lymph nodes; and (5) extrapulmonary involvement.[28]

Epidemiology

The incidence varies with race, sex, and geography, with an average incidence of 11 per 100,00 Caucasians.[6] It is more common in northern Europe, where the incidence is 20 per 100,000, as compared with Japan, where it is 1.3 per 100,000. It is more prevalent in African Americans than white Americans, with a prevalence of 35.5 per 100,000 versus 10.9 per 100,000, respectively. Men and women are equally affected below the age of 40, but above that age, it is twice as common in women.[28] Women are more likely to present with an acute onset and extrapulmonary involvement, and their mortality rates are higher. The incidence peaks in the third and fourth decades for men and the fifth decade for women.

Clinical Manifestations

Symptoms vary depending on the organ systems involved (see **Table 1**); it may even be asymptomatic, found incidentally on chest imaging in up to 5%.[6] Disease onset can be acute, with systemic symptoms including fatigue, fever, arthralgia, and night sweats, or subacute.[28] Acute onset is more commonly seen in younger female patients with less frequent cough and dyspnea. Sarcoidosis affects the lungs in over 90% of cases, with both interstitial lung pathology and obstructive airway disease reported at all sites along the upper and lower respiratory tracts in keeping with a unified airway model.[29]

The nose and sinuses are much less frequently involved than the lower airway, in 1% to 6% of cases.[29] Symptoms are often vague, with obstruction, crusting, and bleeding predominating. Anosmia may be due to the nasal obstruction or be sensorineural in nature. In patients with evidence of CRS, the presence of at least two of crusting, anosmia, and epistaxis has been shown to be highly specific for sarcoid rhinosinusitis, and biopsy should, therefore, be considered in such cases.[30] Sarcoid rhinosinusitis is usually associated with both pulmonary and extrapulmonary disease which tends to be recalcitrant and requires prolonged treatment.[29]

Nasal obstruction is often related to edematous hypertrophic mucosa with polypoid granulomatous nodules typically affecting the anterior septum (**Fig. 4**) and inferior turbinates.[29] There may be a "strawberry skin" appearance created by multiple small pale granulomas across the erythematous granular mucosa.[27] Similar mucosal appearances can be seen within the sinuses themselves. The sinonasal disease may progress with ulceration, crusting, atrophy, and adhesions, especially if traumatized by surgery when a septal perforation may also develop. Cutaneous sarcoidosis can be nonspecific with skin lesions, such as erythema nodosum, typically seen on the shins. Over the nose, face, and ears, there can be a more specific cutaneous manifestation of sarcoid known as lupus pernio (**Fig. 5**), which has a typical red/purple appearance and is often associated with severe sarcoidosis and a poor prognosis.[31]

Elsewhere in the upper airway, similar mucosal changes can occur in the hard and soft palate, occasionally leading to oronasal fistulas.[27] The supraglottis, false cords,

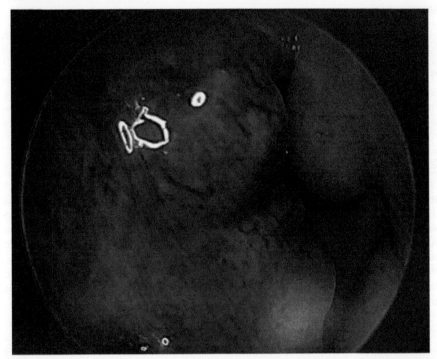

Fig. 4. Endoscopic view of left nasal cavity showing granulomatous sarcoid nodule on the anterior septum.

and subglottis can also be affected, although the vocal cords themselves are typically spared.[29] Dysphonia can occur due to granulomatous mucosal disease from an infiltrative vagal neuropathy or from recurrent laryngeal nerve compression by mediastinal lymphadenopathy.

Investigations

Histology
The diagnosis can be confirmed by biopsy, commonly endobronchial or of skin lesions.[27] Nasal biopsy is positive in 91% of cases if there is macroscopically abnormal

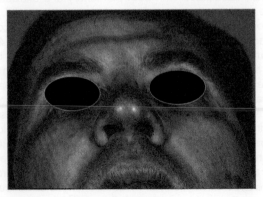

Fig. 5. Lupus pernio of the nasal skin in sarcoidosis.

mucosa, but if the mucosa is not abnormal then biopsy is usually negative (93%).[32] Histology shows typical noncaseating granulomas and is negative for fungi and mycobacteria.[30] The recent guidelines from both the American and British Thoracic Societies advise that biopsy is only required if there is diagnostic uncertainty or in patients with typical long-standing features on imaging.[33]

Serum angiotensin-converting enzyme levels may be raised, as may alkaline phosphatase and both serum and urinary calcium levels, but these tests are not diagnostic with a sensitivity of 60% and specificity of 70%.[6] They are useful screening tests for extrapulmonary disease and may be helpful in monitoring disease activity.[34]

Imaging

CT of the sinuses may be nonspecific with varying degrees of opacification as seen in CRS. This may be due to active granulomatous disease, chronic inflammation, or fibrosis, but nodular mucosal thickening, either within the sinuses or along the septum and inferior turbinates (seen in 21%), is very suggestive of sarcoidosis (**Fig. 6**).[35] Bony erosion is seen in 8% and neo-osteogenesis in 15% of sinuses, and the nasal bones may demonstrate punctate osteolysis or rarefaction.

Staging of Pulmonary Sarcoidosis

Chest x-ray (CXR) showing bilateral hilar lymphadenopathy in conjunction with appropriate clinical features is very suggestive of sarcoidosis, and pulmonary staging is based on the CXR appearances (**Table 2**).[36] Enlarged or calcified lymph nodes, single or multiple lung nodules, and fibrosis may also be seen on CT.[33]

Management

Again, this should be undertaken in a multidisciplinary team setting, but in many cases, no specific treatment is required. Early pulmonary disease may regress spontaneously, with 50% to 90% of stage I and 30% to 70% of stage II disease resolving without treatment.[36] However, 6% to 8% of patients with sarcoidosis have a reduced life expectancy[34] with death due to pulmonary involvement in 70% of sarcoid-related mortality and to cardiac disease in most other cases.[37]

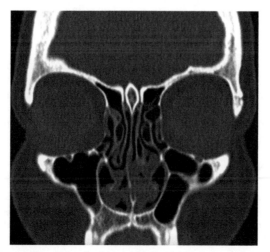

Fig. 6. Coronal CT scan showing soft tissue nodular thickening of the septum and inferior turbinates in sarcoidosis.

Table 2
Pulmonary staging of sarcoidosis based on chest x-ray appearances[36]

Stage 0	Normal CXR
Stage I	Enlarged lymph nodes
Stage II	Enlarged lymph nodes and parenchymal involvement
Stage III	Parenchymal involvement without enlarged lymph nodes or fibrosis
Stage IV	Fibrosis

Systemic Treatment

To reduce treatment-related morbidity, recent guidelines recommend that treatment should be commenced only if there is potential danger of a fatal outcome or permanent disability, or unacceptable loss of quality of life.[34] Although some patients can be managed with nonsteroidal anti-inflammatory agents, oral steroids are the mainstay of systemic treatment, with a tapering dose for several months or longer, depending on the site and severity of the disease. If additional immunosuppressive treatment is required, either for disease control or as a steroid-sparing agent, methotrexate is most commonly used. Mycophenolate mofetil, leflunomide, and azathioprine can also be considered. Hydroxychloroquine is used primarily to treat fatigue, and joint and cutaneous sarcoidosis, but may also be steroid sparing. Biologic agents such as infliximab, a tumor-necrosis factor antagonist, are third-line agents.[38] Despite treatment, lung transplantation may be required in certain cases.

Treatment of Sinonasal Symptoms

Sinonasal symptoms may benefit from any systemic treatment required, but the mainstay of topical treatment for the nose and sinuses are nasal rinses, topical steroids, lubricants, and regular decrusting if necessary. Surgery has little role and should be avoided because of the risk of adhesions and septal perforation, but careful debulking of granulomatous lesions can provide symptomatic relief in select cases, particularly those with nasal obstruction from granulomatous lesions or polyps.[29,39] In a retrospective review of 86 patients with sinonasal sarcoid, surgery was performed in six cases for refractory sinonasal symptoms because of granulomatous lesions obstructing the ostiomeatal complex as well as nasal polyps.[40]

SUMMARY

Granulomatous and vasculitic diseases of the nose and sinuses often present with vague symptoms that mimic more common conditions such as rhinitis and CRS. Patients may therefore present to ENT surgeons in the first instance and it is extremely important to consider the diagnosis in atypical or recalcitrant cases and investigate appropriately. Management should involve a multidisciplinary team; systemic treatment is usually required, and surgery is rarely indicated.

CLINICS CARE POINTS

- Maintain a low threshold of suspicion for granulomatosis with polyangiitis (GPA) and sarcoid, which can mimic general inflammatory diseases of the upper and lower airways in keeping with the unified airway model.
- Crusting and blood-stained nasal discharge should be considered due to a granulomatous disease until proven otherwise.

- Antineutrophil cytoplasmic antibody (ANCA) has low sensitivity, especially in localized or limited GPA, and biopsy may also be inconclusive.
- A combination of clinical findings, serologic tests, imaging, and histology may be required for diagnosis.
- Prompt management within a multidisciplinary team setting is essential to improve morbidity and prognosis and to avoid complications of untreated disease.
- Systemic treatment is usually required and there is little role for sinonasal surgery.

DISCLOSURE

The authors have no commercial or financial conflicts of interest to declare. No funding was received.

REFERENCES

1. Jennette JC, Falk RJ, Bacon PA, et al. 2012 Revised International Chapel Hill Consensus Conference Nomenclature of Vasculitides. Arthritis Rheum 2013; 65:1–11.
2. Ross C, Makhzoum JP, Pagnoux C. Updates in ANCA-associated vasculitis. Eur J Rheumatol 2022. https://doi.org/10.5152/eujrheum.2022.20248.
3. Stone JH, Wegener's Granulomatosis Etanercept Trial Research Group. Limited versus severe Wegener's granulomatosis: baseline data on patients in the Wegener's granulomatosis etanercept trial. Arthritis Rheum 2003;48:2299–309.
4. Leavitt RY, Fauci AS, Bloch DA, et al. The American College of Rheumatology 1990 criteria for the classification of Wegener's granulomatosis. Arthritis Rheum 1990;33:1101–7.
5. Robson JC, Grayson PC, Ponte C, et al. 2022 American College of Rheumatology/European Alliance of Associations for Rheumatology classification criteria for granulomatosis with polyangiitis. Ann Rheum Dis 2022;81:315–20.
6. Fokkens WJ, Lund VJ, Hopkins C, et al. European position paper on rhinosinusitis and nasal polyps 2020. Rhinology 2020;29:1–464.
7. Srouji IA, Andrews P, Edwards C, et al. Patterns of presentation and diagnosis of patients with Wegener's granulomatosis: ENT aspects. J Laryngol Otol 2007;121: 653–8.
8. Kühn D, Hospowsky C, Both M, et al. Manifestation of granulomatosis with polyangiitis in head and neck. Clin Exp Rheumatol 2018;36(Suppl 1):78–84.
9. Felicetti M, Cazzador D, Padoan R, et al. Ear, nose and throat involvement in granulomatosis with polyangiitis: how it presents and how it determines disease severity and long-term outcomes. Clin Rheumatol 2018;37:1075–83.
10. Puéchal X, Iudici M, Pagnoux C, et al, French Vasculitis Study Group. Comparative study of granulomatosis with polyangiitis subsets according to ANCA status: data from the French Vasculitis Study Group Registry. RMD Open 2022;8: e002160.
11. Trimarchi M, Bertazzoni G, Bussi M. Cocaine induced midline destructive lesions. Rhinology 2014;52:104–11.
12. Lloyd G, Lund VJ, Beale T, et al. Rhinologic changes in Wegener's granulomatosis. J Laryngol Otol 2002;116:565–9.
13. D'Anza B, Langford CA, Sindwani R. Sinonasal imaging findings in granulomatosis with polyangiitis (Wegener granulomatosis): A systematic review. Am J Rhinol Allergy 2017;31:16–21.

14. Borner U, Landis BN, Banz Y, et al. Diagnostic value of biopsies in identifying cytoplasmic antineutrophil cytoplasmic antibody-negative localized Wegener's granulomatosis presenting primarily with sinonasal disease. Am J Rhinol Allergy 2012;26:475–80.

15. Masiak A, Zdrojewski Z, Peksa R, et al. The usefulness of histopathological examinations of non-renal biopsies in the diagnosis of granulomatosis with polyangiitis. Reumatologia 2017;5:230–6.

16. Yates M, Watts RA, Bajema IM, et al. EULAR/ERA-EDTA recommendations for the management of ANCA-associated vasculitis. Ann Rheum Dis 2016;75:1583–94.

17. Stone JH, Merkel PA, Spiera R, et al, RAVE-ITN Research Group. Rituximab versus cyclophosphamide for ANCA-associated vasculitis. N Engl J Med 2010; 363:221–32.

18. Jones RB, Tervaert JW, Hauser T, et al. European Vasculitis Study Group. Rituximab versus cyclophosphamide in ANCA-associated renal vasculitis. N Engl J Med 2010;363:211–20.

19. Jayne DRW, Merkel PA, Schall TJ, et al, ADVOCATE Study Group. Avacopan for the Treatment of ANCA-Associated Vasculitis. N Engl J Med 2021;384:599–609.

20. Guillevin L, Pagnoux C, Karras A, et al, French Vasculitis Study Group. Rituximab versus azathioprine for maintenance in ANCA-associated vasculitis. N Engl J Med 2014;371:1771–80.

21. Smith R, Jayne D, Merkel P. A randomized, controlled trial of rituximab versus azathioprine after induction of remission with rituximab for patients with ANCA-associated Vvsculitis and relapsing disease [abstract]. Arthritis Rheumatol 2019;71(suppl 10). Available at: https://acrabstracts.org/abstract/a-randomized-controlled-trial-of-rituximab-versus-azathioprine-after-induction-of-remission-with-rituximab-for-patients-with-anca-associated-vasculitis-and-relapsing-disease/. Accessed May 11, 2022.

22. Cannady SB, Batra PS, Koening C, et al. Sinonasal Wegener granulomatosis: A single-institution experience with 120 cases. Laryngoscope 2009;119:757–61.

23. Erickson VR, Hwang PH. Wegener's granulomatosis: current trends in diagnosis and management. Curr Opin Otolaryngol Head Neck Surg 2007;15:170–6.

24. Ezzat WH, Compton RA, Basa KC, et al. Reconstructive techniques for the saddle nose deformity in granulomatosis with polyangiitis: a systematic review. JAMA Otolaryngol Head Neck Surg 2017;143:507–12.

25. Nouraei SA, Obholzer R, Ind PW, et al. Results of endoscopic surgery and intralesional steroid therapy for airway compromise due to tracheobronchial Wegener's granulomatosis. Thorax 2008;63:49–52.

26. Takagi D, Nakamaru Y, Maguchi S, et al. Otologic manifestations of Wegener's granulomatosis. Laryngoscope 2002;112:1684–90.

27. Alobid I, Guilemany JM, Mullol J. Nasal manifestations of systemic illnesses. Curr Allergy Asthma Rep 2004;4:208–16.

28. Schupp JC, Freitag-Wolf S, Bargagli E, et al. Phenotypes of organ involvement in sarcoidosis. Eur Respir J 2018;51:1700991.

29. Morgenthau AS, Teirstein AS. Sarcoidosis of the upper and lower airways. Expert Rev Respir Med 2011;5:823–33.

30. Reed J, deShazo RD, Houle TT, et al. Clinical features of sarcoid rhinosinusitis. Am J Med 2010;123:856–62.

31. Judson MA. The clinical features of sarcoidosis: a comprehensive review. Clin Rev Allergy Immunol 2015;49:63–78.

32. Wilson R, Lund V, Sweatman M, et al. Upper respiratory tract involvement in sarcoidosis and its management. Eur Respir J 1988;1:269–72.

33. Millward K, Fiddler CA, Thillai M. Update on sarcoidosis guidelines. Curr Opin Pulm Med 2021;27:484–9.
34. Thillai M, Atkins CP, Crawshaw A, et al. BTS Clinical Statement on pulmonary sarcoidosis. Thorax 2021;76:4–20.
35. Joshi R, Zenga J, Getz A, et al. THU0403 Sinonasal sarcoidosis: Review of clinical and imaging features: 7 year experience. Ann Rheum Dis 2013;71:291–2.
36. Scadding JG. Prognosis of intrathoracic sarcoidosis in England. A review of 136 cases after five years' observation. Br Med J 1961;2:1165–72.
37. Ho JSY, Chilvers ER, Thillai M. Cardiac sarcoidosis - an expert review for the chest physician. Expert Rev Respir Med 2019;13:507–20.
38. Crouser ED, Lozanski G, Fox CC, et al. The CD4+ lymphopenic sarcoidosis phenotype is highly responsive to anti-tumor necrosis factor-{alpha} therapy. Chest 2010;137:1432–5.
39. Aloulah M, Manes RP, Ng YH, et al. Sinonasal manifestations of sarcoidosis: a single institution experience with 38 cases. Int Forum Allergy Rhinol 2013I;3:567–72.
40. Kay DJ, Har-El G. The role of endoscopic sinus surgery in chronic sinonasal sarcoidosis. Am J Rhinol 2001;15:249–54.

Immunoglobulin Deficiency and the Unified Airway

Chadi A. Makary, MD[a],*, David W. Jang, MD[b], Patricia Lugar, MD[c]

KEYWORDS

- Chronic rhinosinusitis • Unified airway • Immune deficiencies

KEY POINTS

- Primary immunodeficiency disorders commonly manifest as recurrent sinopulmonary infections, supporting the concept of the unified airway.
- Primary immunoglobulin deficiencies are classified into common variable immunoglobulin deficiency, specific antibody deficiency, IgG subclass deficiency, and selective IgA deficiency.
- Treatment is geared toward decreasing the number of infections and preventing long-term sequelae and complications that may arise from repeated infections.

INTRODUCTION

Immunodeficiency disorders represent a broad spectrum of diseases that can lead to more frequent and more severe infections of the upper and lower airways. These disorders can be primary or secondary in origin. Primary immunodeficiency disorders (PIDs) are caused by intrinsic, inherited defects in the immune system[1] and are varied in cell of origin. Most patients with PIDs have defects in B-cell function (humoral immunity) characterized by a decreased number of B cells, and/or impaired production of protective antibodies or immunoglobulin (Ig). These disorders of Ig production and function commonly manifest as recurrent sinopulmonary infections,[1] supporting the concept of the unified airway.

CLASSIFICATION

The 2015 Practice Parameter for the Diagnosis and Management of Primary Immunodeficiency, under the American Academy of Allergy, Asthma & Immunology, provides

No financial disclosure or conflict of interest to report.
[a] Department of Otolaryngology-Head and Neck Surgery, West Virginia University, One Medical Center Drive, HSC 4th Floor, Morgantown, WV, USA; [b] Department of Head and Neck Surgery & Communication Sciences, Duke University, Durham, NC, USA; [c] Division of Allergy and Immunology, Department of Medicine, Duke University, Durham, NC, USA
* Corresponding author.
E-mail address: Chadi.makary@hsc.wvu.edu

Otolaryngol Clin N Am 56 (2023) 97–106
https://doi.org/10.1016/j.otc.2022.09.007
0030-6665/23/© 2022 Elsevier Inc. All rights reserved.

oto.theclinics.com

a comprehensive classification system for more than 200 known PIDs, including genetic abnormalities and syndromes affecting both cell-mediated and humoral immunity[1]; these are distinct from secondary immunodeficiencies, which are due to known underlying causes such as AIDS, leukemia, and chemotherapy.[1] Among the PIDs, primary Ig deficiencies comprise more than half of all cases and are of particular relevance to the otolaryngologist given the prevalence of upper respiratory manifestations. At present, primary Ig deficiencies are classified into the following conditions:

- Common variable immunoglobulin deficiency (CVID)
- Specific antibody deficiency (SAD)
- IgG subclass deficiency (IGGSD)
- Selective IgA deficiency (SIGAD)

DIAGNOSIS

CVID is the most commonly diagnosed symptomatic primary Ig deficiency.[2,3] CVID is characterized by both low serum Ig levels and an inadequate antibody response.[2] CVID likely represents the end manifestation of multiple but related disease processes, both acquired and genetic. Several single gene mutations with both autosomal dominant and recessive transmission have been associated with CVID, including abnormalities of the CD19, CD20, CD21, and target of antiproliferative antibody-1 genes.[2] However, most cases of CVID are not associated with a single genetic defect and seem to manifest spontaneously at any age.[3] Owing to the unclear pathogenesis of what is likely a heterogeneous group of disorders, the diagnosis of CVID can vary depending on institution and professional society. As proposed by several international groups, commonly accepted diagnostic criteria for CVID are as follows[1]:

- Low serum levels of IgG (at least 2 SDs below mean) in addition to low serum levels of IgM and/or IgA
- Inadequate antibody response to vaccination
- Absence of other known causes of hypogammaglobulinemia
- Clinical symptoms consistent with immune deficiency (ie, recurrent infections, pathognomonic comorbidity)

Each criterion has a level of complexity that can make interpretation of laboratory values, and therefore diagnosis, difficult. Clinical expertise combined with individual patient factors is paramount in making the diagnosis of CVID. Ig levels, for example, depend on age, race, and ethnicity. Although no standard range has been universally adopted, laboratories will typically use 2 SDs below the mean as the lower limit of normal.[2,4] As for specific antibody response to vaccination, the vaccine type and definition of adequate response can vary significantly. Most commonly used is the pneumococcal conjugate vaccine, by which specific antibody titers are measured before and after vaccination. Diphtheria and tetanus vaccines have also been used. Finally, a host of medications, namely, corticosteroids, have been associated with hypogammaglobulinemia, and a careful history is necessary to rule out known causes of low Ig levels to make the diagnosis of CVID. At present, diagnostic genetic testing for CVID is not the standard of care at most institutions. The diagnosis of CVID is often delayed, with Quinti and colleagues[3] reporting a mean delay time of 9 years.

The diagnosis of SAD, IGGSD, and SIGAD are also largely through laboratory data. The diagnosis of SIGAD is made if low levels of IgA are found in isolation, whereas the diagnosis of IGGSD is made when 1 or more of the 4 IgG subclasses are at a low level even in the setting of normal total IgG levels. Neither requires the presence of an

Table 1
Clinical manifestations of primary immunodeficiency disorders

PID	Upper Airway	Lower Airway	Other
CVID	Chronic and recurrent rhinosinusitis (up to 82%) Recurrent otitis media	Bronchitis and pneumonia (up to 75%) Chronic lung disease (30%)	Lupus, rheumatoid arthritis Granulomatous diseases (10%) Malignancies
SAD	Chronic and recurrent rhinosinusitis (most common) Recurrent otitis media	Bronchitis and pneumonia Bronchiectasis	Atopy Connective tissue diseases Autoimmune disorders Hematopoietic
IGGSD	Asymptomatic Chronic and recurrent rhinosinusitis Recurrent otitis media	Asymptomatic Bronchitis and pneumonia Asthma and chronic obstructive pulmonary disease	Atopy Vasculitis Cytopenia
SIGAD	Asymptomatic Chronic and recurrent rhinosinusitis Recurrent otitis media (less common)	Asymptomatic Bronchitis and pneumonia Bronchiectasis Chronic obstructive pulmonary disease	Inflammatory bowel disease Celiac disease Anaphylactic

Abbreviations: CVID, common variable immunoglobulin deficiency; IGGSD, IgG subclass deficiency; PIDs, primary immunodeficiency disorders; SAD, specific antibody deficiency; SIGAD, selective IgA deficiency.

inadequate specific antibody response. SAD, on the other hand, is diagnosed when total IgG levels are normal, but there is an inadequate response to polysaccharide-and/or protein-based vaccination. However, the clinical significance of each of these diagnoses is unclear. For example, SIGAD is the most commonly found Ig deficiency on serology, but the vast majority of patients are asymptomatic. In addition, patients often require serial testing and can meet criteria for more than 1 Ig deficiency over a period.

PATHOGENESIS

The pathogenesis of primary Ig deficiencies is not fully understood but thought to be highly variable. Some cases have been linked to polymorphisms at single gene loci, but most cases are thought to be polygenetic. At a cellular level, B-cell dysfunction is the obvious culprit, but an inadequate helper T-cell response in addition to regulatory T-cell dysfunction has also been implicated in CVID.[5,6] The underlying immune dysfunction at the basis of all the primary Ig deficiencies manifests not only as low Ig levels and recurrent infection but also as noninfectious sequelae such as autoimmunity, chronic inflammatory disease, and lymphoproliferative disorders. As the understanding of the pathogenesis of CVID advances, genetic testing and biomarkers followed by therapeutic targets will likely come to the forefront of diagnosis and management.

EAR, NOSE, AND THROAT (ENT)/UPPER AIRWAY MANIFESTATIONS

Patients with immunodeficiency disorders present with frequent and more severe infections of the upper and lower airways, most commonly sinopulmonary infections **Table 1**. These infections can occur in the setting of both primary and secondary immune dysfunctions. Patients with chronic rhinosinusitis (CRS) with PIDs have a disease that can be refractory to medical and surgical treatment (**Fig. 1**). Patients may also present with recurrent acute rhinosinusitis (RARS), where patients report 4 or more episodes of acute sinusitis requiring multiple courses of antibiotics, sometimes associated with bronchitis or pneumonia.[7] Acute exacerbation of chronic rhinosinusitis, although not fully understood, is also a common manifestation of difficult-to-treat patients with CRS and can be more common in the setting of immunodeficiency disorders.[8] Finally, complications of rhinosinusitis, such as meningitis and orbital infections, can be more severe in patients with PIDs (**Fig. 2**).

Up to 82% of patients with CVID present with CRS or RARS.[9] Other otolaryngologic manifestations of patients with CVID include aphthouslike oral lesions and recurrent otitis media.[9] Common pathogens include encapsulated bacteria mainly *Streptococcus pneumoniae* and *Haemophilus influenzae*.[10] Patients with SIGAD can be asymptomatic depending on whether the deficiency is partial or complete. Spectrum of infection severity can vary.[11] Chronic and recurrent rhinosinusitis are the most common manifestation of SIGAD, followed by otitis media and adenotonsillitis. Upper respiratory viral infections (colds) and laryngitis are more common in these patients. Typical pathogens include encapsulated bacteria, mainly *S pneumoniae* and *H influenzae*.[10] Like SIGAD, IGGSD is relatively common and can be variable in its presentation.[12] Although some patients are asymptomatic, rhinosinusitis and otitis media are the most common presenting infections in these patients. IGGSD is also commonly associated with other primary immunodeficiencies such as SIGAD and SAD as well as immune regulatory disorders seen in atopic disorders, and autoimmunity. Presentation of patients with SAD can overlap with all the other conditions.[1] CRS and RARS are the most common infections in these patients.

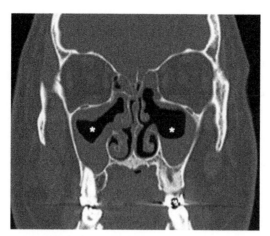

Fig. 1. Computed tomographic (CT) scan of the sinuses, coronal cut, and bony window of an adult patient who continued to have recalcitrant chronic rhinosinusitis despite appropriate medical therapy and despite endoscopic sinus surgery. Scan shows persistent mucosal inflammation and thickening of the maxillary sinuses despite widely opened sinuses (*asterisks*).

NON-ENT MANIFESTATIONS

PIDs can affect the lower airway in a variety of manifestations, including being asymptomatic. Both acute and chronic infectious manifestations are the most common, including bronchitis and pneumonia. Chronic granulomatous changes in the lung

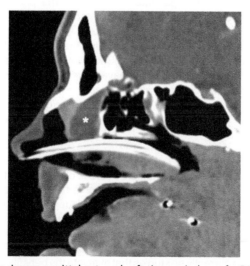

Fig. 2. CT scan of the sinuses, sagittal cut, and soft tissue window of a 21-year-old male who presented with *Streptococcus pneumoniae* meningitis and ventriculitis. Asterisk shows an infected encephalocele and rhinosinusitis. Upon further investigation, patient had history of recurrent rhinosinusitis and bronchitis, and had multiple family members who died of meningitis and pneumonia. He was found to have primary immunodeficiency disorder (hypogammaglobulinemia), and he was started on intravenous Ig replacement therapy.

can occur as well. Chronic lung disease can lead to structural damage to the lungs, which often causes bronchiectasis, interstitial lung disease, and pulmonary fibrosis. PIDs have also been associated with autoimmune disorders, connective tissue disease, and malignancies, namely, lymphoma.

CVID often causes recurrent bronchitis and pneumonias associated with recurrent hospitalizations.[9] By the time patients are diagnosed with CVID, about 30% have chronic lung disease (bronchiectasis or interstitial lung disease).[9] In addition to recurrent pulmonary infections, SAD has been associated with bronchiectasis of unknown origin.[13] Patients with SAD have symptoms suggesting atopy; however, there are no data to support increased incidence of testing-proven atopic diseases in patients with SAD. Patients with SIGAD, in addition to frequent sinopulmonary infections, can develop bronchiectasis and chronic obstructive pulmonary disease (COPD), inflammatory bowel diseases, autoimmune disorders, and anaphylactic reactions to blood products.[14] Patients with IGGSD are found to have higher incidence of atopic diseases, asthma and COPD, and autoimmune disorders such as vasculitis and cytopenias.[15]

TREATMENT

Treatment of primary Ig deficiency is geared toward decreasing the number of infections and to prevent long-term sequelae and complications that may arise from repeated infections. Treatment options for PIDs are limited, and involve vaccination, antibiotic prophylaxis, early culture-directed antibiotic therapy, and Ig replacement therapy.[1,16–18]

Vaccination

There is limited evidence that patients who receive the pneumovax vaccine will develop protective levels in their S pneumoniae titers, which may lead to fewer sinus infections.[19] A recent study showed that the number of health care encounters for CRS significantly decreased in the 2 years following the administration of the pneumococcal vaccine in patients with CRS and RARS with low strep titers.[20] Because a large proportion of patients with CRS and RARS have low baseline S pneumoniae titers, it is important to provide those patients with the vaccine; this alone may be enough to lower the number of sinusitis episodes. When patients do not respond, that is, the repeat titers continue to be low, further treatment options are warranted.

Antibiotics

Patients with PID frequently require multiple courses of antibiotics for acute exacerbation of their CRS or for RARS. Many times, patients have received multiple courses before being diagnosed with PID. In addition, the frequent use of oral antibiotics alters the microbiology. Therefore, it is important to perform cultures on any purulence seen on the nasal examination, and choose antimicrobial therapy based on the cultures.

The role of antibiotic prophylaxis in patients with PIDs to prevent recurrent rhinosinusitis is unclear. There are currently no studies that evaluate the benefits of antibiotic prophylaxis. One study showed that bacteria are commonly present in the sinuses of patients with primary hypogammaglobulinemia suggesting an infectious cause of chronic mucosal inflammation.[21] Based on this, consideration of prophylactic antibiotics was recommended for patients with PIDs. β-Lactams, trimethoprim-sulfamethoxazole, and azithromycin have been suggested as options for prophylactic treatment.

Immunoglobulin Replacement Therapy

There is paucity of data to support the use of Ig replacement therapy in patients with CRS or RARS. The most recent statements from rhinologic societies, ICAR 2021[8] and EPOS 2020,[22] both highlighted the need for further studies to evaluate the role of Ig replacement therapy in patients with sinusitis. A recent systematic review performed by Samargandy and colleagues[16] in 2020 identified only 2 small studies[18,23] that reached opposing conclusions. The study by Walsh and colleagues[18] showed that Ig replacement therapy has a positive impact on CRS symptoms in patients with CVID or SAD, whereas its effect on RARS was unclear. More recently, 2 additional studies have been published showing the beneficial role of Ig replacement in decreasing the number of rhinosinusitis episodes in adults and pediatric patients with PID.[24,25] There is need for more studies looking at the outcome of Ig replacement therapy in patients with RARS, and comparing Ig therapy to other treatment modalities.

Surgery

Endoscopic sinus surgery (ESS) for patients with CRS or RARS in the setting of PID is considered when appropriate medical therapy has failed, or as an adjunct to medical therapy. Surgery is also considered when complications develop, such as orbital or intracranial complications. The goals of surgery are to restore sinus drainage, debride or irrigate the sinuses, and ensure wide opening of the sinuses to allow for optimal delivery of topical medications.

A recent meta-analysis[16] identified multiple studies that showed the benefit of ESS for patients with CRS with immunodeficiencies.[26–32] Several of those studies included patients with primary immunodeficiencies, secondary immunodeficiencies (most commonly HIV patients), and patients with autoimmune disorders. Most of these studies were limited to case series. Khalid and colleagues[28] performed a case-control studies comparing the outcome of ESS in patients with immunodeficiencies. Cases included patients with CRS with immune dysfunction (primary, secondary, autoimmune disorders). Controls included immunocompetent patients with CRS. Both cases and controls showed similar improvement in subjective and objective scores postoperatively. Another study by Miglani and colleagues[30] showed subjective improvement in patients with CRS with immunodeficiency who underwent ESS (decrease in 22-item Sino-nasal Outcome Test [SNOT-22] scores). However, those patients had higher revision ESS rates than patients with CRS who were immunocompetent.[30] One limitation of this study is that investigators did not specify the type of immunodeficiency disorders included. More research is needed to better define the role of ESS in patients with CRS and immunodeficiencies. Studies with larger sample sizes that separate between the different types of immune dysfunction should be conducted to develop practice guidelines.

SUMMARY

Primary Ig deficiencies are a heterogeneous group of disorders with widespread implications for the unified airway. Manifestations can vary greatly, with some patients being asymptomatic, whereas others suffering from acute and chronic life-threatening pathologic conditions of the upper and lower airways. Although the diagnosis of PIDs can be complex, the onus of early diagnosis and initiation of treatment will often fall on the shoulders of the otolaryngologist.

CLINICS CARE POINTS

- Patients presenting with recurrent upper respiratory infections and/or recalcitrant CRS should be evaluated for primary immunodeficiency disorders.
- Early recognition and diagnosis can prevent long-term sequelae and complications that may arise from repeated infections.
- Treatment include culture-directed and/or prophylactic antibiotics, immunoglobulin replacement therapy, and FESS when necessary.
- Multidisciplinary approach between the otolaryngologist and the allergist/immunologist is recommended to ensure high quality care for patients with CRS and PID.

REFERENCES

1. Bonilla FA, Khan DA, Ballas ZK, et al. Practice parameter for the diagnosis and management of primary immunodeficiency. J Allergy Clin Immunol 2015;136(5): 1186–205, e1-78.
2. Bonilla FA, Barlan I, Chapel H, et al. International consensus document (ICON): common variable immunodeficiency disorders. J Allergy Clin Immunol Pract 2016;4(1):38–59.
3. Quinti I, Soresina A, Spadaro G, et al. Long-term follow-up and outcome of a large cohort of patients with common variable immunodeficiency. J Clin Immunol 2007;27(3):308–16.
4. Chapel H, Cunningham-Rundles C. Update in understanding common variable immunodeficiency disorders (CVIDs) and the management of patients with these conditions. Br J Haematol 2009;145(6):709–27.
5. Berbers RM, van der Wal MM, van Montfrans JM, et al. Chronically activated T-cells retain their inflammatory properties in common variable immunodeficiency. J Clin Immunol 2021;41(7):1621–32.
6. Unger S, Seidl M, van Schouwenburg P, et al. The TH1 phenotype of follicular helper T cells indicates an IFN-gamma-associated immune dysregulation in patients with CD21low common variable immunodeficiency. J Allergy Clin Immunol 2018;141(2):730–40.
7. Rosenfeld RM, Piccirillo JF, Chandrasekhar SS, et al. Clinical practice guideline (update): adult sinusitis. Otolaryngol Head Neck Surg 2015;152(2 Suppl):S1–39.
8. Orlandi RR, Kingdom TT, Smith TL, et al. International consensus statement on allergy and rhinology: rhinosinusitis 2021. Int Forum Allergy Rhinol 2021;11(3): 213–739.
9. Gathmann B, Mahlaoui N, Gérard L, et al. Clinical picture and treatment of 2212 patients with common variable immunodeficiency. J Allergy Clin Immunol 2014; 134(1):116–26.
10. Gathmann B, Goldacker S, Klima M, et al. The German national registry for primary immunodeficiencies (PID). Clin Exp Immunol 2013;173(2):372–80.
11. Aytekin C, Tuygun N, Gokce S, et al. Selective IgA deficiency: clinical and laboratory features of 118 children in Turkey. J Clin Immunol 2012;32(5):961–6.
12. Shackelford PG, Granoff DM, Madassery JV, et al. Clinical and immunologic characteristics of healthy children with subnormal serum concentrations of IgG2. Pediatr Res 1990;27(1):16–21.

13. van Kessel DA, van Velzen-Blad H, van den Bosch JM, et al. Impaired pneumococcal antibody response in bronchiectasis of unknown aetiology. Eur Respir J 2005;25(3):482–9.

14. Jorgensen GH, Gardulf A, Sigurdsson MI, et al. Clinical symptoms in adults with selective IgA deficiency: a case-control study. J Clin Immunol 2013;33(4):742–7.

15. Kim JH, Park S, Hwang YI, et al. Immunoglobulin G subclass deficiencies in adult patients with chronic airway diseases. J Korean Med Sci 2016;31(10):1560–5.

16. Samargandy S, Grose E, Chan Y, et al. Medical and surgical treatment outcomes in patients with chronic rhinosinusitis and immunodeficiency: a systematic review. Int Forum Allergy Rhinol 2021;11(2):162–73.

17. Stevens WW, Peters AT. Immunodeficiency in chronic sinusitis: recognition and treatment. Am J Rhinol Allergy 2015;29(2):115–8.

18. Walsh JE, Gurrola JG 2nd, Graham SM, et al. Immunoglobulin replacement therapy reduces chronic rhinosinusitis in patients with antibody deficiency. Int Forum Allergy Rhinol 2017;7(1):30–6.

19. Kashani S, Carr TF, Grammer LC, et al. Clinical characteristics of adults with chronic rhinosinusitis and specific antibody deficiency. J Allergy Clin Immunol Pract 2015;3(2):236–42.

20. Bareiss AK, Kattar N, Tivis R, et al. Health-care utilization for sinusitis after pneumococcal vaccination in patients with low antibody titers. Int Forum Allergy Rhinol 2021. https://doi.org/10.1002/alr.22954.

21. Kainulainen L, Suonpää J, Nikoskelainen J, et al. Bacteria and viruses in maxillary sinuses of patients with primary hypogammaglobulinemia. Arch Otolaryngol Head Neck Surg 2007;133(6):597–602.

22. Fokkens WJ, Lund VJ, Hopkins C, et al. European position paper on rhinosinusitis and nasal polyps 2020. Rhinology 2020;58(Suppl S29):1–464.

23. Williams P, White A, Wilson JA, et al. Penetration of administered IgG into the maxillary sinus and long-term clinical effects of intravenous immunoglobulin replacement therapy on sinusitis in primary hypogammaglobulinaemia. Acta Otolaryngol 1991;111(3):550–5.

24. Behnke J, Jimenez-Herrera P, Peppers B, et al. Outcome of immunoglobulin replacement therapy in children with rhinosinusitis. Int Forum Allergy Rhinol 2021. https://doi.org/10.1002/alr.22921.

25. Makary CA, Behnke J, Peppers B, et al. Outcome of immunoglobulin replacement therapy in adults with rhinosinusitis. Laryngoscope 2022;132(4):732–6.

26. Dao AM, Rereddy SK, Wise SK, et al. Management of non-invasive rhinosinusitis in the immunosuppressed patient population. Laryngoscope 2015;125(8): 1767–71.

27. Friedman M, Landsberg R, Tanyeri H, et al. Endoscopic sinus surgery in patients infected with HIV. Laryngoscope 2000;110(10 Pt 1):1613–6.

28. Khalid AN, Mace JC, Smith TL. Outcomes of sinus surgery in ambulatory patients with immune dysfunction. Am J Rhinol Allergy 2010;24(3):230–3.

29. Lund VJ, MacKay IS. Outcome assessment of endoscopic sinus surgery. J R Soc Med 1994;87(2):70–2.

30. Miglani A, Divekar RD, Azar A, et al. Revision endoscopic sinus surgery rates by chronic rhinosinusitis subtype. Int Forum Allergy Rhinol 2018;8(9):1047–51.

31. Murphy C, Davidson TM, Jellison W, et al. Sinonasal disease and olfactory impairment in HIV disease: endoscopic sinus surgery and outcome measures. Laryngoscope 2000;110(10 Pt 1):1707–10.
32. Sabini P, Josephson GD, Reisacher WR, et al. The role of endoscopic sinus surgery in patients with acquired immune deficiency syndrome. Am J Otolaryngol 1998;19(6):351–6.

Aspirin-Exacerbated Respiratory Disease and the Unified Airway: A Contemporary Review

Benjamin K. Walters, MD[a], John B. Hagan, MD[b],
Rohit D. Divekar, MBBS, PhD[b], Thomas J. Willson, MD[a],
Janalee K. Stokken, MD[c], Carlos D. Pinheiro-Neto, MD, PhD[c],
Erin K. O'Brien, MD[c], Garret Choby, MD[c],*

KEYWORDS

- Chronic rhinosinusitis with nasal polyposis • Asthma • Aspirin intolerance
- Aspirin-exacerbated respiratory disease • Biological agents • Samter's Triad
- NSAID intolerance

KEY POINTS

- Diagnosis of aspirin-exacerbated respiratory disease (AERD) is made when patients fulfill criteria for chronic rhinosinusitis with nasal polyposis and asthma and demonstrate upper and/or lower respiratory symptoms in response to nonsteroidal antiinflammatory drug (NSAID) ingestion.
- The pathophysiology of AERD involves dysregulation of arachidonic acid metabolism, which predisposes to chronic upper and lower airway inflammation and an exaggerated inflammatory response after NSAID ingestion.
- Endoscopic sinus surgery (ESS) is often needed, as symptoms tend to be recalcitrant to conventional medical management, and up-front extended frontal sinus approaches may be appropriate when performed by an experienced surgeon.
- ESS can be followed by aspirin desensitization in particularly symptomatic or revision cases.
- In recalcitrant cases, dupilumab seems to be more efficacious than mepolizumab and omalizumab for reducing nasal polyp burden; however, all 3 have demonstrated efficacy in the management of chronic rhinosinusitis symptoms. Direct comparison trials are needed to further evaluate the relative efficacy of these agents.

Conflicts of Interest: The authors declare no relevant conflicts of interest.
[a] Department of Otolaryngology, San Antonio Military Medical Center, San Antonio, TX, USA;
[b] Department of Allergic Diseases, Mayo Clinic College of Medicine, Rochester, MN, USA;
[c] Department of Otolaryngology – Head & Neck Surgery, Mayo Clinic College of Medicine, Rochester, MN, USA
* Corresponding author. Rhinology and Endoscopic Skull Base Surgery, Chair of Quality, Department of Otorhinolaryngology – Head and Neck Surgery, Joint Appointment; Department of Neurologic Surgery, Mayo Clinic, 200 First St. SW, Rochester, MN 55905.
E-mail address: choby.garret@mayo.edu

BACKGROUND
General Background and Epidemiology

Described in 1967,[1,2] the classic "Samter's Triad" of asthma, chronic rhinosinusitis with nasal polyposis (CRSwNP), and aspirin sensitivity is now referred to as aspirin-exacerbated respiratory disease (AERD) or nonsteroidal antiinflammatory-exacerbated respiratory disease.[3,4]

The estimated rates of AERD in various demographics are listed in **Table 1**.[4–7]

An estimated 1.4 million Americans are currently diagnosed with AERD,[3] although the actual number may be much higher, as any part of the diagnostic triad may be present but not yet recognized. Up to 15% of patients with CRSwNP and asthma are unaware of their sensitivity to aspirin.[4] In women, AERD has a higher incidence, presents earlier, and is often more severe.[4,8–10]

Patient Presentation

AERD typically develops in the third or fourth decade of life, with a median age of presentation of 34 years.[3,11–13] Upper airway symptoms typically precede lower airway symptoms by 1 to 2 years, although asthma is often diagnosed before CRSwNP. Aspirin intolerance generally appears last.[12] Asthma and CRSwNP in these patients tend to be recalcitrant to conventional therapy. Hyposmia, rapid polyp regrowth, and middle ear pathology are common.[12,14]

NSAID intolerance manifests as upper and/or lower respiratory symptoms presenting usually within 30 to 120 minutes after ingestion.[12,13,15] The most common manifestations are bronchoconstriction (88%) and rhinorrhea and/or nasal congestion (42%),[13] although gastrointestinal or cutaneous symptoms may occur.[16,17] Although any cyclooxygenase-1 (COX-1) inhibitor can elicit symptoms, COX-2 selective NSAIDs such as celecoxib are almost always well tolerated.[11,13,18] Inquiring about reactions to alcohol can be useful to screen for NSAID intolerance, as approximately 75% to 83% of patients will report mild upper or, less commonly, lower airway symptoms after ingestion of red wine or other alcoholic drinks.[3,11,19]

DIAGNOSTICS

The diagnostic criteria for AERD include the following:[4]

- Asthma
  - Diagnosed with spirometry with bronchodilator or methacholine challenge to confirm reversible bronchial obstruction[20]
- CRSwNP

Table 1
Estimated rates of aspirin-exacerbated respiratory disease in various demographics

Demographic	Percentage
General population	0.3%–0.9%
Mild-to-moderate asthma	5%–10%
CRSwNP	10%–16%
Severe asthma	15%
CRSwNP + asthma	30%–40%
CRSwNP + severe asthma	78%

○ Diagnosed by clinical history, nasal endoscopy (**Fig. 1**), and computed tomography (**Fig. 2**)[21,22]
- NSAID intolerance
  ○ Diagnosed by clinical history or aspirin challenge[12,13,15]

Using aspirin challenge as the gold standard, clinical history was found to be 96% specific but only 52% sensitive for the diagnosis of NSAID intolerance.[23] Potential reasons to consider recommending an aspirin challenge include the following:[11,24]

- No history of NSAID intake
- Pharmacologic inhibition with antileukotriene or biological agent
- Baseline tolerance from daily NSAID (eg, low-dose [81 mg daily] aspirin)
- Severe baseline asthma and/or CRSwNP, as patient may not recognize acute worsening on NSAID ingestion—although those with a forced expiratory volume (FEV1) lower than 60% to 70% may not be appropriate candidates for an oral challenge[18]

An aspirin challenge is typically an outpatient procedure, and several protocols have been published.[12,15,25] In general, aspirin is given in a controlled fashion using incrementally higher doses every 60 to 90 minutes, starting with 10 to 20 mg and ending when a reaction occurs or when a patient has tolerated a 325 mg dose. Reactions typically occur at low doses, around 20 to 160 mg, which preferentially inhibit COX-1.[25,26] A positive challenge is indicated by a decrease in FEV1 of 15% to 20% or the presence of acute upper or lower respiratory symptoms within 30 to 120 minutes.[3,4,12] Intranasal ketorolac or L-lysine-aminosalicylic acid (if available) is less sensitive but can also be used in those at risk of a severe reaction.[18,27] Antileukotriene agents may be used to decrease the likelihood of a severe reaction for patients with higher reaction risks such as those with a significantly elevated Sino-nasal Outcome Test (SNOT-22) score.[25,26,28,29]

Because patients are often unaware of their NSAID intolerance, there has recently been increased research to identify biomarkers that could help identify patients with AERD earlier in a relatively noninvasive manner. One of the most promising of these is urinary leukotriene E4 (uLTE4), which is the stable end-product of the leukotriene pathway, induces eosinophil recruitment to respiratory tissues,[12,30] and correlates with severity of reactions to aspirin.[31] Serum levels are typically too low to measure; however, urinary levels can be measured in a variety of ways, including

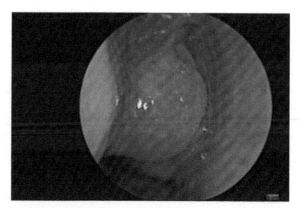

Fig. 1. Nasal endoscopy demonstrating nasal polyposis.

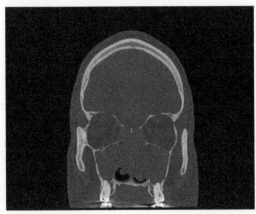

Fig. 2. Computed tomography scan in an patient with AERD demonstrating pansinusitis.

radioimmunoassay and mass spectrometry.[32,33] Liquid-chromatography mass spectrometry (LC-MS) is a reliable, reproducible, and easily accessible commercial assay that is available through many tertiary medical centers and national laboratory chains, although it is ultimately processed through the Mayo clinic as of this writing.[34] A cutoff value of 166 pg/mg creatinine (Cr) predicts aspirin sensitivity with 89% specificity using LC-MS.[35] uLTE4 levels have been found to decrease after endoscopic sinus surgery (ESS) and zileuton therapy, and may correlate with disease severity.[32,36,37] Further research is required to elucidate this biomarker's role in the diagnosis and treatment of AERD.

Pathophysiology

AERD is characterized by dysregulated arachidonic acid metabolism, which results in increased production of proinflammatory leukotrienes and decreased production of antiinflammatory prostaglandins.[38] Arachidonic acid can be metabolized via the COX-1 pathway into prostaglandins and thromboxanes or the 5-lipoxygenase (5-LO) pathway into cysteinyl leukotrienes (cysLTs), which are lipid mediators that cause bronchoconstriction, mucous secretion, eosinophilic inflammation, and increased vascular permeability (**Fig. 3**).[12]

The following have been associated with AERD:

- Overproduction and heightened sensitivity of cysLTs,[39] which are acutely increased even further on COX-1 inhibition[32,33,40]
- Elevated cysLT1 receptor expression in bronchi and nasal polyps[41]
- Baseline preferential metabolism via 5-LO causing increased susceptibility to COX-1 inhibition[18]
- Reduction in prostaglandin E2 (PGE2), causing increased production of LTB4 and activation of eosinophils and mast cells[12,28]
- Increased baseline levels of prostaglandin D2 (PGD2), causing bronchoconstriction and recruitment of eosinophils, basophils, and type 2 innate lymphoid cells (ILC2s) into respiratory tissue[42]
- Platelet-derived augmentation of the 5-LO pathway and increase in arachidonic acid, cysLTs, PGD2, histamine, and tryptase[3,18,43–45]

This complex pathophysiology affords numerous opportunities for developing targeted treatment options.[46]

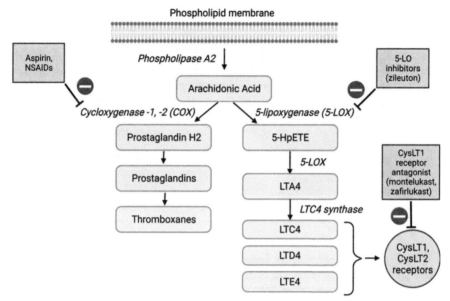

Fig. 3. Arachidonic acid metabolism pathway. (*From* Choby G, Low CM, Levy JM, et al. Urine leukotriene E4: implications as a biomarker in chronic rhinosinusitis. Otolaryngol Head Neck Surg. 2022;166(2):224-232.)

Surgical Management and Outcomes

ESS is one of the mainstays of AERD management in those who remain symptomatic despite appropriate medical therapy and has resulted in the following outcomes:

- Significantly reduced SNOT-22 score[47]
- Improved hyposmia[48]
- NSAID tolerance or decreased reaction severity[49]
- Decreased uLTE4[31,49]
- Increased plasma lipoxin A4 and decreased peripheral eosinophilia[49,50]
- Reduced asthma symptom severity and frequency[51]

Several studies demonstrate higher revision rates after primary ESS in patients with AERD as compared with NSAID-tolerant patients with CRSwNP. A recent meta-analysis demonstrated a revision rate of 27.2% in those diagnosed with AERD, compared with 18.6% in CRSwNP overall.[52] To minimize the risk of recurrence, the current standard for initial surgery is comprehensive ESS, defined as bilateral large maxillary antrostomies, complete ethmoidectomies, sphenoidotomies, and at least Draf IIa frontal sinusotomies, which creates a wide cavity, allowing for optimal delivery of topical steroids.[53–57]

The extent of frontal sinus dissection remains a matter of controversy. Although an endoscopic modified Lothrop procedure (EMLP), also called a Draf III, has historically been performed in revision settings for inflammatory disease,[58] data are emerging that could support earlier EMLP in AERD when performed by an experienced sinus surgeon (**Fig. 4**). A retrospective case series by Bassiouni and colleagues demonstrated a persistent (>3 months) polyp recurrence rate of 55% in patients with AERD treated with a Draf IIa compared with 11% in those treated with Draf III. For their entire cohort of patients with CRSwNP, the recurrence rates were 26% (Draf IIa) versus 16% (Draf

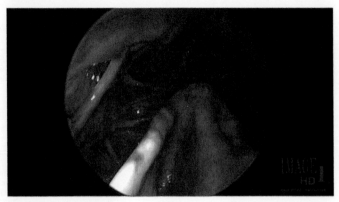

Fig. 4. Nasal endoscopy demonstrating a well-healed common frontal sinus cavity after a Draf III procedure.

III).[59] In a separate cohort of 31 patients undergoing EMLP, the revision rate was 22.5% after an average follow-up of 36 months, and all but one of the revisions was due to polyp recurrence rather than frontal ostium stenosis.[60] However, a similar recurrence rate of 26.2% was reported by Grose and colleagues in a series of 141 patients with AERD after ESS, in which only 6% underwent Draf III and none received postoperative aspirin desensitization (AD).[55] Other nuanced approaches for extended frontal sinus dissection may also be considered, such as bilateral Draf IIb,[61] "cross-court" Draf IIb,[62] or Draf IIb with superior septectomy.[63] Further research is needed to determine the optimal extent of initial frontal sinus surgery in these patients.

Medical Management

The initial medical management of AERD includes a trial of appropriate medical therapy with saline irrigations, topical nasal steroids, and a course of oral corticosteroids, similar to all patients with CRSwNP, as well as standard asthma therapy with inhaled corticosteroids (ICS) with or without a long-acting beta agonist.[3,21] However, these patients are frequently refractory to standard treatment—24% to 51% are oral steroid dependent—thus, further medical management is typically required.[39,64] A low salicylate diet has been reported to show some positive clinical effects in AERD,[65,66] although it is unclear if these findings are directly related to decreasing salicylates.[7] Modifying fatty acid intake (high omega-3/low omega-6) correlated with a decrease in uLTE4 and improvement in SNOT-22 and asthma control questionnaire scores in a small cohort of 10 patients.[67] Because of the paucity of supporting evidence, larger, adequately blinded studies with long-term follow-up periods are needed to determine the sustainability and efficacy of these dietary interventions.

Antileukotriene Therapy

Antileukotrienes have demonstrated modest efficacy for the treatment of aspirin-intolerant asthma. Montelukast is a competitive antagonist at the cysLT1 receptor. As first-line therapy, montelukast is inferior to ICS.[68] However, in oral steroid-dependent aspirin-intolerant asthmatics, adding montelukast has demonstrated a 10.2% improvement in FEV1, reduction in asthma exacerbations, and improvement in quality of life.[69] Zileuton inhibits 5-LO and thus inhibits cysLT production and may also block mast cell activation and PGD2 release indirectly (see **Fig. 3**).[28,70] Zileuton is reported to be more effective than montelukast for AERD in patient surveys and has demonstrated a 20% to 23% improvement in FEV1 within hours, which is greater than what is seen in patients with aspirin-tolerant asthma.[71–73] It has also been associated with decreased uLTE4.[37] The side effects of antileukotriene agents can be significant. Montelukast carries a black box warning for serious mental health side effects including increased suicidality, although this has not been consistently noted in all studies.[74] Zileuton requires monitoring for hepatotoxicity.[75]

Aspirin Desensitization

Currently, standard management of patients with AERD who remain symptomatic despite appropriate standard medical therapy includes comprehensive ESS followed by ongoing topical corticosteroid irrigations and appropriate asthma medication. In cases of revision ESS or particularly severe symptoms, AD may be performed approximately 3 to 4 weeks after ESS.[25,39,50,57,76–78] This window of opportunity following a sinus surgery when the theoretic intensity of aspirin sensitivity risk may be reduced and uLTE4 levels may be low is an optimal time to perform the AD procedure. Progressively higher doses of aspirin are ingested until a reaction is noted, similar to an aspirin challenge. Symptoms typically wane over a 3-hour period, and desensitization is confirmed when patients tolerate a repeat administration of the provocative dose and at least one subsequent dose.[15,16]

AD can be safely carried out by an experienced team in an outpatient setting.[15,79,80] However, adverse reactions to aspirin are anticipated to occur, may be potentially serious, and include laryngeal, upper and lower respiratory, gastrointestinal, and potentially systemic reactions. These reactions can typically be managed with systemic antihistamines, inhaled bronchodilators such as albuterol, proton pump inhibitors, and intramuscular epinephrine and systemic corticosteroids, although recalcitrant symptoms may require use of supplemental oxygen, intravenous fluids, and transfer to an elevated level of care. A leukotriene-modifying agent should be started before desensitization to reduce the risk of a severe reaction.[25] Multiple protocols have been published and are summarized in the American Academy of Allergy, Asthma and Immunology working group guidelines on AD.[25] A 6-month trial is typically recommended to determine clinical effectiveness.[25,38,81] Patients older than 60 years may require lower maintenance doses.[82]

The mechanism of AD is only partially understood, but the following effects are known:

- Decreased cysLT1 receptor expression on nasal polyps[41]
- Reduced sensitivity to inhaled LTE4[83]
- Reduced PGD2[25,26]
- Decreased interleukin-4 (IL-4), IL-13, and STAT6 activity[25]
- Paradoxically increased cysLTs[25,26]

AD, particularly following ESS, has demonstrated the following beneficial effects:

- Decreased need for revision surgery
  - 91% of a University of Pennsylvania cohort who underwent complete ESS and AD and were followed-up for at least 30 months did not require revision surgery.[84]
- Improved SNOT-22
  - A Stanford University cohort who underwent ESS followed by AD had significantly decreased SNOT-22 scores after ESS with even further significant improvement in first 6 months of AD; none needed revision surgery.[85]
- Improvement in FEV1 decreased rescue inhaler and steroid use[86]

- Reduced polyp scores, polyp recurrence, and frequency of acute rhinosinusitis[64,78]
- Reduced alcohol related respiratory symptoms[87]

AD allows patients to tolerate NSAIDs, enabling them to adhere to cardiovascular disease prevention guidelines and minimize narcotic and steroid intake for pain and other inflammatory conditions.[88]

When considering longer term studies, rates of discontinuing aspirin therapy ranges from 9% to 18%[88,89]; this is typically due to ineffectiveness or gastrointestinal effects that can often be easily treated with proton pump inhibition or sucralfate.[25,82,86] Clinically significant gastrointestinal bleeding occurs in less than 1%.[90] Coronary artery vasospasm is a rare occurrence and generally responds to oral steroids.[25] Absolute and relative contraindications to AD are listed in **Table 2**.[25]

Biological Therapy

Several biological agents with proven efficacy for asthma have also demonstrated benefits in CRSwNP, and many studies have included patients with AERD. Dupilumab, mepolizumab, and omalizumab are currently approved by the Federal Drug Administration for CRSwNP and are often used in the "salvage" setting for AERD.[91,92]

Dupilumab is a monoclonal antibody targeting IL-4Ra, the common receptor for IL-4 and IL-13.[92,93] Inhibition of IL-4 reduces immunoglobulin E (IgE) class switching and receptor expression, and inhibition of IL-13 reduces goblet cell metaplasia, mucous secretions, tissue hyperresponsiveness, and chemokine propagation.[94] In a review of 29 different randomized controlled trials (RCTs) for biological agents that included patients with AERD, dupilumab was found to be the most effective for all end points, including need for rescue polyp surgery and SNOT-22 scores.[95] Dupilumab significantly decreases the frequency of severe asthma exacerbations and improves lung function and asthma control, particularly in patients with higher baseline eosinophil levels.[93] It has demonstrated significant reductions in nasal polyp scores (least-squares mean difference vs placebo ranging from −1.8 to −2.5).[87,96–98] Approximately 30% of patients in RCTs evaluating dupilumab for CRSwNP had AERD. Their improvement overall was not inferior to other types of CRSwNP,[97] and one study demonstrated more improvement in nasal polyp score and olfaction in patients with AERD.[96] Patients with AERD who did not benefit from IL-5 inhibition demonstrated significant improvement in SNOT-22 scores and FEV1% predicted after changing to dupilumab.[92] Dupilumab also decreases uLTE4 levels[99] and may reduce the risk of revision surgery when used perioperatively.[100]

Mepolizumab targets IL-5, leading to reduced eosinophil survival and activation.[101] AERD polyps were found in one study to have 3 times more eosinophils and higher

Table 2	
Selected absolute and relative contraindications to aspirin desensitization	
Absolute	**Relative**
Bleeding disorders	Upcoming sinus surgery
History of gastrointestinal or intracranial bleeding	Pregnancy and breastfeeding
Aortic or cerebral aneurysm	Elderly or significant fall risk
Uncontrolled asthma	Peptic ulcer disease
	Eosinophilic esophagitis
	Age < 14 y (risk of Reye syndrome)

levels of IL-5 than aspirin-tolerant patients.[102] Mepolizumab decreases in uLTE4, upGD2, and nasal PGD2, LTB4, and thromboxane levels.[103] Mepolizumab also results in a modest decrease in nasal polyp scores compared with placebo (mean adjusted difference in medians of −0.73).[98,104] In a retrospective review of 22 patients with AERD treated with mepolizumab, there were significant improvements in SNOT-22 scores, and no patients required revision sinus surgery or increases in oral steroids.[102]

Omalizumab targets IgE, which is associated with increased lower airway inflammation and faster polyp regrowth in patients with AERD.[101] Binding of free IgE and subsequent reduction in IgE receptor expression may decrease airway inflammation by reducing eosinophil, basophil, and mast cell activation.[101,105] In patients with AERD, omalizumab causes a significant decrease in uLTE4 and upGD2 metabolite, improves patient-reported nasal symptom scores, and reduces need for systemic steroids.[106–108] An RCT with 16 patients demonstrated a significant decrease in the increase of uLTE4 after aspirin challenge in the treatment group, and 62% developed oral aspirin tolerance.[107] In another study involving 33 patients with AERD on omalizumab, 56% developed aspirin tolerance and another 18% tolerated higher dosages. Polyp size decreased in all patients.[109]

Overall, these results demonstrate that biological agents, particularly dupilumab, represent promising alternatives for refractory cases of AERD, although there are potential limitations to biological therapy. There are no long-term safety data, as most trials have followed-up patients for no more than 1 year, although dropout rates of less than 5% indicate acceptable short-term safety.[110] The cost can be prohibitive and is estimated at around $33,000 to $49,000 USD annually.[88] Biological agents have not been shown to be permanently disease-modifying and will likely need to be continued indefinitely to maintain an effect. Aspirin also needs to be continued indefinitely to maintain effect; however, in comparison, an AD procedure costs an estimated $1700 to $3000, and a typical annual supply of aspirin costs less than $100. Even multiple revision ESS procedures can be completed for a lower cost than a single year of biological therapy.[88] A recent cost-benefit analysis demonstrated that ESS was more cost-effective and should remain the standard of care.[111] There are no current biologics that can prevent all aspirin reactions, so AD is unique in its ability to consistently allow patients to take NSAIDs for needs such as pain, cardioprotection, and inflammation.[110] Despite these limitations, biologics are a valuable alternative for patients who are unable to undergo or do not respond well to surgery and/or AD.

Aspirin-Exacerbated Respiratory Disease and the Unified Airway

The pathophysiology and clinical behavior of AERD provide strong evidence for the unified airway concept. By definition, all patients have both upper and lower airway disease, and both are typically more severe than in aspirin-tolerant patients. Patients with CRSwNP and asthma have greater sinonasal inflammation[112,113] and require more surgeries than those without asthma.[4] Epithelial barrier dysfunction and upregulation of type 2 cytokines are exhibited in both CRSwNP and asthma.[114] Mast cells and degranulated eosinophils, both associated with asthmatic airway inflammation, are abundant in the sinuses of patients with AERD.[26,39,115] Ingestion of alcohol or NSAIDs commonly induces both upper and lower airway symptoms.[19] Patients with AERD have poorer percent-predicted FEV1 than aspirin-tolerant asthmatics with CRSwNP.[4] The presence of NSAID intolerance is associated with significant increases in Lund-Mackay and Lund-Kennedy scores, as well as absolute eosinophil counts and asthma severity.[116,117] There is evidence to suggest that treatment of CRSwNP improves various measures of asthma control, including FEV1, peak expiratory flow, oral steroid dependence, and asthma control test scores,[118–120] although this is not consistent in all studies.[121] AD improves both upper and lower airway symptoms.[89,122] Both the upper and lower airways need to be treated in a coordinated fashion in this disease, which may be one reason why patients have demonstrated better outcomes in a multidisciplinary clinic setting.[57,123]

FUTURE DIRECTIONS

Although our understanding of the pathophysiology of AERD has expanded in the last decade, there is yet much to learn. Early evidence suggests that multiple endotypes of AERD exist and if understood, may explain why some patients fail to respond to or tolerate specific treatments such as AD. Further understanding of these endotypes may guide individualized therapy.[56,101,124]

There has been increasing support for the role of platelets in AERD, which may drive inflammation through thromboxane receptor activation.[125] Prasugrel, a P2Y12 receptor inhibitor that blocks platelet activation as well as transcellular cysLT synthesis, inhibited aspirin reactions in a small subset of patients with AERD with mild upper respiratory symptoms and high baseline platelet activation, indicating that targeting platelets may be useful.[12,126] A phase II clinical trial is currently underway comparing ifetroban, an oral thromboxane receptor antagonist, with placebo in AERD (NCT03028350).

Biologics that target type 2 inflammatory mediators IL-33 and thymic stromal lymphopoietin (TSLP) are currently undergoing investigation. Tezepelumab, an anti-TSLP monoclonal antibody, was recently approved for asthma and has demonstrated improved FEV1, decreased asthma exacerbations, and decreased peripheral eosinophilia in allergy-induced asthma, indicating that it may represent a therapeutic option for AERD.[127–129] Fevipiprant, a selective PGD2 receptor (also known as CRTH2) antagonist, is theoretically promising, as PGD2 works through this receptor to recruit ILC2s, eosinophils, basophils, macrophages, and Th2 cells to sites of tissue inflammation.[130]

Finally, further research is needed to determine optimal and perhaps individualized surgical management including extent of initial frontal sinus surgery and use of adjuncts such as steroid-eluting stents in patients with AERD, particularly in the era of biological therapy.

SUMMARY

AERD is a recalcitrant form of asthma and CRSwNP that presents many treatment challenges. Although it has become clear that comprehensive ESS with postoperative AD allows for reasonable disease control in most patients, this solution does not work for all patients. Complex pathophysiology affords numerous opportunities for specific therapies. Perhaps as endotypes and biomarkers of disease severity are further understood, our vision to provide optimal, coordinated medical and surgical care resulting in ongoing relief for all patients with AERD will become an achievable task.

CLINICS CARE POINTS

- AERD typically presents in the fourth decade of life with upper than lower respiratory symptoms and finally NSAID hypersensitivity.
- Answering "no" to the question "are you allergic to NSAIDs," is not sufficient to exclude AERD—possibilities such as silent desensitization, lack of exposure to NSAIDs, and unrecognized reactions must be considered to avoid a missed diagnosis.

- Aspirin sensitivity may be confirmed with an aspirin challenge in patients with an equivocal history, and biomarkers such as uLTE4 may suggest increased risk of aspirin intolerance.
- Initial treatment of AERD includes standard asthma therapy and appropriate medical treatment of CRSwNP.
- For those whose sinus symptoms persist despite appropriate medical therapy, a comprehensive ESS (with consideration of upfront extended frontal sinus procedures by an experienced sinus surgeon) should be performed.
- All patients should be counseled regarding the risks and benefits of AD, which, when performed, should optimally be carried out 3 to 4 weeks after ESS.
- Biological agents are currently more expensive than ESS and AD and lack long-term safety data but should be considered in patients who fail to respond to or are unable to undergo ESS with or without AD.

REFERENCES

1. Samter M, Beers RF. Concerning the nature of intolerance to aspirin. J Allergy 1967;40:281–93.
2. Samter M, Beers RF. Intolerance to aspirin. Clinical studies and consideration of its pathogenesis. Ann Intern Med 1968;68:975–83.
3. Laidlaw TM, Levy JM. NSAID-ERD Syndrome: the new hope from prevention, early diagnosis and new therapeutic targets. Curr Allergy Asthma Rep 2020; 20(4):10.
4. Stevens WW, Peters AT, Hirsch AG, et al. Clinical characteristics of patients with chronic rhinosinusitis with nasal polyps, asthma, and aspirin exacerbated respiratory disease. J Allergy Clin Immunol 2017;5(4):1061–70.
5. Kshirsagar RS, Chou DW, Wei J, et al. Aspirin-exacerbated respiratory disease: longitudinal assessment of a large cohort and implications of diagnostic delay. Int Forum Allergy Rhinol 2019;10(4):465–73.
6. Stevenson D, Szczeklik A. Clinical and pathologic perspectives on aspirin sensitivity and asthma. J Allergy Clin Immunol 2006;118(4):773–86.
7. White AA, Stevenson DD. Aspirin-exacerbated respiratory disease. N Engl J Med 2018;379(11):1060–70.
8. Szczeklik A, Nizankowska E, Duplaga M. Natural history of aspirin-induced asthma. AIANE Investigators. European network on aspirin-induced asthma. Eur Resp J 2000;16(3):432–6.
9. Ma C, Mehta NK, Nguyen S, et al. Demographic variation in chronic rhinosinusitis by subtype and region: a systematic review. Am J Rhinol Allergy 2022; 36(3):367–77.
10. Roland LT, Wang H, Mehta CC, et al. Longitudinal progression of aspirin-exacerbated respiratory disease: analysis of a national insurance claims database. Int Forum Allergy Rhinol 2019;9(12):1420–3.
11. Buchheit K, Bensko JC, Lewis E, et al. The importance of timely diagnosis of aspirin-exacerbated respiratory disease for patient health and safety. World J Otorhinolaryngol 2020;6(4):203–6.
12. Dominas C, Gadkaree S, Maxfield AZ, et al. Aspirin-exacerbated respiratory disease: A review. Laryngoscope Investig Otolaryngol 2020;5(3):360–7.
13. Haque R, White AA, Jackson DJ, et al. Clinical evaluation and diagnosis of aspirin-exacerbated respiratory disease. J Allergy Clin Immunol 2021;148(2): 283–91.

14. Gudziol V, Michel M, Sonnefeld C, et al. Olfaction and sino-nasal symptoms in patients with CRSwNP and AERD and without AERD: a cross-sectional and longitudinal study. Eur Arch Ororhinolaryngol 2017;274(3):1487–93.

15. DeGregorio GA, Singer J, Cahill K, et al. A one-day, 90-minute aspirin challenge and desensitization protocol in aspirin-exacerbated respiratory disease. J Allergy Clin Immunol 2019;7(4):1174–80.

16. Cahill KN, Murphy K, Singer J, et al. Plasma tryptase elevation during aspirin-induced reactions in aspirin-exacerbated respiratory disease. J Allergy Clin Immunol 2019;143(2):799–803, e792.

17. Blanca-Lopez N, Haroun E, Ruano FJ, et al. ASA challenge in children with hypersensitivity reactions to NSAIDs differentiate between cross-intolerant and selective responders. J Allergy Clin Immunol Pract 2018;6(4):1226–32.

18. Kowalski ML, Agache I, Bavbeck S, et al. Diagnosis and management of NSAID-Exacerbated Respiratory Disease (N-ERD) – a EAACI position paper. Allergy 2019;74(1):28–39.

19. Cardet JC, White AA, Barrett NA, et al. Alcohol-induced respiratory symptoms are common in patients with aspirin exacerbated respiratory disease. J Allergy Clin Immunol Pract 2014;2(2):208–13.

20. Brigham EP, West NE. Diagnosis of asthma: diagnostic testing. Int Forum Allergy Rhinol 2015;5(Suppl 1):S27–30.

21. Orlandi RR, Kingdom TT, Smith TL. International consensus statement on allergy and rhinology: rhinosinusitis 2021. Int Forum Allergy Rhinol 2021;11(3):213–739.

22. Malfitano MJ, Santarelli GD, Gelpi M, et al. A comparison of sphenoid sinus osteoneogenesis in aspirin-exacerbated respiratory disease. Am J Rhinol Allergy 2021;35(2):172–8.

23. Baudrand H, Zaouche S, Dubost R, et al. Aspirin hypersensitivity: characteristics and diagnostic approach [in French]. Rev Mal Respir 2015;32(3):221–8.

24. White AA, Bosso JV, Stevenson DD. The clinical dilemma of "silent desensitization" in aspirin-exacerbated respiratory disease. Allergy Asthma Proc 2013; 34(4):378–82.

25. Stevens WW, Jerschow E, Baptist AP, et al. The role of aspirin desensitization followed by oral aspirin therapy in managging patients with aspirin-exacerbated respiratory disease: a work group report from the rhinitis, rhinosinusitis and ocular allergy committee of the American Academy of Allergy, Asthma & Immunology. J Allergy Clin Immunol 2021;147(3):827–44.

26. Cahill KN. Immunologic effects of aspirin desensitization and high-dose aspirin therapy in aspirin-exacerbated respiratory disease. J Allergy Clin Immunol 2021;148(2):344–7.

27. White AA, Bigby T, Stevenson D. Intranasal ketorolac challenge for the diagnosis of aspirin-exacerbated respiratory disease. Ann Allergy Asthma Immunol 2006;97(2):190–5.

28. Li KL, Lee AY, Abuzeid WM. Aspirin Exacerbated Respiratory Disease: Epidemiology, Pathophysiology, and Management. Med Sci 2019;7(3):45.

29. Waldram J, Walters K, Simon R, et al. Safety and outcomes of aspirin desensitization for aspirin-exacerbated respiratory disease: a single center study. J Allergy Clin Immunol 2018;141(1):250–6.

30. Laitinen LA, Laitinen A, Haahtela T, et al. Leukotriene-E(4) and granulocytic infiltration into asthmatic airways. Lancet 1993;341(8851):989–90.

31. Daffern PJMD, Hugli TE, Stevenson DD. Association of urinary leukotriene E4 excretion during aspirin challenges with severity of respiratory responses. J Allergy Clin Immunol 1999;104(3 Pt 1):559–64.

32. Choby G, O'Brien EK, Smith A, et al. Elevated urine leukotriene E4 is associated with worse objective markers in nasal polyposis patients. Laryngoscope 2020; 131(5):961–6.
33. Choby G, Low CM, Levy JM, et al. Urine leukotriene E4: implications as a biomarker in chronic rhinosinusitis. Otolaryngol Head Neck Surg 2022;166(2): 224–32.
34. Lueke AJ, Meeusen JW, Donato LJ, et al. Analytical and clinical validation of an LC-MS/MS method for urine leukotriene E4: a marker of systemic mastocytosis. Clin Biochem 2016;49(13–14):979–82.
35. Divekar R, Hagan J, Rank M, et al. Diagnostic utility of urinary LTE4 in asthma, allergic rhinitis, chronic rhinosinusitis, nasal polyps, and aspirin sensitivity. J Allergy Clin Immunol 2016;4(4):665–70.
36. Higashi N, Taniguchi M, Mita H, et al. Clinical features of asthmatic patients with increased urinary leukotriene E4 excretion (hyperleukotrienuria): involvement of chronic hyperplastic rhinosinusitis with nasal polyposis. J Allergy Clin Immunol 2004;113(2):277–83.
37. Mohebati A, Milne GL, Zhou XK, et al. Effect of zileuton and celecoxib on urinary LTE4 and PGE-M levels in smokers. Cancer Prev Res (Phila) 2015;6(7):646–55.
38. Hahn J, Appel H, Scheithauer MO, et al. Symptom control of patients with chronic rhinosinusitis with nasal polyps under maintenance therapy with daily acetylsalicylic acid. Am J Rhinol Allergy 2020;34(4):554–63.
39. Bosso JV, Locke TB, Kuan EC, et al. Complete endoscopic sinus surgery followed by aspirin desensitization is associated with decreased overall corticosteroid use. Int Forum Allergy Rhinol 2020;10(9):1043–8.
40. Hagan JB, Laidlaw TM, Divekar R, et al. Urinary leukotriene E4 to determine aspirin intolerance in asthma: a systematic review and meta-analysis. J Allergy Clin Immunol 2016;5(4):990–7.
41. Sousa AR, Parikh A, Scadding G, et al. Leukotriene receptor expression on nasal mucosal inflammatory cells in aspirin-sensitive rhinosinusitis. N Engl J Med 2002;347(19):1493–9.
42. Cahill KN, Bensko JC, Joyce JA, et al. Prostaglandin D(2): a dominant mediator of aspirin-exacerbated respiratory disease. J Allergy Clin Immunol 2015;135(1): 245–52.
43. Laidlaw TM, Boyce JA. Aspirin-exacerbated respiratory disease - new prime suspects. N Engl J Med 2016;374(5):484–8.
44. Antoine C, Murphy RC, Henson PM, et al. Time-dependent utilization of platelet arachidonic acid by the neutrophil in formation of 5-lipoxygenase products in platelet-neutrophil co-incubations. Biochim Biophys Acta 1992;1128(2–3): 139–46.
45. Raiden S, Schettini J, Salamone G, et al. Human platelets produce granulocyte-macrophage colony-stimulating factor and delay eosinophil apoptosis. Lab Investig 2003;83(4):589–98.
46. Bartemes KR, Choby G, O'Brien EK, et al. Mass cytometry reveals unique subsets of T cells and lymphoid cells in nasal polyps from patients with chronic rhinosinusitis (CRS). Allergy 2021;76(7):2222–6.
47. Kuan EC, Kennedy WP, Patel NN, et al. Pre-intervention SNOT-22 scores predict outcomes in aspirin exacerbated respiratory disease. Am J Otolaryngol 2021; 42(5):103025.
48. Spielman DB, Overdevest J, Gudis DA. Olfactory outcomes in the management of aspirin exacerbated respiratory disease related chronic rhinosinusitis. World J Otorhinolaryngol 2020;6(4):207–13.

49. Jerschow E, Edin ML, Chi Y, et al. Sinus surgery is associated with a decrease in aspirin-induced reaction severity in AERD patients. J Allergy Clin Immunol 2019; 7(5):1580–8.
50. Shah SJ, Abuzeid WM, Ponduri A, et al. Endoscopic sinus surgery improves aspirin treatment response in AERD patients. Int Forum Allergy Rhinol 2019; 9(12):1401–8.
51. Adelman J, McLean C, Shaigany K, et al. The role of surgery in management of Samter's Triad: a systematic review. Otolaryngol Head Neck Surg 2016;155(2): 220–37.
52. Loftus CA, Soler ZM, Koochakzadeh S, et al. Revision surgery rates in chronic rhinosinusitis with nasal polyps: a meta-analysis of risk factors. Int Forum Allergy Rhinol 2020;10(2):199–207.
53. DeConde AS, Suh JD, Mace JC, et al. Outcomes of complete vs targeted approaches to endoscopic sinus surgery. Int Forum Allergy Rhinol 2015;5(8): 691–700.
54. Muhonen EG, Goshtasbi K, Papagiannopoulos P, et al. Appropriate extent of surgery for aspirin-exacerbated respiratory disease. World J Otorhinolaryngol 2020;6(4):235–40.
55. Grose E, Lee DJ, Yip J, et al. Surgical outcomes in aspirin-exacerbated respiratory disease without aspirin desensitization. Int Forum Allergy Rhinol 2020; 10(10):1149–57.
56. Schlosser RJ. Aspirin-exacerbated respiratory disease: personalized medical and surgical approaches. Int Forum Allergy Rhinol 2020;10(9):1035–6.
57. Bosso JV, Tripathi SH, Kennedy DW, et al. Multidisciplinary single-center outcomes compared to two-center outcomes for the treatment of aspirin exacerbated respiratory disease. J Allergy Clin Immunol Pract 2021;9(6):2498–500.
58. Shih LC, Patel VS, Choby GW, et al. Evolution of the endoscopic modified Lothrop procedure: A systematic review and meta-analysis. Laryngoscope 2018; 128(2):317–26.
59. Bassiouni A, Wormald PJ. Role of frontal sinus surgery in nasal polyp recurrence. Laryngoscope 2013;123(1):36–41.
60. Morrissey DK, Bassiouni A, Pstaltis AJ, et al. Outcomes of modified endoscopic Lothrop in aspirin-exacerbated respiratory disease with nasal polyposis. Int Forum Allergy Rhinol 2016;6(8):820–5.
61. Patel VS, Choby G, Shih LC, et al. Equivalence in outcomes between Draf 2B vs Draf 3 frontal sinusotomy for refractory chronic frontal rhinosinusitis. Int Forum Allergy Rhinol 2018;8(1):25–31.
62. Choby G, Nayak JV. The "Cross-court draf IIb" procedure for advanced nasal septum or frontal sinus pathology and nasal septum pathology. Laryngoscope 2018;128(7):1527–30.
63. Bhalla V, Sykes KJ, Villwock JA, et al. Draf IIB with superior septectomy: finding the "middle ground. Int Forum Allergy Rhinol 2019;9(3):281–5.
64. Larivee N, Chin CJ. Aspirin desensitization therapy in aspirin-exacerbated respiratory disease: a review. Int Forum Allergy Rhinol 2020;10(4):450–64.
65. Sommer DD, Rotenberg BW, Sowerby LJ, et al. A novel treatment adjunct for aspirin exacerbated respiratory disease: the low-salicylate diet: a multicenter randomized control crossover trial. Int Forum Allergy Rhinol 2016;6(4):385–91.
66. Levy JM, Rudmik L, Peters AT, et al. Contemporary management of chronic rhinosinusitis with nasal polyposis in aspirin exacerbated respiratory disease: an evidence-based review with recommendations. Int Forum Allergy Rhinol 2016; 6(12):1273–83.

67. Schneider TR, Johns CB, Palumbo ML, et al. Dietary fatty acid modification for the treatment of Aspirin-Exacerbated Respiratory Disease: a prospective pilot trial. J Allergy Clin Immunol Pract 2018;6(3):825–31.

68. Zeiger RS, Szefler SJ, Phillips BR, et al. Response profiles to fluticasone and montelukast in mild-to-moderate persistent childhood asthma. J Allergy Clin Immunol 2006;117(1):45–52.

69. Dahlen SE, Malmstron K, Nizankowska E, et al. Improvement of aspirin-intolerant asthma by montelukast, a leukotriene antagonist: a randomized, double-blind, placebo-controlled trial. Am J Resp Crit Care Med 2002; 165(1):9–14.

70. Laidlaw TM, Gakpo D, Bensko JC, et al. Leukotriene-associated rash in aspirin-exacerbated respiratory disease. J Allergy Clin Immunol 2020;8(9):3170–1.

71. Von Ta, White AA. Survey-defined patient experiences with aspirin-exacerbated respiratory disease. J Allergy Clin Immunol Pract 2015;3(5):711–8.

72. Dahlen B, Nizankowska E, Szczeklik A, et al. Benefits from adding the 5-lipoxygenase inhibitor zileuton to conventional therapy in aspirin-intolerant asthmatics. Am J Resp Crit Care Med 1998;147(4 Pt 1):1187–94.

73. Laidlaw TM, Fuentes DJ, Want Y. Efficacy of zileuton in patients with asthma and history of aspirin sensitiity: a retrospective analysis of data from two phase 3 studies. J Allergy Clin Immunol 2017;139(2):1.

74. Sansing-Foster V, Haug N, Mosholder A, et al. Risk of psychiatric adverse events among montelukast users. J Allergy Clin Immunol Pract 2021;9(1): 385–93, e312.

75. Watkins PB, Dube LM, Walton-Bowen K, et al. Clinical pattern of zileuton-associated liver injury: results of a 12-month study in patients with chronic asthma. Drug Saf 2007;30(9):805–15.

76. Ramos CL, Woessner KM. Updates on treatment options in aspirin exacerbated respiratory disease. Curr Opin Allergy Clin Immunol 2022;22(1):50–4.

77. Sweis AM, Locke TB, Ig-Izevbekhai KI, et al. Effectiveness of endoscopic sinus surgery and aspirin therapy in the management of aspirin-exacerbated respiratory disease. Allergy Asthma Proc 2021;42(2):136–41.

78. Ryan L, Segarra D, Tabor M, et al. Systematic review of outcomes for endoscopic sinus surgery and subsequent aspirin desensitization in aspirin-exacerbated respiratory disease. World J Otorhinolaryngol 2020;6(4):220–9.

79. Chen JR, Buchmiller BL, Khan DA. An Hourly Dose-Escalation Desensitization Protocol for Aspirin-Exacerbated Respiratory Disease. J Allergy Clin Immunol Pract 2015;3(6):926–31.

80. Pelletier T, Roizen G, Ren Z, et al. Comparable safety of 2 aspirin desensitization protocols for aspirin exacerbated respiratory disease. J Allergy Clin Immunol Pract 2019;7(4):1319–21.

81. Cooper T, Greig SR, Zhang H, et al. Objective and subjective sinonasal and pulmonary outcomes in aspirin desensitization therapy: a prospective cohort study. Auris Nasus Larynx 2019;46(4):526–32.

82. Locke TB, Swies AM, Gleeson PK, et al. Age as a factor in treatment of aspirin-exacerbated respiratory disease: relationship to required aspirin maintenance dose after desensitization. Int Forum Allergy Rhinol 2020;10(10):1180–1.

83. Arm JP, O'Hickey SP, Spur BW, et al. Airway responsiveness to histamine and leukotriene E4 in subjects with aspirin-induced asthma. Am Rev Respir Dis 1989;140:148–53.

84. Adappa ND, Ranasinghe VJ, Trope M, et al. Outcomes after complete endoscopic sinus surgery and aspirin desensitization in aspirin-exacerbated respiratory disease. Int Forum Allergy Rhinol 2018;8(1):49–53.

85. Cho KS, Soudry E, Psaltis AJ. Long-term sinonasal outcomes of aspirin desensitization in aspirin exacerbated respiratory disease. Otolaryngol Head Neck Surg 2014;151(4):575–81.

86. Chaaban MR, Moffatt D, Wright AE, et al. Meta-analysis exploring sinopulmonary outcomes on aspirin desensitization in aspirin-exacerbated respiratory disease. Otolaryngol Head Neck Surg 2021;164(1):11–8.

87. Arnold M, Kuruvilla M, Levy JM, et al. Dupilumab improves alcohol tolerance in aspirin-exacerbated respiratory disease. Ann Allergy Asthma Immunol 2021;127(3):379–81.

88. Bosso J. Aspirin desensitization for aspirin-exacerbated respiratory disease in the era of biologics: clinical perspective. Int Forum Allergy Rhinol 2021;11(4):822–3.

89. Berges-Gimeno MP, Simon RA, Stevenson DD. Long-term treatment with aspirin desensitization in asthmatic patients with aspirin-exacerbated respiratory disease. J Allergy Clin Immunol 2003;111(1):180–6.

90. Sweis AM, Locke TB, Ig-Izevbekhai KI, et al. Major complications of aspirin desensitization and maintenance therapy in aspirin-exacerbated respiratory disease. Int Forum Allergy Rhinol 2021;11(2):115–9.

91. D'Souza GE, Nwagu U, Barton B, et al. Outcomes of aspirin exacerbated respiratory disease in patients treated with aspirin desensitization and biologics. Int Forum Allergy Rhinol 2021;12(3):306–9.

92. Bavaro N, Gakpo D, Mittal A, et al. Efficacy of dupilumab in patients with aspirin-exacerbated respiratory disease and previous inadequate response to anti-IL-5 or anti-IL-5Ra in a real-world setting. J Allergy Clin Immunol 2021;9(7):2910–2.

93. Castro M, Corren J, Pavord ID, et al. Dupilumab Efficacy and Safety in Moderate-to-Severe Uncontrolled Asthma. N Engl J Med 2018;378(26):2486–96.

94. Barnes P. The cytokine network in chronic obstructive pulmonary disease. Am J Respir Cell Mol Biol 2009;41(6):631–8.

95. Oykhman P, Paramo FA, Bousquet PJ, et al. Comparative efficacy and safety of monoclonal antibodies and aspirin desensitization for chronic rhinosinusitis with nasal polyposis: A systematic review and network meta-analysis. J Allergy Clin Immunol 2022;149(4):1286–95.

96. Laidlaw TM, Mullol J, Fan C, et al. Dupilumab improves nasal polyp burden and asthma control in patients with CRSwNP and AERD. J Allergy Clin Immunol Pract 2019;7(7):2462–5.

97. Bachert C, Han JK, Desrosie M, et al. Efficacy and safety of dupilumab in patients with severe chronic rhinosinusitis with nasal polyps (LIBERTY NP SINUS-24 and LIBERTY NP SINUS-52): results from two multicentre, randomised, double-blind, placebo-controlled, parallel-group phase 3 trials. Lancet 2019;394(10209):1638–50.

98. Wangberg H, Spierling Bagsic SR, Osuna L, et al. Appraisal of the real-world effectiveness of biologic therapies in aspirin-exacerbated respiratory disease. J Allergy Clin Immunol Pract 2021;10(2):478–84.

99. Mustafa SS, Vadamalai K, Scott B, et al. Dupilumab as add-on therapy for chronic rhinosinusitis for nasal polyposis in aspirin exacerbated respiratory disease. Am J Rhinol Allergy 2021;35(3):399–407.

100. Patel P, Bensko JC, Bhattacharyya N, et al. Dupilumab as an adjunct to surgery in patients with aspirin-exacerbated respiratory disease. Ann Allergy Asthma Immunol 2022;128(3):326–8.
101. Buchheit KM, Laidlaw TM, Levy JM. Immunology-based recommendations for available and upcoming biologics in aspirin-exacerbated respiratory disease. J Allergy Clin Immunol 2021;148(2):348–50.
102. Tuttle KL, Buchheit KM, Laidlaw TM, et al. A retrospective analysis of mepolizumab in patients with aspirin-exacerbated respiratory disease. J Allergy Clin Immunol Pract 2018;6(3):1045–7.
103. Buchheit KM, Lewis E, Gakpo D, et al. Mepolizumab targets multiple immune cells in aspirin-exacerbated respiratory disease. J Allergy Clin Immunol 2021; 148(2):574–84.
104. Han JK, Bachert C, Fokkens W, et al. Mepolizumab for chronic rhinosinusitis with nasal polyps (SYNAPSE): a randomised, double-blind, placebo-controlled, phase 3 trial. Lancet Respir Med 2021;9(10):1141–53.
105. Workman AD, Bleier BS. Biologic therapies versus surgical management for aspirin-exacerbated respiratory disease: a review of preliminary data, efficacy, and cost. World J Otorhinolaryngol 2020;6(4):230–4.
106. Hayashi H, Mitsui C, Nakatani E. Omalizumab reduces cysteinyl leukotriene and 9α,11β-prostaglandin F2 overproduction in aspirin-exacerbated respiratory disease. J Allergy Clin Immunol 2016;137(5):1585–7.
107. Hayashi H, Fukutomi Y, Mitsui C, et al. Omalizumab for aspirin hypersensitivity and leukotriene overproduction in aspirin-exacerbated respiratory disease: a randomized controlled trial. Am J Resp Crit Care Med 2020;201(12):1488–98.
108. Gevaert P, Omachi TA, Corren J, et al. Efficacy and safety of omalizumab in nasal polyposis: 2 randomized phase 3 trials. J Allergy Clin Immunol 2020; 146(3):595–605.
109. Quint T, Dahm V, Ramazanova D, et al. Omalizumab-induced aspirin tolerance in nonsteroidal anti-inflammatory drug-exacerbated respiratory disease patients is independent of atopic sensitization. J Allergy Clin Immunol 2021;10(2): 506–16.
110. Laidlaw T. Aspirin desensitization vs biologics for patients with aspirin-exacerbated respiratory disease. Ann Allergy Asthma Immunol 2021;126(2): 118–9.
111. Parasher AK, Gliksman M, Segarra D, et al. Economic Evaluation of Dupilumab Versus Endoscopic Sinus Surgery for the Treatment of Chronic Rhinosinusitis With Nasal Polyps. Int Forum Allergy Rhinol 2021. https://doi.org/10.1002/alr. 22936.
112. Phillips KM, Hoehle LP, Bergmark RW, et al. Chronic rhinosinusitis severity is associated with need for asthma-related systemic corticosteroids. Rhinology 2017;55(3):211–7.
113. Phillips KM, Bergmark RW, Hoehle LP, et al. Chronic rhinosinusitis exacerbations are differentially associated with lost productivity based on asthma status. Rhinology 2018;56(4):323–9.
114. Laidlaw TM, Mullol J, Woessner KM, et al. Chronic rhinosinusitis with nasal polyps and asthma. J Allergy Clin Immunol Pract 2021;9(3):1133–41.
115. Yamashita T, Tsuji H, Maeda N, et al. Etiology of nasal polyps associated with aspirin-sensitive asthma. Rhinol Suppl 1989;8:15–24.
116. Batra PS, Tong LY, Citardi MJ. Analysis of Comorbidities and Objective Parameters in Refractory Chronic Rhinosinusitis. Laryngoscope 2013;123:S1–11.

117. Bochenek G, Szafraniec K, Kuschill-Dziurda J, et al. Factors associated with asthma control in patients with aspirin-exacerbated respiratory disease. J Respir Med 2015;109(5):588–95.

118. Schlosser RJ, Smith TL, Mace J, et al. Asthma quality of life and control after sinus surgery in patients with chronic rhinosinusitis. Allergy 2017;72(3):483–91.

119. Ragab S, Scadding GK, Lund VJ, et al. Treatment of chronic rhinosinusitis and its effects on asthma. Eur Resp J 2006;28(1):68–74.

120. Ikeda K, Tanno N, Tamura G, et al. Endoscopic sinus surgery improves pulmonary function in patients with asthma associated with chronic sinusitis. Ann Otol Rhinol Laryngol 1999;108:355–9.

121. Lourijsen ES, Reitsma S, Vleming M, et al. Endoscopic sinus surgery with medical therapy versus medical therapy for chronic rhinosinusitis with nasal polyps: a multicentre, randomised, controlled trial. Lancet 2022;10(4):337–46.

122. Ledford DK, Wenzel SE, Lockey RF. Aspirin or Other Nonsteroidal Inflammatory Agent Exacerbated Asthma. J Allergy Clin Immunol Pract 2014;2(6):653–7.

123. Li KL, Fang CH, Ferastraoaru D, et al. Patient Satisfaction and Efficiency Benefits of a Novel Multidisciplinary Rhinology and Allergy Clinic. Ann Otol Rhinol Laryngol 2020;129(7):699–706.

124. Bochenek G, Kuschill-Dziurda J, Szafraniec K, et al. Certain subphenotypes of aspirin-exacerbated respiratory disease distinguished by latent class analysis. J Allergy Clin Immunol 2014;133(1):98–103.

125. Laidlaw TM, Kidder MS, Bhattacharyya N, et al. Cysteinyl leukotriene overproduction in aspirin-exacerbated respiratory disease is driven by platelet-adherent leukocytes. Blood 2012;119(16):3790–8.

126. Laidlaw TM, Cahill KN, Cardet JC, et al. A trial of P2Y12 receptor inhibition with prasugrel identifies a potentially distinct endotype of patients with aspirin-exacerbated respiratory disease. J Allergy Clin Immunol 2018;143(1):316–24.

127. Corren J, Parnes JP, Wang L, et al. Tezepelumab in Adults with Uncontrolled Asthma. N Engl J Med 2017;377(10):936–46.

128. Menzies-Gow A, Corren J, Bourdin A, et al. Tezepelumab in Adults and Adolescents with Severe, Uncontrolled Asthma. N Engl J Med 2021;384(19):1800–9.

129. Gauvreau GM, O'Byrne PM, Boulet LP, et al. Effects of an anti-TSLP antibody on allergen-induced asthmatic responses. N Engl J Med 2014;370(22):2102–10.

130. Cahill K. Fevipiprant in CRSwNP and comorbid asthma: wrong target population or wrong PGD2 receptor? J Allergy Clin Immunol 2022. https://doi.org/10.1016/j.jaci.2022.03.001.

Unified Airway—Cystic Fibrosis

Do-Yeon Cho, MD[a,b,c], Jessica W. Grayson, MD[a], Bradford A. Woodworth, MD[a,b],*

KEYWORDS

- Sinusitis • Chronic sinusitis • Cystic fibrosis • CFTR • CFTR modulators
- Acquired CFTR dysfunction • Endoscopic sinus surgery

KEY POINTS

- Cystic fibrosis (CF) affects the upper and lower airways and is one of the most common autosomal recessive disorders.
- Chronic rhinosinusitis (CRS) with CF exhibits distinctive characteristics compared with other CRS phenotypes regarding its pathogenesis, clinical course, and treatment.
- Paranasal sinuses serve as a reservoir for bacterial transmission to the lower airways; therefore, controlling sinonasal infections is a high priority for improving pulmonary outcomes.
- Endoscopic sinus surgery improves the quality of life in patients with symptomatic CF and may have the benefit of decreasing bacterial transmission to the lower airway.
- Cystic fibrosis transmembrane conductance regulator (CFTR) modulators address the underlying CFTR defect by improving the trafficking and function of the protein channel and are a highly effective treatment of CF-CRS.
- Regardless of the mechanism underlying (congenital or acquired) CFTR dysfunction, increasing transepithelial Cl⁻ secretion and apical fluid hydration in CRS are appealing options for therapeutic intervention.

INTRODUCTION

Cystic fibrosis (CF) is one of the most common genetic disorders, affecting approximately 1 in 2500 Caucasians annually.[1] This multisystem disease caused by mutations in the cystic fibrosis transmembrane conductance regulator (CFTR) gene is characterized by defective transport of the anions (chloride [Cl⁻] and bicarbonate) across airway epithelia, which leads to abnormally viscous secretions in the airways and other organ

a Department of Otolaryngology - Head & Neck Surgery, University of Alabama at Birmingham, 1155 Faculty Office Tower 510 20th Street South, Birmingham, AL 35233, USA; b Gregory Fleming James Cystic Fibrosis Research Center, University of Alabama at Birmingham, Birmingham, AL, USA; c Department of Surgery, Division of Otolaryngology, Veteran Affairs Medical Center, Birmingham, AL, USA
* Corresponding author.
E-mail address: bwoodworth@uabmc.edu

Otolaryngol Clin N Am 56 (2023) 125–136
https://doi.org/10.1016/j.otc.2022.09.009
0030-6665/23/© 2022 Elsevier Inc. All rights reserved.

systems.[2] Secretion in the airways usually serves to dispel outside particles and pollutants through mucociliary clearance (MCC). This mechanism is widely considered the airway's primary innate defense against bacterial infections. The most common genetic mutation is F508del CFTR, where improper protein folding and processing within the respiratory epithelia leads to ineffective anion secretion. Individuals with thick mucus are at an increased risk of MCC disruption and chronic, recurrent bacterial infections in the upper and lower airways, including severe chronic rhinosinusitis (CRS).

PATHOPHYSIOLOGY OF CYSTIC FIBROSIS TRANSMEMBRANE CONDUCTANCE REGULATOR DYSFUNCTION

The epithelial lining of the sinonasal cavities is composed of airway surface liquid (ASL) containing a low viscosity periciliary fluid layer (sol) around the respiratory cilia and a superficial mucus (gel) layer, which functions to sweep inhaled particles into the digestive tract through coordinated MCC.[3] CFTR functions as a Cl^- and bicarbonate transporter and is critical to sustaining adequate height of the ASL. Decreased CFTR-mediated Cl^- secretion across the mucosal surface contributes to the development of airway disease by depletion of ASL, which, in turn, may hinder effective MCC by increasing viscosity and adhesion of mucus and cause persistent infection and/or inflammation[4]; this is readily observed in patients with CF with absent CFTR function.

An enriched understanding of the role of CFTR in the maintenance of normal epithelial function has revealed that mild, and variable CFTR mutations, play a causative role in many diseases not classically associated with CF.[5] CFTR-related diseases, due to either partial function from heterozygosity or acquired CFTR dysfunction, encompass well-known pathological disorders that seem to be influenced by CFTR genotype, including chronic obstructive pulmonary disease, allergic bronchopulmonary aspergillosis, idiopathic bronchiectasis, and CRS.[3] For example, Wang and colleagues[6] performed genetic testing on 147 non-CF patients with severe CRS and discovered a 7% incidence of CFTR mutations compared with the presence of 2% in 123 healthy controls. In another study of 58 children with CRS, 12% carried a single CF mutation, which was much higher than the expected frequency of 4%.[7] Despite not having classic features of CF, heterozygosity for CFTR mutations confer significant risk for the development of CRS. Furthermore, acquired CFTR dysfunction with decreased CFTR-mediated Cl^- secretion across human sinonasal epithelia from CRS subjects compared with normal controls has been identified in vitro and ex vivo.[8,9] Ex vivo samples of CRS epithelium also exhibit decreased mucous strand velocity consistent with dysfunctional mucous transport from acquired CFTR dysfunction.[10] Furthermore, multiple perturbations (cigarette smoke,[11–19] hypoxia,[20–30] viral and bacterial exoproducts such as influenza M2 protein and lipopolysaccharide[31–35]) induce an acquired CFTR dysfunction in the sinonasal cavities and lower airways.

Acquired CFTR deficiency contributing to the propagation of chronic infection in CRS differs substantially from prevailing models regarding the pathogenesis of CRS.[36–40] The possibility of dysfunctional Cl^- transport in CRS suggests new avenues relevant to the field of rhinology; in particular, perturbations that decrease CFTR-mediated transport have important implications for understanding impaired MCT in numerous upper and lower respiratory infectious illnesses.

THE UNIFIED AIRWAY IN CYSTIC FIBROSIS

The idea of the unified airway model considers the entire respiratory system to represent a functional unit that consists of the nasal cavity, sinuses, laryngotracheal airway, and distal lung.[41,42] The upper and lower airways are composed of the same pseudostratified, ciliated, columnar epithelium, so they are both affected by the same inflammatory and infectious processes. This intimate connection has become increasingly recognized and explored.[42] The prevalence of asthma among patients with CRS (approximately 20%) is much greater than observed in the general population and is much higher (42%) in those who undergo ESS.[43,44] Treatment of upper airway inflammation also seems to affect pulmonary outcomes in asthma because successful management of CRS results in decreased asthma medication, improved pulmonary function, and fewer exacerbations.[45] Analogous to the relationship between CRS and asthma, aggressive CRS treatment in CF may improve pulmonary outcomes.[42]

The acute intensification of sinus symptoms preceding a pulmonary exacerbation is an anecdotal finding noted in patients with CF that may suggest transmission of bacterial infection from the sinus cavities to the distal lung. Support for this association includes findings that establish the presence of similar bacteria in CF sinus and pulmonary cultures.[46–49] Johansen and colleagues[48] found that most patients with CF were discovered to have sinus colonization with the identical genotype of *Pseudomonas aeruginosa* affecting the lung. Other research has confirmed that cultures of induced sputum were similar to sinonasal cultures removed during ESS.[50] In cases of lung transplantation in patients with CF, a close association between posttransplantation bronchoalveolar lavage and sinus cultures has been acknowledged, with similarities in both genotype and gene expression phenotypes of the recovered pathogens.[46,51,52] These findings indicate the sinuses serve as a bacterial reservoir for transmitting the disease to the lower airways, making control of sinonasal infections a high priority for improving pulmonary outcomes and emphasizing the importance of improving our understanding of CF sinus pathogenesis.[53]

CLINICAL MANAGEMENT

The approach to patients with CF is complex, and optimal management requires the collaboration and expertise of a multidisciplinary team to carefully weigh different therapeutic alternatives and reduce the overall burden of care for patients with CF.[54] Based on a recent systematic review, nasal saline, CFTR modulators, and endoscopic sinus surgery are supportive in managing patients with CF-CRS. These interventions receive a grade of *Recommend* for use in patients with CF.[54] Intranasal corticosteroid and topical antibiotics are considered optional, but clinical judgment and experience are essential in caring for patients with this uniquely challenging disorder.[54] Furthermore, a recent Cystic Fibrosis Foundation Multidisciplinary Consensus Statement arrived at a grade of recommendation for 16 questions based on an updated review of all available evidence (**Table 1**).[55]

Currently, there are no absolute criteria for when to intervene with ESS in CF-CRS; thus, most clinicians make decisions for therapy based on experience and patient complaints. A low incidence of self-reported symptoms despite radiographic and endoscopic evidence of sinus disease in most patients with CF underscores the problems of establishing appropriate indications for surgical management. However, persistent symptoms despite a course of antibiotics (either during inpatient admission or provided on an outpatient basis) are a consistent indication for surgical intervention. Despite a lack of randomized controlled trials, evidence suggests that ESS does impart a significant reduction of sinonasal symptoms. A systematic review of sinus surgery outcomes noted that patients with CF report improvement in quality of life after ESS but at a lower rate and for a shorter duration than non–CF-CRS patients.[56] ESS also resulted in significant benefit in both sinus symptoms and quality of life in

Table 1		
Cystic fibrosis foundation recommendations		
#	**CFF Recommendations**	**Vote**
1	The CFF recommends that CF infection control guidelines be followed for children and adults with CF being seen by an otolaryngology team.	100.00%
2	The CFF recommends otolaryngology consultation for children and adults with CF with persistent ear, nose, and throat symptoms.	100.00%
3	The CFF recommends the administration of a sinonasal quality-of-life tool to children and adults with CF (eg, SN-5 for ages 6–12 y and SNOT-22 for ages 13 y or older), to identify sinonasal symptoms.	93.10%
4	The CFF recommends nasal saline irrigation for children and adults with CF with signs or symptoms of CRS.	100.00%
5	The CFF recommends the treatment of allergic rhinitis, including topical nasal corticosteroids, to improve nasal symptoms in children and adults with CF and concomitant allergic rhinitis.	100.00%
6	The CFF recommends endoscopic sinus surgery for children and adults with CF who have symptomatic CRS refractory to appropriate medical therapy.	100.00%
7	The CFF recommends that perioperative airway clearance therapy be continued as tolerated in children and adults with CF who undergo endoscopic sinus surgery for CRS.	100.00%
8	The CFF recommends baseline hearing study for ototoxic monitoring for all children and adults with CF in anticipation of receiving ototoxic therapies.	96.55%
9	The CFF recommends ototoxic monitoring annually for children and adults with CF who are exposed to ototoxic medications.	100.00%
10	The CFF recommends ototoxic monitoring following each course of intravenous ototoxic medications for children and adults with CF who already have any hearing loss.	89.66%
11	The CFF recommends voice evaluation and management for children and adults with CF and dysphonia (hoarseness).	100.00%
12	The CFF recommends against the routine use of systemic corticosteroids for CF-CRS in children and adults.	100.00%
13	The CFF recommends against the routine use of intranasal corticosteroids administered by nebulizers in children and adults with CF-CRS.	96.55%
14	The CFF recommends against performing routine endoscopic sinus surgery for children and adults with CF for the sole indication of declining lung function.	100.00%
15	The CFF recommends against performing routine adenoidectomy alone for the treatment of CRS in children with CF.	89.66%
16	The CFF recommends against performing routine balloon sinuplasty for children and adults with CF-CRS.	100.00%

The strongest positive statements of the multidisciplinary committee are recommendations for or against specific interventions. These recommendations generally apply to most of the patients.

Abbreviations: CF, cystic fibrosis; CF-CRS, cystic fibrosis–related chronic rhinosinusitis; CFF, Cystic Fibrosis Foundation; CRS, chronic rhinosinusitis; SN-5, 5-question Sinus and Nasal Quality of Life Survey; SNOT-22, 22-question Sino-Nasal Outcome Test.

From Kimple AJ, Senior BA, Naureckas ET et al. Cystic Fibrosis Foundation otolaryngology care multidisciplinary consensus recommendations. International forum of allergy & rhinology 2022, with permission.

children with CF according to a meta-analysis.[57] Although the amount of surgery is not standardized, more extensive surgery in the maxillary sinuses to improve access (modified endoscopic medial maxillectomy[58,59] or maxillary mega-antrostomy[60,61]) increases the clearance of mucus via better access for physical debridement in the clinic, exposure for saline irrigations, and improved delivery of therapeutics (ie, tobramycin, budesonide) (**Figs. 1** and **2**).

CYSTIC FIBROSIS TRANSMEMBRANE CONDUCTANCE REGULATOR MODULATORS

CFTR modulators deserve special mention, as they have revolutionized the treatment of CF disease. Modulators improve the function of the CFTR protein through several distinct mechanisms. Ivacaftor is a channel potentiator that was first approved for individuals with CF harboring at least one copy of the G551D mutation in 2012.[62] G551D CFTR is present at the plasma apical membrane in normal quantities but has dysfunctional channel opening. Ivacaftor acts as a channel potentiator, increasing the probability that the channel will be open to improve the transport of Cl⁻. This drug conferred significant clinical improvement on all aspects of CF disease, including an average gain of lung function of 10% and improvement in sinonasal quality of life.[62–64] Subsequent small molecule CFTR channel "correctors" were developed in order to improve the function of the most common mutation, F508del.[65] F508del causes "misfolding" of the CFTR protein in the endoplasmic reticulum, which is recognized as dysfunctional and destroyed by the cell's internal machinery. CFTR channel correctors process F508del to the cell surface in sufficient quantities to affect the manifestations of the disease. Ivacaftor is provided at the same time to improve F508del channel opening. The combination of the correctors, tezacaftor and elexacaftor, with ivacaftor resulted in a marked improvement in CF morbidity and mortality with improved lung function greater than 14% FEV1 and improved sinonasal quality of life in clinical trials.[54,66–68]

CL⁻ SECRETAGOGUES FOR ACQUIRED CYSTIC FIBROSIS TRANSMEMBRANE CONDUCTANCE REGULATOR DYSFUNCTION IN CHRONIC RHINOSINUSITIS

Because MCT is influenced by the transepithelial movement of Cl⁻, there is increasing interest in the use of agents that stimulate Cl⁻ secretion for the treatment of diseases caused by dysfunctional MCC in acquired CFTR defects (such as chronic obstructive pulmonary disease, asthma, and CRS).[8,12,13,69,70] Although several drugs targeting CFTR (CFTR modulators) have been approved by the Food and Drug Administration

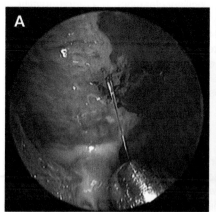 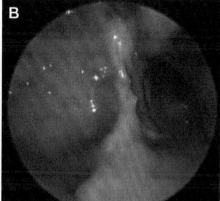

Fig. 1. Transnasal 30-degree endoscopic view of a CF maxillary antrostomy opening with thick, insipissated mucopurulence (*A*) and corresponding image in the clinic following modified medial maxillectomy and aggressive topical therapy (*B*). The maxillary sinus floor is flush with the nasal cavity floor with wide exposure for saline irrigations, topical therapeutics, and endoscopic debridement in the clinic.

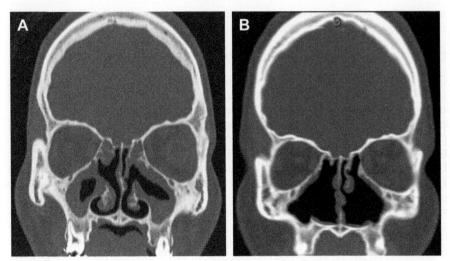

Fig. 2. Coronal CT scan through the mid-maxillary sinus before (*A*) and after (*B*) modified endoscopic medial maxillectomy and aggressive topical therapeutic irrigations.

for CF disease, compounds from natural products are also being explored, ranging from extracts of South Pacific sponges to plants in local health food stores, as CFTR modulators are not available for the non-CF population.[71,72] For example, genistein, curcumin, and resveratrol have been evaluated for their potential as adjunct therapies for patients with CF, as they can stimulate CFTR, thereby increasing Cl⁻ transport.[73–75] Similarly, resveratrol, genistein, quercetin, and hesperidin are in preclinical studies for their potential as CFTR activators in CRS.[20,76–80] The commercial product Sinupret (Bionorica, Neumarkt, Germany) is marketed as mucolytics and has proved beneficial in treating sinusitis. These products are rich in genistein and other flavonoids and were demonstrated to activate CFTR-mediated Cl⁻ secretion in respiratory epithelia.[24,81] We have previously shown that this compound improves sinus potential difference and markers of mucociliary clearance in a rabbit preclinical model of sinusitis.[26] An alternative pathway for Cl⁻ transport, the calcium-activated chloride channel, has also been investigated for therapeutic activation in CF and other airway diseases with Uridine-5′-triphosphate and other analogues.[82,83] We recently identified that Korean red ginseng aqueous extract stimulates Cl⁻ secretion in a sustained fashion in both wild-type and CFTR⁻/⁻ murine sinonasal epithelial cells and augments markers of MCT, suggesting translational therapeutic potential in both CF and non-CF chronic airway disease.[84]

SUMMARY

Sinus cavities can act as a bacterial reservoir for transmitting bacteria to the lower airways. Therefore, controlling sinonasal infections is a high priority for improving pulmonary outcomes. Based on the currently available evidence, nasal saline, ESS, and CFTR modulators are recommended to manage CF-CRS when appropriate. Although multiple causes contribute to the pathogenesis of CRS without CF, acquired CFTR dysfunction has important implications for understanding impaired MCT in numerous upper and lower respiratory diseases. Furthermore, there is increased interest in using agents that stimulate Cl⁻ secretion to treat chronic airway diseases caused by dysfunctional MCC such as CRS.

CLINICS CARE POINTS

- Based on a recent systematic review, nasal saline, CFTR modulators, and endoscopic sinus surgery are indicated in the management of patients with CF-CRS.
- Modified endoscopic medial maxillectomy or maxillary mega-antrostomy increases the clearance of mucus through better access for physical debridement in the clinic as well as exposure to saline irrigations and the topical delivery of therapeutics (ie, tobramycin, budesonide).
- The combination of the correctors (tezacaftor and elexacaftor) and a potentiator (ivacaftor) resulted in a marked improvement in CF morbidity and mortality with improved lung function greater than 14% FEV1 and improved sinonasal quality of life in clinical trials.

DISCLOSURES

B A. Woodworth, M.D. is a consultant for Cook Medical, Smith and Nephew, and Medtronic.

FUNDING SUPPORT

This work was supported by National Institute of Diabetes and Digestive and Kidney Diseases (5P30DK072482) and National Institutes of Health (NIH)/National Heart, Lung, and Blood Institute (1 R01 HL133006-05) to BW and NIH/National Institute of Allergy and Infectious Diseases (K08AI146220, 1R21AI168894-01), Triological Society Career Development Award, and Cystic Fibrosis Foundation K08 Boost Award (CHO20A0-KB) to DYC.

REFERENCES

1. Moller W, Haussinger K, Ziegler-Heitbrock L, et al. Mucociliary and long-term particle clearance in airways of patients with immotile cilia. Respir Res 2006;7:10.
2. Tipirneni KE, Woodworth BA. Medical and surgical advancements in the management of cystic fibrosis chronic rhinosinusitis. Curr Otorhinolaryngol Rep 2017;5:24–34.
3. Chaaban MR, Kejner A, Rowe SM, et al. Cystic fibrosis chronic rhinosinusitis: a comprehensive review. Am J Rhinol Allergy 2013;27:387–95.
4. Birket SE, Chu KK, Liu L, et al. A functional anatomic defect of the cystic fibrosis airway. Am J Respir Crit Care Med 2014;190:421–32.
5. Knowles MR, Durie PR. What is cystic fibrosis? N Engl J Med 2002;347:439–42.
6. Wang X, Moylan B, Leopold DA, et al. Mutation in the gene responsible for cystic fibrosis and predisposition to chronic rhinosinusitis in the general population. JAMA 2000;284:1814–9.
7. Raman V, Clary R, Siegrist KL, et al. Increased prevalence of mutations in the cystic fibrosis transmembrane conductance regulator in children with chronic rhinosinusitis. Pediatrics 2002;109:E13.
8. Cho DY, Hwang PH, Illek B. Effect of L-ascorbate on chloride transport in freshly excised sinonasal epithelia. Am J Rhinol Allergy 2009;23:294–9.
9. McCormick J, Hoffman K, Thompson H, et al. Differential chloride secretory capacity in transepithelial ion transport properties in chronic rhinosinusitis. Am J Rhinol Allergy 2020;34:830–7.
10. Tipirneni KE, Zhang S, Cho DY, et al. Submucosal gland mucus strand velocity is decreased in chronic rhinosinusitis. Int Forum Allergy Rhinology 2018;8:509–12.

11. Courville CA, Tidwell S, Liu B, et al. Acquired defects in CFTR-dependent beta-adrenergic sweat secretion in chronic obstructive pulmonary disease. Respir Res 2014;15:25.

12. Dransfield MT, Wilhelm AM, Flanagan B, et al. Acquired cystic fibrosis transmembrane conductance regulator dysfunction in the lower airways in COPD. Chest 2013;144:498–506.

13. Rab A, Rowe SM, Raju SV, et al. Cigarette smoke and CFTR: implications in the pathogenesis of COPD. Am J Physiol Lung Cell Mol Physiol 2013;305:L530–41.

14. Raju SV, Jackson PL, Courville CA, et al. Cigarette smoke induces systemic defects in cystic fibrosis transmembrane conductance regulator function. Am J Respir Crit Care Med 2013;188:1321–30.

15. Raju SV, Tate JH, Peacock SK, et al. Impact of heterozygote CFTR mutations in COPD patients with chronic bronchitis. Respir Res 2014;15:18.

16. Sloane PA, Shastry S, Wilhelm A, et al. A pharmacologic approach to acquired cystic fibrosis transmembrane conductance regulator dysfunction in smoking related lung disease. PLoS One 2012;7:e39809.

17. Alexander NS, Blount A, Zhang S, et al. Cystic fibrosis transmembrane conductance regulator modulation by the tobacco smoke toxin acrolein. Laryngoscope 2012;122:1193–7.

18. Virgin FW, Azbell C, Schuster D, et al. Exposure to cigarette smoke condensate reduces calcium activated chloride channel transport in primary sinonasal epithelial cultures. Laryngoscope 2010;120:1465–9.

19. Cohen NA, Zhang S, Sharp DB, et al. Cigarette smoke condensate inhibits transepithelial chloride transport and ciliary beat frequency. Laryngoscope 2009;119:2269–74.

20. Woodworth BA. Resveratrol ameliorates abnormalities of fluid and electrolyte secretion in a hypoxia-Induced model of acquired CFTR deficiency. Laryngoscope 2015;125(Suppl 7):S1–13.

21. Tipirneni KE, Grayson JW, Zhang S, et al. Assessment of acquired mucociliary clearance defects using micro-optical coherence tomography. Int Forum Allergy Rhinology 2017;7:920–5.

22. Banks C, Freeman L, Cho DY, et al. Acquired cystic fibrosis transmembrane conductance regulator dysfunction. World J Otorhinolaryngol Head Neck Surg 2018;4:193–9.

23. Guimbellot JS, Fortenberry JA, Siegal GP, et al. Role of oxygen availability in CFTR expression and function. Am J Respir Cell Mol Biol 2008;39:514–21.

24. Zhang S, Skinner D, Hicks SB, et al. Sinupret activates CFTR and TMEM16A-dependent transepithelial chloride transport and improves indicators of mucociliary clearance. PLoS One 2014;9:e104090.

25. Lim DJ, McCormick J, Skinner D, et al. Controlled delivery of ciprofloxacin and ivacaftor via sinus stent in a preclinical model of Pseudomonas sinusitis. Int Forum Allergy Rhinology 2020;10:481–8.

26. Cho DY, Skinner D, Mackey C, et al. Herbal dry extract BNO 1011 improves clinical and mucociliary parameters in a rabbit model of chronic rhinosinusitis. Int Forum Allergy Rhinology 2019;9:629–37.

27. Cho D-Y, Mackey C, Van Der Pol WJ, et al. Sinus microanatomy and microbiota in a rabbit model of rhinosinusitis. Front Cell Infect Microbiol 2018;7:540.

28. Cho DY, Lim DJ, Mackey C, et al. Preclinical therapeutic efficacy of the ciprofloxacin-eluting sinus stent for Pseudomonas aeruginosa sinusitis. Int Forum Allergy Rhinology 2018;8:482–9.

29. Lim DJ, Skinner D, West JM, et al. In vitro evaluation of a novel oxygen-generating biomaterial for chronic rhinosinusitis therapy. Int Forum Allergy Rhinology 2022; 12:181–90.

30. Blount A, Zhang S, Chestnut M, et al. Transepithelial ion transport is suppressed in hypoxic sinonasal epithelium. Laryngoscope 2011;121:1929–34.

31. Chiu AG, Palmer JN, Woodworth BA, et al. Baby shampoo nasal irrigations for the symptomatic post-functional endoscopic sinus surgery patient. Am J Rhinol 2008;22:34–7.

32. Cho DY, Skinner D, Hunter RC, et al. Contribution of short chain fatty acids to the growth of pseudomonas aeruginosa in rhinosinusitis. Front Cell Infect Microbiol 2020;10:412.

33. Cho DY, Zhang S, Lazrak A, et al. LPS decreases CFTR open probability and mucociliary transport through generation of reactive oxygen species. Redox Biol 2021;43:101998.

34. Cho DY, Zhang S, Skinner DF, et al. Ivacaftor restores delayed mucociliary transport caused by Pseudomonas aeruginosa-induced acquired cystic fibrosis transmembrane conductance regulator dysfunction in rabbit nasal epithelia. Int Forum Allergy Rhinology 2022;12:690–8.

35. Londino JD, Lazrak A, Noah JW, et al. Influenza virus M2 targets cystic fibrosis transmembrane conductance regulator for lysosomal degradation during viral infection. FASEB J 2015;29:2712–25.

36. Kern RC, Conley DB, Walsh W, et al. Perspectives on the etiology of chronic rhinosinusitis: an immune barrier hypothesis. Am J Rhinol 2008;22:549–59.

37. Schleimer RP, Kato A, Peters A, et al. Epithelium, inflammation, and immunity in the upper airways of humans: studies in chronic rhinosinusitis. Proc Am Thorac Soc 2009;6:288–94.

38. Bernstein JM, Ballow M, Schlievert PM, et al. A superantigen hypothesis for the pathogenesis of chronic hyperplastic sinusitis with massive nasal polyposis. Am J Rhinol 2003;17:321–6.

39. Perloff JR, Palmer JN. Evidence of bacterial biofilms in a rabbit model of sinusitis. Am J Rhinol 2005;19:1–6.

40. Khalid AN, Woodworth BA, Prince A, et al. Physiologic alterations in the murine model after nasal fungal antigenic exposure. Otolaryngology–Head Neck Surg 2008;139:695–701.

41. Krouse JH, Brown RW, Fineman SM, et al. Asthma and the unified airway. Otolaryngol Head Neck Surg 2007;136:S75–106.

42. Illing EA, Woodworth BA. Management of the upper airway in cystic fibrosis. Curr Opin Pulm Med 2014;20:623–31.

43. Senior BA, Kennedy DW, Tanabodee J, et al. Long-term impact of functional endoscopic sinus surgery on asthma. Otolaryngol Head Neck Surg 1999; 121:66–8.

44. Hamilos DL. Chronic sinusitis. J Allergy Clin Immunol 2000;106:213–27.

45. Batra PS, Kern RC, Tripathi A, et al. Outcome analysis of endoscopic sinus surgery in patients with nasal polyps and asthma. Laryngoscope 2003;113:1703–6.

46. Munck A, Bonacorsi S, Mariani-Kurkdjian P, et al. Genotypic characterization of Pseudomonas aeruginosa strains recovered from patients with cystic fibrosis after initial and subsequent colonization. Pediatr Pulmonol 2001;32:288–92.

47. Koch C. Early infection and progression of cystic fibrosis lung disease. Pediatr Pulmonol 2002;34:232–6.

48. Johansen HK, Aanaes K, Pressler T, et al. Colonisation and infection of the paranasal sinuses in cystic fibrosis patients is accompanied by a reduced PMN response. J Cyst Fibros 2012;11:525–31.

49. Aanaes K, von Buchwald C, Hjuler T, et al. The effect of sinus surgery with intensive follow-up on pathogenic sinus bacteria in patients with cystic fibrosis. Am J Rhinol Allergy 2013;27:e1–4.

50. Lavin J, Bhushan B, Schroeder JW Jr. Correlation between respiratory cultures and sinus cultures in children with cystic fibrosis. Int J Pediatr Otorhinolaryngol 2013;77:686–9.

51. Ciofu O, Johansen HK, Aanaes K, et al. P. aeruginosa in the paranasal sinuses and transplanted lungs have similar adaptive mutations as isolates from chronically infected CF lungs. J Cyst Fibros 2013;12:729–36.

52. Mainz JG, Naehrlich L, Schien M, et al. Concordant genotype of upper and lower airways P aeruginosa and S aureus isolates in cystic fibrosis. Thorax 2009;64: 535–40.

53. Chang EH. New insights into the pathogenesis of cystic fibrosis sinusitis. Int Forum Allergy Rhinol 2014;4:132–7.

54. Spielman DB, Beswick DM, Kimple AJ, et al. The management of cystic fibrosis chronic rhinosinusitis: An evidenced-based review with recommendations. Int Forum Allergy Rhinology 2022;12(9):1148–83.

55. Kimple AJ, Senior BA, Naureckas ET, et al. Cystic Fibrosis foundation otolaryngology care multidisciplinary consensus recommendations. Int Forum Allergy Rhinology 2022;12(9):1089–103.

56. Georgalas C, Cornet M, Adriaensen G, et al. Evidence-based surgery for chronic rhinosinusitis with and without nasal polyps. Curr Allergy Asthma Rep 2014; 14:427.

57. Vlastarakos PV, Fetta M, Segas JV, et al. Functional endoscopic sinus surgery improves sinus-related symptoms and quality of life in children with chronic rhinosinusitis: a systematic analysis and meta-analysis of published interventional studies. Clin Pediatr 2013;52:1091–7.

58. Virgin FW, Rowe SM, Wade MB, et al. Extensive surgical and comprehensive postoperative medical management for cystic fibrosis chronic rhinosinusitis. Am J Rhinol Allergy 2012;26:70–5.

59. Woodworth BA, Parker RO, Schlosser RJ. Modified endoscopic medial maxillectomy for chronic maxillary sinusitis. Am J Rhinol 2006;20:317–9.

60. McCormick JP, Hicks MD, Grayson JW, et al. Endoscopic management of maxillary sinus diseases of dentoalveolar origin. Oral Maxillofacial Surg Clin N Am 2020;32:639–48.

61. Cho DY, Hwang PH. Results of endoscopic maxillary mega-antrostomy in recalcitrant maxillary sinusitis. Am J Rhinol 2008;22:658–62.

62. Ramsey BW, Davies J, McElvaney NG, et al. A CFTR potentiator in patients with cystic fibrosis and the G551D mutation. N Engl J Med 2011;365:1663–72.

63. Chang EH, Tang XX, Shah VS, et al. Medical reversal of chronic sinusitis in a cystic fibrosis patient with ivacaftor. Int Forum Allergy Rhinol 2015;5:178–81.

64. Hayes D Jr, McCoy KS, Sheikh SI. Improvement of sinus disease in cystic fibrosis with ivacaftor therapy. Am J Respir Crit Care Med 2014;190:468.

65. Lee SE, Farzal Z, Daniels MLA, et al. Cystic Fibrosis Transmembrane Conductance Regulator Modulator Therapy: A Review for the Otolaryngologist. Am J Rhinol Allergy 2020;34:573–80.

66. Beswick DM, Humphries SM, Balkissoon CD, et al. Machine learning evaluates improvement in sinus computed tomography opacification with CFTR modulator therapy. Int Forum Allergy Rhinol 2021;11:953–4.

67. DiMango E, Overdevest J, Keating C, et al. Effect of highly effective modulator treatment on sinonasal symptoms in cystic fibrosis. J Cyst Fibros 2021;20:460–3.

68. Douglas JE, Civantos AM, Locke TB, et al. Impact of novel CFTR modulator on sinonasal quality of life in adult patients with cystic fibrosis. Int Forum Allergy Rhinol 2021;11:201–3.

69. Raju SV, Lin VY, Liu L, et al. The Cystic fibrosis transmembrane conductance regulator potentiator ivacaftor augments mucociliary clearance abrogating cystic fibrosis transmembrane conductance regulator inhibition by cigarette smoke. Am J Respir Cell Mol Biol 2017;56:99–108.

70. Solomon GM, Fu L, Rowe SM, et al. The therapeutic potential of CFTR modulators for COPD and other airway diseases. Curr Opin Pharmacol 2017;34:132–9.

71. Dey I, Shah K, Bradbury NA. Natural compounds as therapeutic agents in the treatment cystic fibrosis. J Genet Syndr Gene Ther 2016;7(1):284.

72. Carlile GW, Keyzers RA, Teske KA, et al. Correction of F508del-CFTR trafficking by the sponge alkaloid latonduine is modulated by interaction with PARP. Chem Biol 2012;19:1288–99.

73. Springsteel MF, Galietta LJ, Ma T, et al. Benzoflavone activators of the cystic fibrosis transmembrane conductance regulator: towards a pharmacophore model for the nucleotide-binding domain. Bioorg Med Chem 2003;11: 4113–20.

74. Galietta LJ, Springsteel MF, Eda M, et al. Novel CFTR chloride channel activators identified by screening of combinatorial libraries based on flavone and benzoquinolizinium lead compounds. J Biol Chem 2001;276:19723–8.

75. Caci E, Folli C, Zegarra-Moran O, et al. CFTR activation in human bronchial epithelial cells by novel benzoflavone and benzimidazolone compounds. Am J Physiol Lung Cell Mol Physiol 2003;285:L180–8.

76. Zhang S, Blount AC, McNicholas CM, et al. Resveratrol enhances airway surface liquid depth in sinonasal epithelium by increasing cystic fibrosis transmembrane conductance regulator open probability. PLoS One 2013;8:e81589.

77. Conger BT, Zhang S, Skinner D, et al. Comparison of cystic fibrosis transmembrane conductance regulator (CFTR) and ciliary beat frequency activation by the CFTR Modulators Genistein, VRT-532, and UCCF-152 in primary sinonasal epithelial cultures. JAMA Otolaryngol Head Neck Surg 2013;139:822–7.

78. Zhang S, Smith N, Schuster D, et al. Quercetin increases cystic fibrosis transmembrane conductance regulator-mediated chloride transport and ciliary beat frequency: therapeutic implications for chronic rhinosinusitis. Am J Rhinol Allergy 2011;25:307–12.

79. Alexander NS, Hatch N, Zhang S, et al. Resveratrol has salutary effects on mucociliary transport and inflammation in sinonasal epithelium. Laryngoscope 2011; 121:1313–9.

80. Azbell C, Zhang S, Skinner D, et al. Hesperidin stimulates cystic fibrosis transmembrane conductance regulator-mediated chloride secretion and ciliary beat frequency in sinonasal epithelium. Otolaryngol Head Neck Surg 2010;143: 397–404.

81. Virgin F, Zhang S, Schuster D, et al. The bioflavonoid compound, sinupret, stimulates transepithelial chloride transport in vitro and in vivo. Laryngoscope 2010; 120:1051–6.

82. Tarran R, Button B, Boucher RC. Regulation of normal and cystic fibrosis airway surface liquid volume by phasic shear stress. Annu Rev Physiol 2006;68:543–61.
83. Mall MA, Galietta LJ. Targeting ion channels in cystic fibrosis. J Cyst Fibros 2015; 14:561–70.
84. Cho DY, Skinner D, Zhang S, et al. Korean Red Ginseng aqueous extract improves markers of mucociliary clearance by stimulating chloride secretion. J Ginseng Res 2021;45:66–74.

Pediatric Unified Airway
Chronic Rhinosinusitis and Lower-Airway Disease

Carly Mulinda, BA, Nathan Yang, MD, David A. Gudis, MD*

KEYWORDS

- Pediatric chronic rhinosinusitis • Pediatric chronic sinusitis
- Endoscopic sinus surgery • Asthma • Cystic fibrosis • Adenoids
- Primarily ciliary dyskinesia • Unified airway

KEY POINTS

- The unified airway concept provides a framework for the understanding and management of interrelated sinonasal and bronchopulmonary conditions. The upper and lower airways often function as an integrated system.
- Medical management of pediatric chronic rhinosinusitis may include a combination of systemic and/or intranasal corticosteroids, nasal saline, and/or antibiotics when bacterial infection is suspected.
- Optimizing management of chronic rhinosinusitis has been shown to improve asthma, cystic fibrosis, and primary ciliary dyskinesia.

INTRODUCTION

Rhinosinusitis, or inflammation of the nasal cavity and paranasal sinuses, is a major cause of morbidity within the pediatric population, resulting in missed days of school and decreased quality of life (QoL).[1,2] The condition is typically classified temporally as acute (less than 1 month), subacute (1 to 3 months), or chronic (more than 90 days).

Pediatric chronic rhinosinusitis (PCRS) is defined as the presence of sinonasal inflammation lasting for at least 90 consecutive or more days in a child 18 years or younger. Diagnosis requires 2 or more of the following symptoms: cough, nasal discharge, nasal obstruction, and facial pressure and/or pain. Objective findings of PCRS must also be evident on anterior rhinoscopy, nasal endoscopy, or computed tomography (CT) imaging.[3] PCRS can be further subdivided according to phenotype (with or without nasal polyps) and/or endotype (Th2-mediated vs non-Th2-mediated). Approximately 8% of children are affected by this disease, most commonly

Department of Otolaryngology–Head and Neck Surgery, Columbia University Irving Medical Center, New York–Presbyterian Hospital, New York, NY, USA
* Corresponding author. 180 Fort Washington Avenue, Suite 850, New York, NY 10032.
E-mail address: Dag62@cumc.columbia.edu

Otolaryngol Clin N Am 56 (2023) 137–146
https://doi.org/10.1016/j.otc.2022.09.010
0030-6665/23/© 2022 Elsevier Inc. All rights reserved.
oto.theclinics.com

children aged 5 to 15 years.[4] In the pediatric population, diagnosis is complicated by conditions like adenoid disease and allergic rhinitis, whose symptoms like nasal discharge and facial pressure overlap with those of PCRS.

Although adult and pediatric chronic rhinosinusitis (CRS) have some shared pathophysiology, including epithelial barrier dysfunction, there are special considerations for pediatric CRS, particularly in young children.[4] Studies have demonstrated that PCRS in children less than 12 years of age tends to be driven by the activity of neutrophils, macrophages, and CD4+ lymphocytes, rather than the eosinophils more commonly seen in older children and adults.[4,5] Furthermore, the nasal cavities of children 12 years of age and younger may be obstructed by adenoids, which are typically present only until young adulthood.[6] Moreover, nasal polyps have an estimated 0.1% incidence in children, and their presence may raise suspicion for underlying systemic disease, such as cystic fibrosis (CF), primary ciliary dyskinesia (PCD), and immunodeficiency.[7]

PCRS is closely related to multiple systemic diseases, including asthma, CF, and PCD. Although PCRS may worsen the bronchopulmonary manifestations of these diseases, the converse is also true, an interrelationship explained by the concept of the unified airway. Herein, the authors describe the relationship between PCRS, a sinonasal inflammatory disease, and other diseases affecting the upper- and lower-respiratory tract in the pediatric population.

ADENOID DISEASE

Although CRS and PCRS share many pathophysiologic features, the presence of the adenoid pad in the pediatric population is a key distinction. The adenoids are lymphatic tissue located on the posterior wall of the nasopharynx behind the soft palate. In infancy, these tissues are essential to the immune system, building immunologic memory to antigens encountered through the oral and nasal cavities and secreting immunoglobulin A (IgA) on reintroduction to those antigens. Adenoids peak in size between ages 2 and 6 years. They begin to gradually decrease in size after the age of 6 until puberty and may be nearly absent by adulthood.[8]

Dysfunction of the adenoid tissue has been shown to significantly influence the pathogenesis of PCRS in children less than 12 years of age.[6] Adenoids have been implicated in the development of PCRS through their role as bacterial reservoirs, their obstruction of the nasopharynx, and the associated reduction in secretory IgA. Studies have shown that the adenoids harbor the same bacteria that contribute to the pathogenesis of CRS. *Haemophilus influenzae*, *Streptococcus pneumoniae*, and *Moraxella catarrhalis* are most frequently isolated from adenoid surfaces of pediatric patients with CRS.[9] Elwany and colleagues[10] cultured the bacteria in both the adenoid core and the middle meatal cavity of pediatric patients with recurrent rhinosinusitis. The study found that the adenoid core cultures held a positive predictive value of 91.5 and a negative predictive value of 84.3 for the bacterial census of the middle meatus.

Bacterial colonization results in chronic inflammation of the upper airway. This chronic inflammatory state is known to alter the ciliated epithelium of the nasal mucosa, disrupting mucociliary clearance of the sinuses.[11] Because of their proximity to the paranasal sinuses and the narrow nasopharynx of children, adenoid hypertrophy may also physically prevent adequate postnasal drainage, amplifying inflammation and increasing susceptibility to microbial colonization. Although increased size may worsen mucociliary clearance, PCRS has been shown to progress independently of adenoid size, suggesting that its function as a bacterial reservoir has an impact equal to if not greater than physical size.[2]

Researchers have also connected biofilms and reduction in secretory IgA to adenoids' contribution to PCRS. In an analysis of adenoids removed after adenoidectomies, Coticchia and colleagues[12] found that 94.9% of adenoid surface area of pediatric patients with CRS were infected with bacterial biofilm, as opposed to the 1.9% adenoid surface area of pediatric patients being treated for obstructive sleep apnea. Biofilms are of clinical significance to the treatment of refractory PCRS, as they reduce the efficacy of antimicrobial pharmacotherapy through expression and transmission of antimicrobial resistance genes.[13] In addition, the adenoids of children with PCRS are known to secrete a reduced amount of secretory IgA, which normally operates as an immune defense against bacteria that attempt to infect upper-respiratory epithelium.[14]

Direct visualization of the adenoids and sinus drainage pathways is best achieved through nasal endoscopy, granting clinicians the opportunity to rule out alternative diagnoses and take bacterial cultures, if necessary. Clinical findings specific to adenoid disease include persistent rhinorrhea and excessive mouth breathing. When suspecting PCRS, noncontrast CT imaging is indicated by failure of medical treatment, particularly performed with axial, coronal, and sagittal views. However, provider hesitance to order CT imaging owing to radiation exposure risk frequently leads to unnecessarily prolonged medical treatment with antibiotics. In the absence of endoscopy, plain lateral neck radiographs may be obtained to assess adenoid size.[15]

Medical management is the recommended initial treatment of PCRS. Intranasal corticosteroids (INCS) and daily nasal saline irrigation (NSI) have been shown to improve QoL in as few as 6 weeks.[13] In addition to symptom improvement, NSI has also been shown to significantly improve CT scan Lund-McKay scores.[16] INCS are commonly used, as their safety and efficacy have been demonstrated in pediatric allergic rhinitis and adult CRS. If bacterial infection is suspected, empiric antibiotics should be administered. Given the most common pathogens in PCRS, high-dose amoxicillin or clindamycin is the standard treatment, but there is no consensus on duration of treatment.[15] The American Academy of Otolaryngology–Head and Neck Surgery (AAO-HNS) recommends a minimum of 10 days of antibacterial treatment.[17]

In PCRS refractory to medical management, surgical intervention is often beneficial. Adenoidectomy is the first-line surgical therapy for persistent PCRS in young children. In addition to being a routine and well-tolerated procedure, adenoidectomy has been shown to significantly improve PCRS symptoms in younger patients. In a meta-analysis studying the efficacy of adenoidectomy alone in refractory PCRS, Brietzke and Brigger[6] found that adenoidectomy improved sinusitis symptoms in 70% of patients (mean age of 5.8 years), supporting its efficacy in younger children. The AAO-HNS consensus statement reported a strong consensus regarding the efficacy of adenoidectomy alone in children 6 years and younger but could not reach consensus regarding children aged 6 to 13 years.[17] However, Mahomva and colleagues[18] more recently assessed the efficacy of adenoidectomy alone in children 7 to 18 years of age (mean, 8.6 years) and found significant symptom improvement, suggesting its efficacy among older children. Adenoidectomy is commonly combined with tonsillectomy, but there is widespread consensus that tonsillectomy alone is an ineffective treatment for PCRS.[5,17]

Adjuvant treatments can also be performed at the time of adenoidectomy. Balloon catheter dilation and maxillary sinus irrigation are safe in the pediatric population and can be useful in the treatment of PCRS. In a meta-analysis of literature regarding PCRS treatment, Patel and colleagues[19] found that paranasal sinus balloon catheter dilation during adenoidectomy had better success than adenoidectomy alone. Ramadan and Cost[20] found that children with severe CRS who received a maxillary sinus wash during adenoidectomy had more symptom improvement (87.5%) than those with adenoidectomy alone (60.7%). Although the preferred surgical treatment in adult CRS, endoscopic sinus surgery (ESS), is reserved for PCRS refractory to adenoidectomy, complicated sinusitis, nasal polyps, or fungal sinusitis, ESS is safe within the pediatric population and can be considered at any age.[21]

ASTHMA

Asthma is a chronic inflammatory disease of the lower airway characterized by bronchial hyperresponsiveness, bronchial inflammation, and reversible endobronchial obstruction. It is a heterogeneous disease with variable risk factors, triggers, severity, and treatment responses. The most common symptoms include cough, dyspnea, chest tightness, and wheezing. Initially, airway obstruction is reversible with standard treatment, but chronic inflammation leads to irreversible modification of the lower airway, a phenomenon known as "airway remodeling."

Asthma is the most common chronic pediatric disease in the United States, responsible for nearly 800,000 emergency department visits and 75,000 hospitalizations for children annually.[22] Although the exact cause of asthma is unclear, multiple risk factors have been identified, including genetic predisposition and various social determinants of health.[23] One prospective study of 259 children reported that respiratory infections, specifically of viral cause, in infancy and early childhood increased the risk of asthma development.[24] The microbiome has also been implicated in asthma development by altering the integrity of the airway barrier.[25]

Like CRS, asthma is a heterogeneous disease with variable phenotypes. However, both disease processes may be divided into 2 general endotypes: Th2-predominant and non-Th2 predominant. Th2-predominant asthma and CRS are characterized by a type of inflammation driven by T-helper cells and characterized by high levels of interleukin-4 (IL-4), IL-5, and IL-13 inflammation. In asthma, the cascade results in release of histamines and leukotrienes, which cause bronchoconstriction. Clinically, distinction between both endotypes allows anticipation of response to corticosteroids, as Th2-predominant disease has a more favorable response.[26]

As seen in adults, PCRS frequently coexists with asthma, especially poorly controlled asthma. In a study of 294 asthmatic children (mean, 7.3 years), 7.5% were found to have both occult sinusitis on nasal endoscopy and poorly controlled asthma.[27] Fuller and colleagues[28] found radiologic evidence of sinusitis in 27% of children admitted with status asthmaticus. Similarly, Anfuso and colleagues[29] reported that children with both PCRS and asthma exhibit higher adenoid levels of fibroblast growth factor-2, epidermal growth factor, growth-related oncogenes, and sinus levels of tumor necrosis factor-alpha compared with children with asthma and no PCRS.

Consistent with the unified airway concept, asthma and CRS have been suggested to share similar pathologic processes in different target tissues. When both diseases are caused by type 2 inflammatory reactions and sustained by predominantly eosinophilic and T-cell lymphocytic infiltration, desquamation of the upper- and lower-airway epithelium, mucus gland hyperplasia, and basement membrane thickening can occur.[26] Furthermore, it has been hypothesized that CRS and asthma may interact through the hematogenous spread of cytokines released from inflammation at 1 portion of the airway, stimulating the systemic release of eosinophils and other type 2 inflammatory cells from the bone marrow.[30]

CRS in patients with asthma has been linked to significantly worse QoL and lung function than those with asthma without CRS.[31] CRS is also a known risk factor for recurrent asthma exacerbations.[32] In an analysis of children with severe and persistent asthma, children with concomitant CRS (16.3%) substantially outnumbered those without CRS (3.8%).[33] Asthma is correlated with worse recurrence rates in adult patients with CRS who undergo ESS, but similar studies are lacking in the pediatric population.[34]

Data show that medical and surgical treatment of PCRS substantially reduces asthma symptoms in children and adults with coexisting asthma and PCRS.[35] In 1984, Rachelefsky and colleagues[36] demonstrated that resolution of sinusitis led to the normalization of pulmonary function tests (PFTs) in 67% of the children with concomitant asthma and PCRS and led to discontinuation of bronchodilators in 79% of the children. Treatment of PCRS with antibiotics has also been shown in multiple studies to reduce bronchial hyperresponsiveness.[37,38] In a study of children with both asthma and PCRS, Friedman and colleagues[39] found that treatment with bronchodilators and antibiotics led to greater improvement in PFTs than treatment with bronchodilators alone. The impact of PCRS treatment with INCS on asthma is not clear. Some studies of patients with concomitant asthma and PCRS showed no improvement of asthma after treating CRS with INCS.[40] Emerging data on biologics targeting type 2 inflammatory mediators, like dupilumab, show efficacy in improving both asthma and CRS with nasal polyposis in adults, but there is still sparse literature on the use of biologics in children.[41]

The surgical treatment of PCRS with ESS has a strong association with improvement in asthma symptoms. In a study of steroid-dependent children with asthma and PCRS who underwent ESS, Manning and colleagues[42] reported fewer missed school days and hospitalizations as well as reduced steroid dependency/usage and improved lower-airway symptoms. Within a sample of 52 pediatric patients, Parson and Phillips[43] found that PCRS treatment with functional ESS resulted in fewer emergency room visits and monthly asthma exacerbations as well as a 96% reduction in asthma symptoms.

CYSTIC FIBROSIS

CF is an autosomal recessive disorder characterized by multiorgan dysfunction, classically of the pulmonary and gastrointestinal system. Genetic mutation of the *CFTR* gene alters cystic fibrosis transmembrane conductance regulator (CFTR) proteins, which are key components of ATP-gated sodium ion channels in cell membranes. Secretion of chloride ions outside of cells is greatly reduced, leading to intracellular water retention and viscous mucus production. In the lower-respiratory tract of patients with CF, impaired mucociliary clearance facilitates pulmonary colonization with opportunistic bacteria, recurrent pulmonary infections, and diminished lung function.

Although pulmonary disease is the dominant clinical manifestation of CF, CRS is a cardinal condition of CF. Common presentation of PCRS in CF includes purulent nasal discharge, nasal congestion, and headache.[44] Sinonasal pathologic condition can be identified through imaging in nearly 100% of patients with CF, generated by bacterial colonization and inflammation stimulated by mucus accumulation.[45] In children who present with bilateral nasal polyposis and signs of sinonasal disease, screening for CF is often clinically indicated.[46] The sinuses of children with CF serve as a bacterial reservoir for *Staphylococcus aureus* and *Pseudomonas aeruginosa*. Bacteria in the sinuses may migrate to the lungs, providing a source for chronic reinfection of the lower airways.[47,48] Although PCRS is known to significantly reduce health-related QoL in non-CF patients, the effect of CRS on CF in children and adults is still being elucidated.[46] Studies have demonstrated a correlation between worsening sinonasal QoL and forced expiratory volume in 1 second in children 12 years with CF, whereas only 20% of children with CF complain of PCRS symptoms.[49,50]

Treatment of bacterial sinusitis is integral to the prevention of pulmonary reinfection with CF-pathogenic bacteria.[47] Empiric antibiotics, namely aminoglycosides alone or with macrolides, are frequently administered to eradicate colonization of S aureus and P aeruginosa in the lungs and sinuses of children with CF.[51] Although effective, ototoxicity is a known side effect of these medications with the potential to hinder a child's speech, language, and social development.[6] Patients with CF PCRS may also benefit from NSI and/or intranasal steroids.[51]

In cases of complicated CRS, including CF CRS, ESS has been shown to be a safe and effective treatment for children. Indications for ESS in the management of CF CRS include worsening pulmonary function, refractory sinonasal symptoms, and increased pulmonary exacerbations.[52] Aanæs[47] evaluated the efficacy of ESS and adjuvant therapy in a prospective study of 58 patients with CF aged 6 to 45 years who underwent ESS and were colonized by P aeruginosa, Burkholderia multivorans, and/or Achromobacter xylosoxidans. Adjuvant therapy consisted of colistin sinus irrigation during surgery, a 2-week course of broad-spectrum intravenous antibiotics, and a regimen of colistin sinus irrigations, nasal saline, and topical nasal steroid spray for at least 6 months. When classified by lung function status, the group of patients with "intermittent colonization" (mean, 17 years) had a reduction from 83% to 25% in postoperative CF-pathogenic–positive bacterial sinus cultures. In a 2016 cohort study of 106 patients with CF aged 6 to 50 years (mean age of 19 years) who had undergone ESS and the same adjuvant treatment, Aanæs found significantly improved lung infection status and delayed chronic CF-pathogenic lung infection at 3-year follow-up. The "intermittent colonization" cohort exhibited the largest improvement in lung infection status.[48] It can be concluded that pediatric ESS with adjuvant medical treatment is the optimal management of refractory CF PCRS.

PRIMARY CILIARY DYSKINESIA

PCD is an autosomal recessive disorder characterized by dysfunctional cilia and impaired mucociliary clearance. Mucus retention results in recurrent bacterial infections of the upper and lower airways and progressively worsening pulmonary function, most commonly bronchiectasis. Common symptoms of PCD include sinusitis, chronic productive cough, recurrent otitis media, and recurrent bronchitis.[53] In addition, recurrent otitis media with effusion may lead to conductive hearing loss in adolescents with PCD. Because of its nonspecific presentation, PCD diagnosis is often delayed to a mean age of 4.4 years.[54]

CRS affects more than 50% of patients with PCD secondary to immotility of ciliated epithelium in the sinonasal tract and mucus accumulation. Like CF, PCD should be included in the differential diagnosis for children who present with sinonasal symptoms and nasal polyps, as nasal polyposis occurs in an estimated 15% of children with PCD.[55] Children with PCD are particularly vulnerable to more severe sinonasal conditions. In 2021, Zawawi and colleagues[56] examined QoL of 47 children with PCD-PCRS in a cross-sectional study, finding that the PCD cohort reported worse sinonasal symptoms and worse QoL than controls with PCRS and without PCD. By the age of 10, children with PCD undergo an average of 25 separate courses of antibiotics, significantly more than their healthy peers.[57]

Antibiotics are a mainstay of medical management of PCD-PCRS. In pediatric patients with PCD, it is recommended to collect cultures of sputum or cough swabs every 3 months.[53] High-dose empiric oral antibiotics treating the most common PCRS pathogens should be administered to treat worsening sinonasal or pulmonary disease. Topical NSI may be used to assist with mucociliary clearance, although no literature yet exists to formally endorse its use in PCD. Although formal studies are still needed in children with PCD, oral corticosteroids may prove useful in reducing inflammation, CRS symptoms, and nasal polyp size, as sputum collected from children with PCD is predominantly neutrophilic.[53,58] However, the risk of growth suppression should be considered.

PCD has also been shown to improve following ESS. In 2016, Alanin and colleagues[59] studied 24 patients with PCD with severe CRS (mean age of 24 years, ranging from 10 to 65 years) who underwent ESS with bronchoalveolar lavage and adjuvant therapy. Nine patients were less than 18 years of age, but were not separately statistically analyzed. Adjuvant treatment included NSI, topical nasal steroids, a 2-week course of oral antibiotics, and, if positive for *P aeruginosa* at surgery, 6 months of local colistin. Bacterial cultures at ESS showed bacterial growth positive for the most common PCD pathogens, *P aeruginosa*, *H influenzae*, and *S pneumoniae*, in 8 of 9 children. At 12-month follow-up, patients reported significantly improved symptoms and QoL, suggesting ESS as a means of improving lung function and QoL in PCD-PCRS.[59]

SUMMARY

Pediatric CRS affects the QoL and severity of associated systemic diseases with bronchopulmonary manifestations. The unified airway concept provides a framework through which clinicians can optimize treatment of comorbid pediatric diseases affecting both the upper- and the lower-respiratory tract.

CLINICS CARE POINTS

- The anatomy of pediatric sinuses suggests targeting treatment to sites that may serve as bacterial reservoirs, such as the adenoids.
- Adenoidectomy and endoscopic sinus surgery are safe and effective treatments of refractory pediatric chronic rhinosinusitis.
- Consistent with the unified airway concept, treatment of pediatric chronic rhinosinusitis improves symptoms and quality of life of patients with concomitant asthma, cystic fibrosis, and primary ciliary dyskinesia.

DISCLOSURE

The authors have no conflicts of interest to disclose.

REFERENCES

1. Cheng BT, Xu M, Hassan S, et al. Children and young adults with chronic rhinosinusitis have higher rates of chronic school absenteeism. Int Forum Allergy Rhinol 2021;11(10):1508–12. https://doi.org/10.1002/alr.22823.
2. Anamika A, Chakravarti A, Kumar R. Atopy and Quality of Life in Pediatric Chronic Rhinosinusitis. Am J rhinology Allergy 2019;33(5):586–90.
3. Fokkens WJ, Lund VJ, Hopkins C, et al. European Position Paper on Rhinosinusitis and Nasal Polyps 2020. Rhinology 2020;58(Suppl S29):1–464.
4. Chan KH, Abzug MJ, Coffinet L, et al. Chronic rhinosinusitis in young children differs from adults: a histopathology study. J Pediatr 2004;144(2):206–12, 2012;130(5):1087-1096.e10.

5. Driscoll PV, Naclerio RM, Baroody FM. CD4+ lymphocytes are increased in the sinus mucosa of children with chronic sinusitis. Arch Otolaryngol Head Neck Surg 1996;122(10):1071–6.

6. Brietzke SE, Brigger MT. Adenoidectomy outcomes in pediatric rhinosinusitis: a meta-analysis. Int J Pediatr Otorhinolaryngol 2008;72(10):1541–5.

7. Heath J, Hartzell L, Putt C, et al. Chronic Rhinosinusitis in Children: Pathophysiology, Evaluation, and Medical Management. Curr Allergy Asthma Rep 2018; 18(7):37.

8. Snidvongs K, Sangubol M, Poachanukoon O. Pediatric Versus Adult Chronic Rhinosinusitis. Curr Allergy Asthma Rep 2020;20(8):29.

9. Davcheva-Chakar M, Kaftandzhieva A, Zafirovska B. Adenoid Vegetations - Reservoir of Bacteria for Chronic Otitis Media with Effusion and Chronic Rhinosinusitis. Pril (Makedon Akad Nauk Umet Odd Med Nauki) 2015;36(3):71–6.

10. Elwany S, El-Dine AN, El-Medany A, et al. Relationship between bacteriology of the adenoid core and middle meatus in children with sinusitis. J Laryngol Otol 2011;125(3):279–81.

11. Maurizi M, Ottaviani F, Paludetti G, et al. Adenoid hypertrophy and nasal mucociliary clearance in children. A morphological and functional study. Int J Pediatr Otorhinolaryngol 1984;8(1):31–41.

12. Coticchia J, Zuliani G, Coleman C, et al. Biofilm surface area in the pediatric nasopharynx: Chronic rhinosinusitis vs obstructive sleep apnea. Arch Otolaryngol Head Neck Surg 2007;133(2):110–4.

13. Belcher R, Virgin F. The Role of the Adenoids in Pediatric Chronic Rhinosinusitis. Med Sci (Basel) 2019;7(2):35.

14. Eun YG, Park DC, Kim SG, et al. Immunoglobulins and transcription factors in adenoids of children with otitis media with effusion and chronic rhinosinusitis. Int J Pediatr Otorhinolaryngol 2009;73(10):1412–6.

15. Foster J, Belcher R, Lipscomb B, et al. Adenoid disease and chronic rhinosinusitis. In: Gudis DA, Schlosser RJ, editors. The unified airway: rhinologic disease and respiratory disorders. Springer; 2020. p. 33–8.

16. Pham V, Sykes K, Wei J. Long-term outcome of once daily nasal irrigation for the treatment of pediatric chronic rhinosinusitis. Laryngoscope 2014;124(4):1000–7.

17. Brietzke SE, Shin JJ, Choi S, et al. Clinical consensus statement: pediatric chronic rhinosinusitis. Otolaryngol Head Neck Surg 2014;151(4):542–53.

18. Mahomva C, Anne S, Roxbury C. Efficacy of Adenoidectomy for the Management of Chronic Rhinosinusitis in Children Older Than 7 Years of Age. Ann Otol Rhinol Laryngol 2021;131(8):868–73.

19. Patel VA, O'Brien DC, Ramadan J, et al. Balloon Catheter Dilation in Pediatric Chronic Rhinosinusitis: A Meta-analysis. Am J Rhinol Allergy 2020;34(5):694–702.

20. Ramadan HH, Cost JL. Outcome of adenoidectomy versus adenoidectomy with maxillary sinus wash for chronic rhinosinusitis in children. Laryngoscope 2008; 118(5):871–3.

21. Gudis DA, Soler ZM. Update on pediatric sinus surgery: indications and outcomes. Curr Opin Otolaryngol Head Neck Surg 2017;25(6):486–92.

22. Centers for Disease Control and Prevention. Most Recent Asthma Data. 2017. Available at: https://www.cdc.gov/asthma/most_recent_data.htm. Accessed April 26, 2022.

23. Perez MF, Coutinho MT. An Overview of Health Disparities in Asthma. Yale J Biol Med 2021;94(3):497–507.

24. Jackson DJ, Gangnon RE, Evans MD, et al. Wheezing rhinovirus illnesses in early life predict asthma development in high-risk children. Am J Respir Crit Care Med 2008;178(7):667–72.
25. Gitomer SA, Ramakrishnan V. Microbiome of the unified airway. In: Gudis DA, Schlosser RJ, editors. The unified airway: rhinologic disease and respiratory disorders. New York: Springer; 2020. p. 1–15.
26. Busse WW, Lemanske RF Jr. Asthma. N Engl J Med 2001;344(5):350–62.
27. Marseglia GL, Caimmi S, Marseglia A, et al. Occult sinusitis may be a key feature for non-controlled asthma in children. J Biol Regul Homeost Agents 2012;26(1 Suppl):S125–31.
28. Fuller CG, Schoettler JJ, Gilsanz V, et al. Sinusitis in status asthmaticus. Clin Pediatr (Phila) 1994;33(12):712–9.
29. Anfuso A, Ramadan H, Terrell A, et al. Sinus and adenoid inflammation in children with chronic rhinosinusitis and asthma. Ann Allergy Asthma Immunol 2015; 114(2):103–10.
30. Poddighe D, Brambilla I, Licari A, et al. Pediatric rhinosinusitis and asthma. Respir Med 2018;141:94–9.
31. Ek A, Middelveld RJ, Bertilsson H, et al. Chronic rhinosinusitis in asthma is a negative predictor of quality of life: results from the Swedish GA(2)LEN survey. Allergy 2013;68(10):1314–21.
32. ten Brinke A, Sterk PJ, Masclee AA, et al. Risk factors of frequent exacerbations in difficult-to-treat asthma. Eur Respir J 2005;26(5):812–8.
33. Matsuno O, Ono E, Takenaka R, et al. Asthma and sinusitis: association and implication. Int Arch Allergy Immunol 2008;147(1):52–8.
34. Sella GCP, Tamashiro E, Sella JA, et al. Asthma Is the Dominant Factor for Recurrence in Chronic Rhinosinusitis. J Allergy Clin Immunol Pract 2020;8(1):302–9.
35. Tosca MA, Cosentino C, Pallestrini E, et al. Improvement of clinical and immunopathologic parameters in asthmatic children treated for concomitant chronic rhinosinusitis. Ann Allergy Asthma Immunol 2003;91(1):71–8.
36. Rachelefsky GS, Katz RM, Siegel SC. Chronic sinus disease with associated reactive airway disease in children. Pediatrics 1984;73(4):526–9.
37. Oliveira CA, Solé D, Naspitz CK, et al. Improvement of bronchial hyperresponsiveness in asthmatic children treated for concomitant sinusitis. Ann Allergy Asthma Immunol 1997;79(1):70–4.
38. Tsao CH, Chen LC, Yeh KW, et al. Concomitant chronic sinusitis treatment in children with mild asthma: the effect on bronchial hyperresponsiveness. Chest 2003; 123(3):757–64.
39. Friedman R, Ackerman M, Wald E, et al. Asthma and bacterial sinusitis in children. J Allergy Clin Immunol 1984;74(2):185–9.
40. American Lung Association–Asthma Clinical Research Centers' Writing Committee, Dixon AE, Castro M, et al. Efficacy of nasal mometasone for the treatment of chronic sinonasal disease in patients with inadequately controlled asthma. J Allergy Clin Immunol 2015;135(3):701–9.e5.
41. Licari A, Castagnoli R, Marseglia A, et al. Dupilumab to Treat Type 2 Inflammatory Diseases in Children and Adolescents. Paediatr Drugs 2020;22(3):295–310.
42. Manning SC, Wasserman RL, Silver R, et al. Results of endoscopic sinus surgery in pediatric patients with chronic sinusitis and asthma. Arch Otolaryngol Head Neck Surg 1994;120(10):1142–5.
43. Parsons DS, Phillips SE. Functional endoscopic surgery in children: a retrospective analysis of results. Laryngoscope 1993;103(8):899–903.

44. Kang SH, Dalcin Pde T, Piltcher OB, et al. Chronic rhinosinusitis and nasal polyposis in cystic fibrosis: update on diagnosis and treatment. J Bras Pneumol 2015; 41(1):65–76.
45. Gentile VG, Isaacson G. Patterns of sinusitis in cystic fibrosis. Laryngoscope 1996;106(8):1005–9.
46. Virgin FW. Clinical chronic rhinosinusitis outcomes in pediatric patients with cystic fibrosis. Laryngoscope Investig Otolaryngol 2017;2(5):276–80.
47. Aanæs K. Bacterial sinusitis can be a focus for initial lung colonisation and chronic lung infection in patients with cystic fibrosis. J Cyst Fibros 2013; 12(Suppl 2):S1–20.
48. Alanin MC, Aanaes K, Høiby N, et al. Sinus surgery postpones chronic Gram-negative lung infection: cohort study of 106 patients with cystic fibrosis. Rhinology 2016;54(3):206–13.
49. Robertson JM, Friedman EM, Rubin BK. Nasal and sinus disease in cystic fibrosis. Paediatr Respir Rev 2008;9(3):213–9.
50. Friedman EM, Stewart M. An assessment of sinus quality of life and pulmonary function in children with cystic fibrosis. Am J Rhinol 2006;20(6):568–72.
51. Kimple AJ, Senior BA, Naureckas ET, et al. Cystic Fibrosis Foundation otolaryngology care multidisciplinary consensus recommendations. Int Forum Allergy Rhinol 2022;12(9):1089–103.
52. Tumin D, Hayes D Jr, Kirkby SE, et al. Safety of endoscopic sinus surgery in children with cystic fibrosis. Int J Pediatr Otorhinolaryngol 2017;98:25–8.
53. Barbato A, Frischer T, Kuehni CE, et al. Primary ciliary dyskinesia: a consensus statement on diagnostic and treatment approaches in children. Eur Respir J 2009;34(6):1264–76.
54. Coren ME, Meeks M, Morrison I, et al. Primary ciliary dyskinesia: age at diagnosis and symptom history. Acta Paediatr 2002;91(6):667–9.
55. Min YG, Shin JS, Choi SH, et al. Primary ciliary dyskinesia: ultrastructural defects and clinical features. Rhinology 1995;33(4):189–93.
56. Zawawi F, Shapiro AJ, Dell S, et al. Otolaryngology Manifestations of Primary Ciliary Dyskinesia: A Multicenter Study. Otolaryngol Head Neck Surg 2022; 166(3):540–7.
57. Sommer JU, Schäfer K, Omran H, et al. ENT manifestations in patients with primary ciliary dyskinesia: prevalence and significance of otorhinolaryngologic comorbidities. Eur Arch Otorhinolaryngol 2011;268(3):383–8.
58. Alanin MC. Primary ciliary dyskinesia. In: Gudis DA, Schlosser RJ, editors. The unified airway: rhinologic disease and respiratory disorders. New York: Springer; 2020. p. 185–94.
59. Alanin MC, Aanaes K, Høiby N, et al. Sinus surgery can improve quality of life, lung infections, and lung function in patients with primary ciliary dyskinesia. Int Forum Allergy Rhinol 2017;7(3):240–7.

Upper Airway Cough Syndrome

Angela M. Donaldson, MD, FARS

KEYWORDS

- UACS • Chronic cough • Rhinitis • Chronic rhinosinusitis • Postnasal drip

KEY POINTS

- Upper airway cough syndrome (UACS) is a common cause of chronic cough, often associated with rhinitis or chronic rhinosinusitis.
- UACS is diagnosed after ruling out other causes of cough.
- Empiric treatment with H1 receptor antihistamines and decongestants is both therapeutic and diagnostic.

INTRODUCTION

Chronic cough impacts 4% to 10% of the adult population and is one of the most common chief complaints in ambulatory care centers.[1,2] Chronic cough is defined as a daily cough for greater than 8 weeks in adults and greater than 4 weeks in children. The most common causes of chronic cough are postnasal drip, asthma, and gastroesophageal reflux disease (GERD). When patient variables such as smoking and angiotensin-converting enzyme (ACE) inhibitor use are eliminated, these three idiopathic causes of chronic cough are associated with 90% of chronic cough etiologies.[3] Upper airway cough syndrome (UACS), formerly known as postnasal drip syndrome, is a diagnosis of exclusion in which chronic cough is associated with allergic rhinitis, nonallergic rhinitis, and chronic rhinosinusitis. It can also be diagnosed without other related conditions. UACS is one of the most common causes of chronic cough with a prevalence between 9% and 82%. This broad range in prevalence is primarily because of the slow adaptation of the term into clinical practice and the difference in treatment patterns between different countries. There is a relative agreement that in nonsmokers, UACS is considered the first or second most common cause of chronic cough in the world.[2,4] UACS is also frequently associated with other conditions that may cause a chronic cough. Irwin and colleagues found in up to 42% of patients, the cough is associated with three or more etiologies.[2,4,5]

Disclosures: none.
Department of Otolaryngology Head & Neck Surgery, Mayo Clinic Florida, 4500 San Pablo Road, Jacksonville, FL, USA
E-mail address: Donaldson.angela@mayo.edu

Otolaryngol Clin N Am 56 (2023) 147–155
https://doi.org/10.1016/j.otc.2022.09.011
0030-6665/23/© 2022 Elsevier Inc. All rights reserved.
oto.theclinics.com

Postnasal drip syndrome (PNDS) was first described by Dobell in 1866.[6] Frank published on this condition in 1794, but it was not until 1974 that the condition was noted as a common cause of chronic cough. It was originally described as a deep-seated fullness or sensation of mucus in the back of the nasopharynx or pharynx leading to cough and intermittent expectorant of mucus. The use of the term "postnasal drip syndrome" (PNDS) and recognition of its clinical importance in patient care was not immediately accepted. For many European physicians at the time, this condition had a high prevalence in the United States but was not often seen in the United Kingdom, and was even termed "American catarrh" within European medical societies. However, by the start of the twentieth century, the term postnasal drip syndrome was recognized as a medical condition in the European literature. PNDS was a well-accepted terminology until the American College of Chest Physicians (ACCP) guidelines in 2006 recommended that the term be changed to UACS.[3] Although it was initially thought that purulent nasal secretions were the cause of chronic cough, several studies demonstrated that other etiologies including inflammation and irritation of the upper airway structures could trigger a cough without the presence of postnasal drip. It was this controversy in the literature that led to the ACCPs decision to change the term to UACS. Today, there are still disagreements regarding the proper terminology to describe postnasal drip sensation associated with cough. The European Respiratory Society (ERS) does not characterize postnasal drip as a syndrome. It believes postnasal drip cannot fully explain the cough or why some patients with postnasal drip do not cough. Currently, the ERS guidelines describe UACS and PNDS as "rhinitis/rhinosinusitis" or upper airway disease caused cough.

Some of the challenges to effectively recognizing UACS as a potential cause of cough include a lack of objective findings and/or diagnostic testing. Additionally, the sensation of postnasal drip is subjective with no clear mechanism to quantify the amount. However, even with these limitations, the literature consistently demonstrates that UACS is a common cause of chronic cough. In this article, the author discusses the clinical and diagnostic findings frequently found in UACS. The author also discusses treatment options and hypothesis for the pathogenesis of this syndrome.

DISCUSSION

The diagnosis of UACS is made by history, physical examination, radiology findings, and most importantly, response to medical therapy. In addition to cough, symptoms of UACS include clearing of the throat, nasal drainage, and the sensation of mucus dripping into the throat. Clinical details such as timing and character of cough have not been found to hold diagnostic value.[3] Physical examination findings may be suggestive of UACS. These include mucus or secretions in the nasopharynx and oropharynx. Cobblestoning of the oropharyngeal mucosa has also been documented in patients with UACS. Mucous secretions in the naso- or oropharynx may not be present at the time of the examination. Therefore, inquiring about current symptoms before physical examination may complement the examination findings. Currently, there is no objective testing or clinical findings pathognomic of UACS. Therefore, the clinical history is relied on to determine if empiric treatment or further work-up is appropriate. A chest x-ray should be performed for patients with greater than 4 weeks of cough to rule out other pulmonary conditions. Computer tomography may be performed if history and nasal endoscopy are concerning for chronic rhinosinusitis (CRS). Empiric therapy leading to resolution of cough is both diagnostic and therapeutic. However, given that first-generation antihistamines impact the upper airway and central nervous system, the actual cause of cough cannot be confirmed with the resolution of symptoms after empiric treatment.

| **Box 1** |
| **Types of rhinitis** |
| Nonallergic Rhinitis
• Vasomotor Rhinitis
• Nonallergic Rhinitis with Eosinophilia |
| Rhinitis due to Anatomic Abnormalities |
| Rhinitis due to Physical or Chemical Irritants |
| Occupational Rhinitis |
| Rhinitis Medicamentosa |
| Rhinitis of Pregnancy |

Differential Diagnosis

There is some variability in the definition of rhinitis in the literature. Based on definitions from the Allergic Rhinitis and its Impact on Asthma and the American Academy of Allergy, Asthma, and Immunology, rhinitis is described as one or more symptoms present for greater than 4 weeks including nasal congestion, rhinorrhea (anterior or posterior), sneezing, or itching.[2] Two of the more common types of rhinitis are allergic rhinitis and nonallergic rhinitis. Allergic rhinitis is an immunoglobulin E (IgE)-mediated response to aeroallergens which leads to a histamine release. The diagnosis is confirmed using skin prick testing or radioallergosorbent testing. Nonallergic rhinitis is diagnosed in patients with symptoms for at least 1 hour per day, with no signs of nasal infection and negative skin prick or serum testing for aeroallergens. Nonallergic rhinitis conditions such as vasomotor rhinitis and nonallergic rhinitis with eosinophilia (NARES) are often found in UACS patients. Vasomotor rhinitis is primarily a clinical diagnosis associated with clear rhinorrhea and boggy nasal mucosa triggered by thermal changes, odorants, spicy foods, and alcohol ingestion. In NARES, eosinophils in nasal secretions are present and methacholine testing is negative.

There are several other forms of rhinitis which do not have a specific histamine response and may also be associated with UACS (**Box 1**). In addition, anatomic abnormalities such as septal deviation, inferior turbinate hypertrophy, and nasal valve collapse may place patients at risk for rhinitis leading to subsequent rhinosinusitis.

Chronic rhinosinusitis can be associated with chronic cough and UACS, however, the exact role CRS plays in chronic cough is not clearly understood. Evidence of an association between cough and CRS is supported by a radiologic study which looked at sinus plain films findings and the relationship between the presence of sinusitis and cough. They found a positive predictive value of 81% and a negative predictive value of 95% in patients with chronic cough and excess sputum production with abnormal sinus imaging studies. This study suggested chronic rhinosinusitis was responsible for the chronic cough.[7] There are significant limitations to this study based on current advances in radiologic technology and definitive CRS diagnostic guidelines. A later study failed to show causality between sinus mucosal thickening suggestive of CRS and chronic cough.[8] Future studies using updated CRS guidelines and computer topography are needed to confirm this association. CRS is also associated with other cough-related conditions such as asthma and bronchiectasis. Patients with UACS and asthma or bronchiectasis should be worked up to ensure their lower airway conditions are controlled.

Theoretic Pathogenesis of Upper airway cough syndrome

One of the initial theories regarding the association between postnasal drip symptoms and cough hypothesized that secretions originated in the sinonasal cavity and drained down into the lungs triggering a cough. This idea has been challenged by both observational cohort and experimental studies. The pathogenesis of UACS is now postulated to be secondary to factors including postnasal drip, chronic airway inflammation, and sensory neural hypersensitivity. Airway inflammation and neural sensitivity can be localized to both the upper airway and lower airway. However, the exact mechanism which leads to chronic cough has not been clearly delineated in the literature.

Therapeutic Options

If UACS is associated with a specific condition, such as GERD, uncontrolled asthma, or bronchiectasis, then treatment should be targeted toward that underlying condition. However, if there is no clear etiology, empiric therapy should be instituted. UACS secondary to rhinitis or CRS may require additional therapy if symptoms are not controlled with empiric treatment.

Much like the acceptance of UACS as a diagnosis, many countries have different preferences for the first-line treatment of this condition. In the United States, decongestants are recommended as part of dual therapy regardless of associated conditions such as allergic rhinitis, nonallergic rhinitis, and chronic rhinosinusitis. Decongestants are thought to limit the secretory responses to inflammatory cytokines. For patients with allergic rhinitis (AR), new-generation (nonsedating) antihistamines such as cetirizine, loratadine, and fexofenadine are recommended, whereas those with non-allergic rhinitis (NAR) or CRS should be treated with first-generation (sedating) antihistamines. It is suggested that the anticholinergic effect of first-generation antihistamines plays a significant role in NAR and CRS patients compared with those with AR. Lee and colleagues performed a systematic review to examine chronic cough treatment outcomes with the use of nonsedating antihistamines. Based on four RCTs, patients with asthma and allergic rhinitis are less likely to respond to nonsedating antihistamines compared with non-asthmatic AR patients.[9] The national guidelines published by various respiratory and allergy and immunology societies from European, German, Italian, and British respiratory societies have various recommendations for first-line therapy, from monotherapy to listing of multiple medication options. Specific national and international recommendations can be found in **Table 1**.

UACS associated with conditions other than allergic rhinitis may have additional treatment options if antihistamines and decongestant (A/d) therapy fails. Vasomotor rhinitis with an associated cough should improve with A/d due to the anticholinergic effects of first-generation antihistamines. If patients have a contraindication to this therapy or desire alternative delivery of medication, ipratropium bromide nasal spray can be used. Post-viral cough due to viral upper respiratory infection may also benefit from first-generation A/ds. However, if this fails, montelukast has been shown to improve post-viral cough. Chronic rhinosinusitis symptoms should be treated with nasal saline, topical nasal corticosteroids, and short-term antibiotics, if appropriate.[10] Endoscopic sinus surgery may be required if there is failure of medical therapy.

Currently, there are no data supporting a specific dosage and time duration for medical therapy with nonsedating or sedating H1-histamine receptor antagonist. This makes the decision to treat empirically with a sedating antihistamine more challenging given the potential side effects of fatigue, vision change, and cognitive impairment. Although there is no standard duration of medical therapy, two studies have investigated cough

Table 1 Treatment recommendations for upper airway cough syndrome based on country	
United States	AR: Nonsedating antihistamine/decongestant NAR: Sedating antihistamine/decongestant CRS: Sedating antihistamine/decongestant; nasal steroid spray, antibiotics if appropriate
United Kingdom	AR: Nasal steroid spray
Europe	AR: Nonsedating antihistamine/decongestant
Japan[24]	AR: Nasal steroid spray/antihistamine UACS only nasal steroid spray
Australia	AR: Antihistamine CRS: Nasal steroid spray/antibiotic if appropriate
China	AR: Nasal steroid spray/antihistamine, decongestant if appropriate NAR: Sedating antihistamine/decongestant CRS: Nasal steroid spray; sedating antihistamine/decongestant; macrolide therapy; antibiotic if appropriate

score improvement at separate times. Ciprandi and colleagues looked at 20 patients with cough and AR defined as rhinoconjunctivitis. Patients were treated with loratadine for 4 weeks with assessment of cough frequency and intensity. They noted significant improvement in both variables compared with placebo by the end of the study period.[11] Shioya and colleagues looked at patients with chronic cough and associated eosinophilic bronchitis or atopic cough. They found a significant improvement in cough symptoms with the use of nonsedating antihistamine at 1 week.[12]

Postnasal Drip

Postnasal drip is considered to be an external stimulus which leads to nasal inflammation. One hypothesis suggest that nasal inflammation triggered by postnasal drip leads to signaling of the spinal trigeminal tract and nucleus tractus solitaries (nTS), through the nasociliary nerve of the trigeminal nerve. The nTS is believed to be activated by afferent stimulation from the nucleus of the spinal trigeminal tract leading to signaling of the vagus nerve in the lower airway and generation of a neurogenic inflammation and cough.[13] Evidence of this mechanism was noted in a previous animal study, which found that the degree of nasal inflammation positively correlated with cough.[14]

Conversely, evidence supporting postnasal drip as a cause of chronic cough from a clinical standpoint has been more controversial. It has been reported that a subset of patients with UACS do not complain of postnasal drip, whereas other studies have noted that only a small number of patients with PND complain of cough. Ohara and colleagues looked at 108 patients with rhinitis/rhinosinusitis who complained of symptoms of postnasal drip. In this patient population, only 21% of patients complained of cough. Additionally, of the 23 patients who reported cough symptoms, only 8% had concomitant postnasal drip.[15] Bardin placed radionuclide material in the maxillary sinus and 24 hours later identified the areas in which the radionuclide had migrated. This material was detected in multiple locations including the maxillary sinus, nasopharynx, esophagus, and gastrointestinal tract. However, none of the participants were noted to have radionuclide in their pulmonary aspirate.[16] This study suggests that the chronic cough noted in UACS is not triggered by sinonasal secretions that are aspirated into the lungs. Importantly, this suggestion does not consider those with a risk of aspiration, such as elderly patients and those with a history of cerebrovascular accident.

Sensory Neural Hypersensitivity

Cough reflex is initiated by the vagal sensory neurons located on the nodose and jugular ganglion of the airway. The sensory nerve fibers terminate in and under the airway epithelium and detect irritant signaling entering the airway. Some have theorized that upper airway secretions signal a chemical, thermal, or mechanical response which elicits the cough seen in UACS. Irritant signaling is predominately mediated by unmyelinated C-fibers. These C-fibers are sensitive to a large number of chemical and inhaled mediators, including capsaicin. Capsaicin receptors are found on transient receptor potential vanilloid 1 (TRPV1) which is highly expressed on sensory afferent nerve fibers of the airway. These nerve fibers innervate both the upper and lower airways.[17] Capsaicin and histamine are both mediators that increase cough sensitivity, but do not directly produce cough. In allergic rhinitis patients, capsaicin stimulates rhinitis symptoms more than in healthy controls leading to subsequent increase in cough sensitivity.[18,19] Mechanical stimulants are mediated by myelinated A-delta cough receptors. These receptors are responsive to rapid changes in pH, and some suggest that the repeated mechanical act of coughing leads to airway inflammation.[17] Mechanical and physical stimuli release growth factors such as transforming growth factor beta2, epidermal growth factor, and nerve growth factor.[18] Increased levels of these growth factors have been correlated with an upregulation in the expression of TRPV1 and cough sensitivity.

Chronic Inflammation

It is hypothesized that chronic inflammation, especially of the lower airway, is a cause of cough in UACS. Niimi and colleagues reviewed the literature on the histologic structure of patients with various causes of lower airway inflammation and chronic cough. This review noted an increase in mast cells, neutrophils, and lymphocytes infiltrates compared with healthy controls. From this observation, Niimi and colleagues suggested that the chronic cough seen is UACS was associated with long-term airway inflammation.[20] Hara and colleagues replicated the effect of chronic cough using guinea pigs. Mechanically induced airway collapse resulted in airway inflammation with an increase in capsaicin cough sensitivity and bronchoalveolar lavage (BAL) neutrophil count.[21] However, this study was limited due to the lack of pathology to correlate with the elevation in neutrophils seen in the BAL.

Some studies suggest that chronic inflammation of the pharynx and tonsils are associated with UACS. These studies theorize that persistent and repetitive exposure to nasal secretions leads to localized inflammation. This hypothesis was weakened after a study by Yu and colleagues looking at patients with UACS versus healthy patients and those with rhinitis/sinusitis without cough. Patients were given different concentrations of capsaicin to induce a cough. This threshold was lowest in UACS patients. Once lidocaine was used to anesthetize the region in order to block the afferent stimulation, UACS patients still required lower concentrations of capsaicin to induce a cough, suggesting cough hypersensitivity localized to the lower airway.[22] Additionally, Bucca and colleagues evaluated the impact of laryngeal hyperresponsiveness (LHR) on patients with asthma, GERD, and rhinitis/CRS (UACS), by looking for vocal cord adduction on an inhaled histamine challenge. The histamine challenge led to local inflammation from stimulated secretions with 76% of patients with UACS demonstrating LHR.[23]

Future Directions

Recently, a new paradigm of clinical cough was proposed. Cough hypersensitivity syndrome (CHS) which is triggered by thermal, mechanical, or chemical exposure, is a clinical entity in which cough is the most significant symptom. It encompasses many of the diseases and conditions commonly associated with chronic cough including asthma, GERD, medications, and chronic lung disease. UACS is also considered to be within the paradigm of CHS.[24,25] Future studies focused on diagnostic testing to differentiate the impact of various conditions within CHS on chronic cough would be beneficial. Targeted therapy to specific receptors, such as TRVP1, may also improve symptoms in patients refractory to antihistamine and decongestant therapy.

SUMMARY

UACS, formerly known as postnasal drip syndrome, is one of the most common causes of chronic cough. This syndrome was described over 100 years ago but there is still no objective physical examination or pathognomonic findings that can help diagnose the condition. UACS is thus a diagnosis of exclusion, when asthma, GERD, and other commone conditions have been ruled out. Empiric treatment with H1 receptor antagonist and decongestant is both diagnostic and therapeutic. However, there are variations in treatment recommendations based on the country. The pathogenesis is also unclear as UACS is frequently associated with other conditions, such as allergic rhinitis, nonallergic rhinitis, and chronic rhinosinusitis. Additionally, other comorbidities including asthma and gastroesophageal reflux disease often make the determination of the impact of UACS on chronic cough more difficult.

CLINICS CARE POINTS

- Upper airway cough syndrome (UACS) is a clinical diagnosis of exclusion with no diagnostic testing or objective findings.
- Diagnosis is confirmed based on resolution of symptoms with treatment.
- Treatment includes dual therapy with H1 receptor antihistamines and decongestants. However, recommendations may vary based on the country.
- UACS can be isolated or secondary to rhinitis or chronic rhinosinusitis.
- UACS associated with nonallergic rhinitis and chronic rhinosinusitis should be treated with first-generation (sedating) antihistamines because of its anticholinergic effects.
- UACS associated with allergic rhinitis should be treated with nonsedating (second-generation) antihistamines. Other AR medications including intranasal corticosteroid sprays, nasal antihistamine spray, and leukotriene inhibitors may be considered.
- UACS may be associated with other conditions including gastroesophageal reflux disease, asthma, and bronchiectasis.

REFERENCES

1. Song WJ, Chang YS, Faruqi S, et al. The global epidemiology of chronic cough in adults: a systematic review and meta-analysis. Eur Respir J 2015;45(5):1479–81.
2. Dąbrowska M, Arcimowicz M, Grabczak EM, et al. Chronic cough related to the upper airway cough syndrome: one entity but not always the same. Eur Arch Otorhinolaryngol 2020;277(10):2753–9.
3. Pratter MR. Chronic upper airway cough syndrome secondary to rhinosinus diseases (previously referred to as postnasal drip syndrome): ACCP evidence-based clinical practice guidelines. Chest 2006;129(1 Suppl):63S–71S.

4. Irwin RS, French CL, Chang AB, et al. CHEST Expert Cough Panel*. Classification of Cough as a Symptom in Adults and Management Algorithms: CHEST Guideline and Expert Panel Report. Chest 2018;153(1):196–209.

5. Watelet JB, Van Zele T, Brusselle G. Chronic cough in upper airway diseases. Respir Med 2010;104(5):652–7.

6. Sanu A, Eccles R. Postnasal drip syndrome. Two hundred years of controversy between UK and USA. Rhinology 2008;86.

7. Irwin RS, Curley FS, French FL. Chronic cough: the spectrum and frequency of causes, key components of the diagnostic evaluation, and outcome of specific therapy. Am Rev Respir Dis 1990;141:640–7.

8. Pratter MR, Bartter T, Lotano R. The role of sinus imaging in the treatment of chronic cough in adults. Chest 1999;116(5):1287–91.

9. Lee JH, Lee JW, An J, et al. Efficacy of non-sedating H1-receptor antihistamines in adults and adolescents with chronic cough: a systematic review. World Allergy Organ J 2021;14(8):100568.

10. Orlandi RR, Kingdom TT, Smith TL, et al. International consensus statement on allergy and rhinology: rhinosinusitis 2021. Int Forum Allergy Rhinol 2021;11(3): 213–739.

11. Ciprandi G, Buscaglia S, Catrullo A, et al. Loratadine in the treatment of cough associated with allergic rhinoconjunctivitis. Ann Allergy Asthma Immunol 1995; 75(2):115–20.

12. Shioya T, Satake M, Kagaya M, et al. Antitussive effects of the H1-receptor antagonist epinastine in patients with atopic cough (eosinophilic bronchitis). Arzneimittelforschung 2004;54(4):207–12.

13. Yu L, Xu X, Lv H, et al. Advances in upper airway cough syndrome. Kaohsiung J Med Sci 2015;31(5):223–8.

14. Brozmanova M, Bartos V, Plank L, et al. Experimental allergic rhinitis-related cough and airway eosinophilia in sensitized guinea pigs. J Physiol Pharmacol 2007;58(Suppl 5 Pt 1):57–65.

15. O'Hara J, Jones NS. "Post-nasal drip syndrome": most patients with purulent nasal secretions do not complain of chronic cough. Rhinology 2006;44(4):270–3.

16. Bardin PG, Van Heerden BB, Joubert JR. Absence of pulmonary aspiration of sinus contents in patients with asthma and sinusitis. J Allergy Clin Immunol 1990; 86:82–8.

17. Lucanska M, Hajtman A, Calkovsky V, et al. Upper airway cough syndrome in pathogenesis of chronic cough. Physiol Res 2020;69(Suppl 1):S35–42.

18. Kowalski ML, Dietrich-Miłobedzki A, Majkowska-Wojciechowska B, et al. Nasal reactivity to capsaicin in patients with seasonal allergic rhinitis during and after the pollen season. Allergy 1999;54(8):804–10.

19. O'Hanlon S, Facer P, Simpson KD, et al. Neuronal markers in allergic rhinitis: expression and correlation with sensory testing. Laryngoscope 2007;117(9): 1519–27.

20. Niimi A, Torrego A, Nicholson AG, et al. Nature of airway inflammation and remodeling in chronic cough. J Allergy Clin Immunol 2005;116(3):565–70.

21. Hara J, Fujimura M, Ueda A, et al. Effect of pressure stress applied to the airway on cough-reflex sensitivity in Guinea pigs. Am J Respir Crit Care Med 2008; 177(6):585–92.

22. Yu L, Xu X, Wang L, et al. Capsaicin-sensitive cough receptors in lower airway are responsible for cough hypersensitivity in patients with upper airway cough syndrome. Med Sci Monit 2013;19:1095–101.

23. Bucca CB, Bugiani M, Culla B, et al. Chronic cough and irritable larynx. J Allergy Clin Immunol 2011;127(2):412–9.
24. Morice AH, Millqvist E, Belvisi MG, et al. Expert opinion on the cough hypersensitivity syndrome in respiratory medicine. Eur Respir J 2014;44:1132–48.
25. Yasuda, K. Upper airway cough syndrome may be the main cause of chronic cough in Japan: a cohort study, Fam Pract, Volume 38, 6, December 2021, Pages 751–757.

Unified Airway Disease

Medical Management

Eamon Shamil, MBBS, MRes, FRCS (ORL-HNS)[a,b,*],
Claire Hopkins, DM, FRCS (ORL-HNS)[a,c]

KEYWORDS

- Chronic rhinosinusitis • Nasal polyps • Asthma • Unified airway disease

KEY POINTS

- Patients with type 2 inflammatory disease commonly have concurrent disease in the upper and lower airways, namely chronic rhinosinusitis with nasal polyps and asthma.
- Systemic oral corticosteroids are commonly used to treat both conditions—physicians must be mindful of the potential cumulative risk of adverse events.
- Biologics targeting type 2 inflammation will likely have a beneficial effect on both upper and lower airways, although the magnitude of the effect may differ between both.

INTRODUCTION

Chronic rhinosinusitis (CRS) and asthma are inflammatory disorders of the upper and lower airways, respectively. They have a shared pathophysiology, and hence the description *"unified airway disease."* Their relationship is bidirectional, and they frequently coexist[1]; 20% to 25% of patients with CRS have asthma, whereas to 5% to 10% of asthmatics have CRS.[2] The prevalence of asthma is even higher if patients have CRS with nasal polyps (CRSwNP; range 40%–60%), which is associated with more severe asthma and poorer lung function,[3,4] a lower forced expiratory flow per second (FEV) and a steeper slope of FEV1 against age, equivalent to smoking 1 to 2 packs of cigarettes per day.[5]

The underlying pathophysiology that mediates most cases of CRSwNP and asthma is characterized by eosinophilia and elevated levels of the proeosinophilic cytokines interleukin (IL)-4, IL-5, IL-13, and immunoglobulin E (IgE).[6] This is termed type 2 pattern of inflammation, and is seen in 80% of Caucasian patients with CRSwNP, and up to 94% of patients with comorbid asthma[7]; a combination of nasal polyps, asthma, and a blood eosinophil greater than 300 cells/mm^3 further increases the likelihood.[7]

[a] Guy's and St Thomas' NHS Foundation Trust, London, United Kingdom; [b] ENT Department, Guy's Hospital, Great Maze Pond, London SE1 9RT, United Kingdom; [c] King's College London, United Kingdom
* Corresponding author.
E-mail address: eamon.shamil@nhs.net

Otolaryngol Clin N Am 56 (2023) 157–168
https://doi.org/10.1016/j.otc.2022.09.012
0030-6665/23/© 2022 Elsevier Inc. All rights reserved.
oto.theclinics.com

Non-type 2 inflammation is more commonly linked with CRS without nasal polyps (CRSsNP), and in CRSwNP in patients from Asian countries,[8] which is driven by neutrophils and IL-17 subunits, although this is changing over time.[8–10] There is also a group of patients who phenotypically have CRSsNP, but endotypically have type 2 inflammatory disease. This group accounts for 30% to 55% of patients with type 2 inflammation and is associated with the loss of smell and asthma.[11–13]

In summary, type 2 inflammatory disease can manifest as CRS with or without polyps, and should be considered in any patient with hyposmia and comorbid asthma. Current guidelines advocate CRS treatment decisions based on biological endotype, namely type 2 or non-type 2 inflammation,[14] whereas much of the evidence base on which their recommendations are based have usually grouped all CRS patients together, or defined patients by presence or absence of nasal polyps.[15]

In this article, we will discuss the range of medical therapies for CRS in the setting of combined upper and lower airway disease. Where it exists, we will discuss how treatment of the upper airway affects the control of lower airway disease. These treatments discussed include intranasal corticosteroids (INCSs), oral corticosteroids (OCSs), antibiotics, and biological therapies. We will report where data or recommendations refer to specific subgroups based on endotype, if possible, or phenotype.

INTRANASAL CORTICOSTEROIDS AND NASAL IRRIGATION

INCSs and nasal saline irrigation are considered the first-line treatment of mild CRSwNP.[14,16] Nasal saline irrigation is recommended in most guidelines because it is inexpensive and has a low side-effect profile; however, evidence from randomized control trials (RCTs) is limited.[17]

Second generation INCSs, such as fluticasone and mometasone, are safe for long-term use, without treatment breaks, as their systemic bioavailability is less than 1%,[18] whereas first-generation INCSs, such as beclomethasone, are best avoided, particularly in patients taking inhaled corticosteroids.

A Cochrane review showed that patients who use INCS experience moderate symptom improvement in terms of nasal obstruction, rhinorrhea, and loss of sense of smell.[19] Higher doses of INCSs, often given in the form of drops, may further improve disease severity but the evidence quality is low.[18] There is a low incidence of adverse events, with nasal irritation and epistaxis being the most common. However, problems arise around poor patient compliance, and ineffective dosing. A retrospective review, which evaluated more than 19,000 patients in Canada, found that the overall INCS utilisation was 20% of the population, with a mean dose of just 2.4 bottles per year.[20] Thus, patient education regarding the importance of continued use of their medication, along with the correct delivery techniques is essential. In our experience, patients are often concerned about long-term topical steroid side effects, particularly when taking additional steroid-based medications for asthma, so taking time to allay these fears may pay long-term dividends.

A small number of studies have sought to determine if CRS treatment with INCSs can improve asthma control. In a multicenter, double-blind, placebo-controlled RCT of 388 adults and children with inadequately controlled asthma and chronic rhinitis or sinusitis,[21] Dixon and colleagues[21] found that 24 weeks of INCSs (mometasone) had a small effect at reducing asthma and sinus symptom scores, without improving lung function, asthma quality of life or episodes of poorly controlled asthma. Therefore, although INCSs form an essential component of treating CRSwNP, their impact on asthma may be limited. Patients with CRSwNP are more likely to have severe comorbid asthma, so their lower airway should be closely monitored for deterioration and managed in a multidisciplinary setting with a respiratory physician.

Different methods have been used in order to enhance topical nasal steroid delivery including irrigation, exhalation delivery systems (EDSs) and sinus-eluting stents.[18] A meta-analysis has shown high-volume, low-pressure nasal steroid irrigation to be effective and safe in patients with varying CRS endotypes and phenotypes.[22] A multicenter RCT found that mometasone delivered by high-volume nasal irrigation (240 mL) achieved better postoperative endoscopic and radiological control, in CRS patients at 12 months, compared with the same dose delivered as a nasal sprays.[23] The effectiveness of INCSs is enhanced in patients after surgery, with steroid irrigations used primarily in postoperative patients to achieve delivery into the open cavities.[23,24] However, a recent RCT has shown that budesonide irrigation also benefited patients with no history of surgery, more than patients after surgery.[25] There is no evidence to suggest suppression of the hypothalamic–pituitary–adrenal axis in patients receiving mometasone[26] (4 mg daily for 12 weeks) or budesonide[27] (2 mg daily for 12 months), via nasal irrigation.

The EDS with fluticasone (EDS-FLU) improves distribution of INCS in the upper posterior regions of the nasal cavity when compared with conventional spray pump delivery and achieved improvement in nasal congestion, polyp grade and quality of life,[28,29] in patients who were considered uncontrolled on standard INCS. Adverse events were similar to nasal sprays, including epistaxis, erythema, and acute sinusitis.

Steroid-eluting sinus stents may be sited into the sinonasal cavity before or after endoscopic sinus surgery. The majority of studies have tested their postoperative effect; a meta-analysis of seven industry-funded trials showed reduced postoperative intervention, revision sinus surgery, nasal polyp recurrence, and frontal sinus stenosis.[30] The follow-up period was short, and independent studies with longer term follow-up are recommended. In the setting of patients with nasal polyp recurrence after endoscopic sinus surgery, the RESOLVE I and II sham-controlled RCTs showed that mometasone eluting ethmoid sinus stents reduced the need for further surgery, with improvement in nasal obstruction and smell[31–34]; they also had a good safety profile. Evidence is now emerging for the use of steroid-eluting stents in CRS patients before considering sinus surgery. A phase 1 study showed that steroid-eluting stents inserted in patients with CRSwNP and CRSsNP, *without* a history of sinus surgery, had improvement in SNOT-22 quality of life questionnaire at 24 weeks.[35]

SYSTEMIC ORAL CORTICOSTEROIDS

Systemic OCSs have been shown to downregulate eosinophils and their associated mediators IL-4 and IL-5, which incurs a benefit in type-2 CRSwNP; they are less effective in nontype-2 nasal polyps and CRSsNP.[36] Therefore, a short course of systemic OCSs may be considered in patients with CRSwNP, when INCSs and saline irrigation has failed. Short-term courses of OCSs (<4 weeks) reduce polyp size, symptom severity and improve health-related quality of life, as described by a Cochrane review of eight placebo-controlled RCTs.[37] The ideal dose and duration of OCS is unclear but dosages in the region of 0.5 mg/kg/day, with a maximum daily dose of 60 mg for 5 to 21 days have been used in trials. However, the benefit of systemic steroids is short-lived in many patients, with little or no improvement 3 to 6 months after the end of the course of OCSs.[37]

Immediate adverse events include a higher incidence of gastrointestinal side effects, mood disturbance and insomnia. Repeated use must be carefully weighed up against potential cumulative risks of adverse events. A large retrospective cohort study of patients with asthma who had been prescribed OCSs, found a dose-dependent relationship for adverse outcomes; a cumulative lifetime exposure of as little as 4 courses (1 gram) of OCSs is enough to increase the risk of adverse events, including type 2 diabetes.[20,38] A longitudinal study, which evaluated patients for more than four years, investigated the effect of inhaled and systemic OCSs on bone density in asthmatic patients. Those who had more than 2.5 courses (3–14 days) per year suffered larger loss in bone mineral density.[39] Another concern of patients is the risk of immunosuppression and infection associated with OCS; a review of more than 4000 patients showed that cumulative doses of 700 mg or a daily dose of 10 mg prednisolone has no increased risk of infection complications.[40] One study has suggested that the risk of OCSs exceeds endoscopic sinus surgery when prescribed more frequently than once every year, in the setting of concurrent CRSwNP and asthma.[41]

Short-term relief from OCS may be sought after during major life events, such as wedding or high-stakes examinations, but may leave patients frustrated with poor symptom control for large parts of the year. OCS can also be used to avoid the need for further sinus surgery, where this is the patient's preference, or if they are unfit for a general anaesthetic. Studies have suggested that OCS can help avoid surgery in patients with CRSwNP.[42,43]

Prescribing systemic OCS should be individualized to a patient's clinical history and comorbidities, with a comprehensive discussion regarding the benefits and risks described above. Clinicians must consider that patients may receive short-courses for both upper and lower airways. When a patient is prescribed two or more courses of OCS in a single year, alternatives such as sinus surgery or biologics should be considered.

ANTIBIOTICS

The significance of the sinus microbiome as a direct driver of CRS and asthma is unclear. Questions remain about its link with acute exacerbations and secondary inflammation. There is evidence to suggest that patients with CRS are more likely to have greater airway remodelling and *Staphylococcus aureus* colonization. *S aureus* exotoxins act as superantigens may be isolated in up to 50% of CRSwNP.[44] Nasal colonization of same microorganism has also been linked to asthma pathogenesis through a meta-analysis.[45]

Although the main role of antibiotics in current guidelines is for acute exacerbations of CRS,[14] there is some evidence to support their use to help achieve better disease control outside of acute infections.

There have been various studies evaluating the effect of doxycycline or macrolides in CRSwNP, in patients with and without a history of sinus surgery. An RCT evaluating the use of 12 weeks of doxycycline in CRSwNP patients who had undergone endoscopic sinus surgery found that doxycycline improved quality of life outcomes and Lund-Kennedy scores[46]; patients who showed improvement tended to have normal pretreatment IgE and eosinophil counts, and a significantly lower prevalence of asthma and non-steroidal anti-inflammatory drug (NSAID)-exacerbated respiratory disease (which are associated with type 2 inflammatory disease). Another RCT compared 3 weeks of doxycycline was compared with oral steroids in a placebo-controlled RCT in CRSwNP (including, but not exclusively, postoperative patients), and shown to achieve a small but more durable reduction in polyp size compared with methylprednisolone.[47] Macrolides have also been studied in CRSwNP; long-term postoperative therapy (up to 12 weeks) has also been shown to reduce early polyp recurrence at 24 weeks compared with placebo.[48]

Wallwork and colleagues published a double-blind RCT that excluded patients with nasal polyposis. They showed macrolide benefit in CRS was only seen after 12 weeks of therapy but importantly, this was not sustained 12 weeks after cessation.[49] There was a greater effect in patients with normal levels of IgE, suggesting that benefit would be less likely to be found in patients with Type 2 inflammation.

Currently, long-term antibiotics have a limited role in the ongoing management of CRSwNP; prescribers should consider the impact on antibiotic resistance. The ongoing placebo-controlled RCT, Management for Adults with Chronic RhinOsinusitis (MACRO), will help to establish the role of long-term macrolides and sinus surgery, in CRS with and without nasal polyps.[50]

BIOLOGICS

The shared underlying pathophysiology of CRSwNP and asthma provides the rationale for biologics, which provide a targeted, systemic treatment against the type 2 inflammatory pathway in patients who have failed optimal medical $\pm$ surgical therapy. A recent pragmatic RCT comparing medical treatment (excluding biologics) and sinus surgery for CRSwNP, highlighted the relatively poor outcomes of conventional treatment strategies, with only 4% of those patients receiving medical treatment being controlled at 12 months, whereas 63% were uncontrolled.[51] Patients with CRSwNP and comorbid asthma are more likely to be uncontrolled, concerning both their upper and lower airway diseases, when compared with those without comorbidity.[52]

Currently there are three U.S. Food and Drug Administration (FDA)-approved and European Medicines Agency (EMA)-approved biologics for use in patients with severe CRSwNP: dupilumab, mepolizumab, and omalizumab.[53–55]

Dupilumab is an anti-IL-4 receptor-alpha monoclonal antibody. It has been shown to improve nasal polyp score, nasal congestion, loss of smell, Sino-Nasal Outcome Test-22 (SNOT-22) scores, radiological disease severity, serum IgE, and tissue eosinophil count in patients with severe CRSwNP enrolled in the SINUS24 and SINUS52 trials[56–58]; FEV1 and asthma control were also improved.[56] Patients who experienced nasal polyp recurrence most quickly (less than 3 years postoperatively), derived greater benefit than those who had surgery 10 years ago. The QUEST study also evaluated the effect of dupilumab given fortnightly for 1 year in patients with severe asthma and comorbid CRS (with and without nasal polyps).[59] Patients experienced an improvement in general health, quality of life, smell, and nasal obstruction from 12 weeks; this was sustained at 52 weeks.[59] Patients previously considered difficult to treat (eg, those with NSAID-exacerbated respiratory disease,[60] severe asthma, or multiple surgeries) have been shown to benefit from dupilumab. Real-life registry data support significant improvement in disease control and reduced the need for sinonasal surgery.[61]

Mepolizumab is an anti-IL-5 monoclonal antibody. The SYNAPSE study found that nasal polyp score and nasal congestion improved with mepolizumab; patients who had one sinus surgery saw some improvement in smell, whereas those with more than two earlier sinus surgeries did not derive benefit.[62] A Cochrane review of 137 patients who were treated with mepolizumab, concluded that although SNOT-22 scores improved at 6 months, there was uncertainty about the difference in disease severity.[58]

Reslizumab and benralizumab also target the IL-5-alpha receptor, although neither of them are currently licenced for use in CRSwNP. In two RCTs of patients with inadequately controlled asthma and self-reported CRSwNP, reslizumab reduced acute exacerbations of asthma and improved FEV1 during 52 weeks[63,64]; however, these studies did not assess CRSwNP-related outcomes and relied on self-reporting a diagnosis of CRSwNP. The OSTRO phase 3 RCT demonstrated limited clinical effectiveness of benralizumab in CRSwNP patients who had previous OCS and/or sinus surgery[65]; specifically there was no improvement in SNOT-22 scores, the use of

OCS and time to first sinus surgery, although there was improvement in sense of smell and nasal polyp score.

Omalizumab, an anti-IgE monoclonal antibody, has been shown to significantly reduce nasal congestion, polyp size, and SNOT-22 at 24 weeks in two randomized phase 3 trials.[66] A Cochrane review of 329 patients who were treated with omalizumab reported improvement in SNOT-22 scores at six months, although there was no evidence on disease severity.[58]

In terms of adverse events, omalizumab, mepolizumab, and dupilumab are well tolerated, with little difference in adverse events compared with the placebo group.[58] Dupilumab is most commonly associated with injection site reaction/swelling in 6%.[54] For mepolizumab, adverse events include oropharyngeal pain in 8%, and arthralgia in 6% of patients.[53,62] The commonest adverse events of omalizumab are headaches in 8% and injection site reaction in 5.2% of patients.[54]

Biologics are now incorporated into treatment guidelines for severe, uncontrolled type 2 inflammatory disease, including European Position Paper on Rhinosinusitis and Nasal Polyps (EPOS) 2020,[14] and European Forum for Research and Education in Allergy and Airway Disease (EUFOREA).[67] Such guidelines recognize the added benefit of treating those with comorbid asthma, and the importance of managing patients in a multidisciplinary setting. Current guidance attempts to define markers for type 2 inflammation (eg, tissue eosinophils 10/HPF or greater or blood eosinophils 250 mm or greater,[3] total IgE 100kU/L or greater); however, further research is required to accurately predict those who will respond ahead of trial of treatment.

There are currently no head-to-head studies comparing the biologics and the patient groups and outcomes vary between studies making comparison difficult. However, both the Cochrane review and a recent network meta-analysis suggest that based on safety and efficacy, dupilumab is currently the best choice for patients with CRSwNP.[58,68]

Clinically, there seems to be a mismatch between the effectiveness of some of the other biologics in the upper and lower airways; we have observed that while many patients report significant improvement in asthma control, they remain uncontrolled with respect to their sinus disease. A recent Mayo Clinic review of patients with biologics for asthma with comorbid CRS found that 17% of patients receiving mepolizumab, reslizumab, or benralizumab still required sinus surgery, whereas 28% of those receiving omalizumab underwent surgery after starting their biologic therapy.[57] One study evaluating patients undergoing treatment with mepolizumab found reduced tissue eosinophil counts but elevated sinonasal tissue levels of type 2 cytokines including IL-4, IL-5, and IL-13, suggesting the possibility of a local inflammatory feedback look that may explain the limited clinical responses seen.[69] It is likely that "downstream" inhibition of the type 2 pathway by a single agent may be suboptimal as redundancy of the pathway exists; although one receptor is inhibited, another may become activated.

One of the major limitations of biologic therapy for CRSwNP is lack of cost-effectiveness relative to current treatment pathways, due to the high cost per injection and apparent lack if any disease modifying effect.[70] Once treatment is withdrawn, recurrence of nasal polyps and symptoms occur, although there may be scope to reduce the maintenance dose of a biologic in a patient with controlled disease.[61,71] A Markov model from the United States, which compared dupilumab and endoscopic sinus surgery, predicted that the biologic is 10 times more expensive per quality-adjusted life-year (QALY); the limitations of the study include an underestimate of the direct and indirect cost of surgery, and not accounting for indirect benefits of biologics such as reduced costs from better asthma control, or fewer complications due to less administration of systemic OCS.[72] A cost-effectiveness analysis comparing dupilumab with sinus surgery followed by aspirin desensitization in patients with CRSwNP and AERD also found dupilumab was less cost-effective.[73] For this reason, most guidelines recommend the use of biologics in patients with recurrent disease after endoscopic sinus surgery.

FUTURE DIRECTIONS

Further data from head-to-head clinical trials comparing different biologics with each other, as well as combinations of biologics with surgery, will help guide future therapy and determine their place in treatment algorithms. Biomarkers will also help to prognosticate the administration of biologics, in a manner that is individual to a patient's underlying pathophysiology. This can potentially reduce costs by avoiding administration of biologics that would not work a particular patient, and by reducing the burden of failed medical therapy, potentially therefore increasing market access. Ongoing research will help to identify the optimum point of inhibition of the inflammatory cascade and facilitate the development of future interventions that will achieve adequate disease control of both the upper and lower airways.

SUMMARY

Unified airway disease describes the type 2 inflammation that drives CRSwNP and co-morbid asthma. These patients are more likely to have uncontrolled disease. A clinical algorithm for the multidisciplinary management of the upper and lower airways driven by type 2 inflammation will help identify patients who are likely to benefit from biologics. Head-to-head clinical trials comparing different biologics are required.

SUMMARY

Concurrent CRSwNP in the upper airway, and asthma in the lower airway, often have a shared underlying pathophysiology, namely type 2 inflammation; hence, the term "unified airway disease." The combination of CRSwNP and asthma is associated with uncontrolled disease. The range of treatment of CRSwNP includes INCSs, nasal saline irrigation, OCS, antibiotics, and biologics. Biologics, such as dupilumab, target the type 2 inflammatory pathway, with improvement in upper and lower airway disease control. Head-to-head studies are required to compare different biologics, and establish the magnitude of effect. A combined clinical algorithm for the management of the upper and lower airways in type 2 inflammation will be beneficial, especially for patients with uncontrolled disease who may benefit from biologics.

CLINICS CARE POINTS

- Patients with CRSwNP and comorbid asthma are more likely to be uncontrolled, concerning both their upper and lower airway diseases, when compared with those without comorbidity
- INCS benefit patients with CRSwNP, with limited evidence on the impact of asthma
- Systemic OCS are commonly used to treat both CRSwNP and asthma; physicians should be mindful of the potential cumulative risk of adverse events
- Long-term antibiotics have a limited role in the management of CRSwNP; physicians should consider the effect on antibiotics resistance
- Biologics targeting the type 2 inflammatory disease pathway benefit both the upper and lower airways, although the magnitude of effect may differ between both

DISCLOSURE

- E. Shamil reveals no potential conflict of interest relevant to this article.
- C. Hopkins has received lecture fees from Olympus and fees for serving on an advisory board from Sanofi, GlaxoSmithKline, and Astra Zeneca. No other potential conflict of interest relevant to this article was reported.

REFERENCES

1. Ryu G, Min C, Park B, et al. Bidirectional association between asthma and chronic rhinosinusitis: Two longitudinal follow-up studies using a national sample cohort. Sci Rep 2020;10(1):1–10.
2. Jarvis D, Newson R, Lotvall J, et al. Asthma in adults and its association with chronic rhinosinusitis: the GA2LEN survey in Europe. Allergy 2012;67(1):91–8.
3. Novelli F, Bacci E, Latorre M, et al. Comorbidities are associated with different features of severe asthma. Clin Mol Allergy 2018;16(1). https://doi.org/10.1186/S12948-018-0103-X.
4. Bilodeau L, Boulay MÈ, Prince P, et al. Comparative clinical and airway inflammatory features of asthmatics with or without polyps. Rhinology 2010;48(4):420–5.
5. Obaseki D, Potts J, Joos G, et al. The relation of airway obstruction to asthma, chronic rhinosinusitis and age: results from a population survey of adults. Allergy 2014;69(9):1205.
6. Van Zele T, Claeys S, Gevaert P, et al. Differentiation of chronic sinus diseases by measurement of inflammatory mediators. Allergy 2006;61(11):1280–9.
7. Bachert C, Marple B, Hosemann W, et al. Endotypes of chronic rhinosinusitis with nasal polyps: pathology and possible therapeutic implications. J Allergy Clin Immunol Pract 2020;8(5):1514–9.
8. Zhang N, Van Zele T, Perez-Novo C, et al. Different types of T-effector cells orchestrate mucosal inflammation in chronic sinus disease. J Allergy Clin Immunol 2008;122(5):961–8.
9. Liu Y, Zeng M, Liu Z. Th17 response and its regulation in inflammatory upper airway diseases. Clin Exp Allergy 2015;45(3):602–12.
10. Ghogomu N, Kern R. Chronic rhinosinusitis: the rationale for current treatments. Expert Rev Clin Immunol 2017;13(3):259–70.
11. Stevens WW, Peters AT, Tan BK, et al. Associations between inflammatory endotypes and clinical presentations in chronic rhinosinusitis. J Allergy Clin Immunol Pract 2019;7(8):2812–20.e3.
12. Tomassen P, Vandeplas G, Van Zele T, et al. Inflammatory endotypes of chronic rhinosinusitis based on cluster analysis of biomarkers. J Allergy Clin Immunol 2016;137(5):1449–56.e4.
13. Delemarre T, Holtappels G, De Ruyck N, et al. Type 2 inflammation in chronic rhinosinusitis without nasal polyps: Another relevant endotype. J Allergy Clin Immunol 2020;146(2):337–43.e6.
14. Fokkens W.J., Lund V.J., Hopkins C., et al., European Position Paper on Rhinosinusitis and Nasal Polyps 2020, Rhinology, 58 (Suppl S29), 2020, 1-464.
15. Avdeeva K, Fokkens W. Precision medicine in chronic rhinosinusitis with nasal polyps. Curr Allergy Asthma Rep 2018;18(4). https://doi.org/10.1007/S11882-018-0776-8.
16. Hopkins C. Chronic rhinosinusitis with nasal polyps. N Engl J Med 2019;381(1):55–63.

17. Chong LY, Head K, Hopkins C, et al. Saline irrigation for chronic rhinosinusitis. Cochrane Database Syst Rev 2016;2016(4). https://doi.org/10.1002/14651858. CD011995.pub2.
18. Chong LY, Head K, Hopkins C, et al. Different types of intranasal steroids for chronic rhinosinusitis. Cochrane Database Syst Rev 2016;2016(4). https://doi.org/10.1002/14651858.CD011993.pub2.
19. Chong LY, Head K, Hopkins C, et al. Intranasal steroids versus placebo or no intervention for chronic rhinosinusitis. Cochrane Database Syst Rev 2016; 2016(4). https://doi.org/10.1002/14651858.CD011996.pub2.
20. Rudmik L, Xu Y, Liu M, et al. Utilization patterns of topical intranasal steroid therapy for chronic rhinosinusitis: a canadian population-based analysis. JAMA Otolaryngol Head Neck Surg 2016;142(11):1056–62.
21. Dixon AE, Castro M, Cohen RI, et al. Efficacy of nasal mometasone for the treatment of chronic sinonasal disease in patients with inadequately controlled asthma. J Allergy Clin Immunol 2015;135(3):701–9.e5.
22. Jiramongkolchai P, Patel S, Schneider JS. Use of off-label nasal steroid irrigations in long-term management of chronic rhinosinusitis. Ear Nose Throat J 2021; 100(5):329–34.
23. Harvey RJ, Snidvongs K, Kalish LH, et al. Corticosteroid nasal irrigations are more effective than simple sprays in a randomized double-blinded placebo-controlled trial for chronic rhinosinusitis after sinus surgery. Int Forum Allergy Rhinol 2018;8(4):461–70.
24. Kalish L, Snidvongs K, Sivasubramaniam R, et al. Topical steroids for nasal polyps. Cochrane Database Syst Rev 2012;12:CD006549.
25. Tait S, Kallogjeri D, Suko J, et al. Effect of budesonide added to large-volume, low-pressure saline sinus irrigation for chronic rhinosinusitis: a randomized clinical trial. JAMA Otolaryngol Head Neck Surg 2018;144(7):605.
26. Brown HJ, Batra PS, Eggerstedt M, et al. The possibility of short-term hypothalamic-pituitary-adrenal axis suppression with high-volume, high-dose nasal mometasone irrigation in postsurgical patients with chronic rhinosinusitis. Int Forum Allergy Rhinol 2022;12(3):249–56.
27. Smith KA, French G, Mechor B, et al. Safety of long-term high-volume sinonasal budesonide irrigations for chronic rhinosinusitis. Int Forum Allergy Rhinol 2016; 6(3):228–32.
28. Sindwani R, Han JK, Soteres DF, et al. NAVIGATE I: randomized, placebo-controlled, double-blind trial of the exhalation delivery system with fluticasone for chronic rhinosinusitis with nasal polyps. Am J Rhinol Allergy 2019;33(1): 69–82.
29. Leopold DA, Elkayam D, Messina JC, et al. NAVIGATE II: Randomized, double-blind trial of the exhalation delivery system with fluticasone for nasal polyposis. J Allergy Clin Immunol 2019;143(1):126–34.e5.
30. Goshtasbi K, Abouzari M, Abiri A, et al. Efficacy of steroid eluting stents in management of chronic rhinosinusitis following endoscopic sinus surgery: updated meta-analysis. Int Forum Allergy Rhinol 2019;9(12):1443.
31. Kern RC, Stolovitzky JP, Silvers SL, et al. A phase 3 trial of mometasone furoate sinus implants for chronic sinusitis with recurrent nasal polyps. Int Forum Allergy Rhinol 2018;8(4):471–81.
32. Forwith KD, Han JK, Stolovitzky JP, et al. RESOLVE: bioabsorbable steroid-eluting sinus implants for in-office treatment of recurrent sinonasal polyposis after sinus surgery: 6-month outcomes from a randomized, controlled, blinded study. Int Forum Allergy Rhinol 2016;6(6):573–81.

33. Han JK, Forwith KD, Smith TL, et al. RESOLVE: a randomized, controlled, blinded study of bioabsorbable steroid-eluting sinus implants for in-office treatment of recurrent sinonasal polyposis. Int Forum Allergy Rhinol 2014;4(11):861–70.

34. Han JK, Kern RC. Topical therapies for management of chronic rhinosinusitis: steroid implants. Int Forum Allergy Rhinol 2019;9(S1):S22–6.

35. Douglas RG, Psaltis AJ, Rimmer J, et al. Phase 1 clinical study to assess the safety of a novel drug delivery system providing long-term topical steroid therapy for chronic rhinosinusitis. Int Forum Allergy Rhinol 2019;9(4):378–87.

36. Wen W, Liu W, Zhang L, et al. Increased neutrophilia in nasal polyps reduces the response to oral corticosteroid therapy. J Allergy Clin Immunol 2012;129(6): 1522–8.e5.

37. Head K, Chong LY, Hopkins C, et al. Short-course oral steroids as an adjunct therapy for chronic rhinosinusitis. Cochrane Database Syst Rev 2016;2016(4). https://doi.org/10.1002/14651858.CD011992.pub2.

38. Sullivan PW, Ghushchyan VH, Globe G, et al. Oral corticosteroid exposure and adverse effects in asthmatic patients. J Allergy Clin Immunol 2018;141(1): 110–6.e7.

39. Matsumoto H, Ishihara K, Hasegawa T, et al. Effects of inhaled corticosteroid and short courses of oral corticosteroids on bone mineral density in asthmatic patients : a 4-year longitudinal study. Chest 2001;120(5):1468–73.

40. Stuck AE, Minder CE, Frey FJ. Risk of infectious complications in patients taking glucocorticosteroids. Rev Infect Dis 1989;11(6):954–63.

41. Leung RM, Smith TL, Kern RC, et al. Should oral corticosteroids be used in medical therapy for chronic rhinosinusitis? A risk analysis. Laryngoscope 2021; 131(3):473–81.

42. Lal D, Scianna JM, Stankiewicz JA. Efficacy of targeted medical therapy in chronic rhinosinusitis, and predictors of failure. Am J Rhinol Allergy 2009;23(4): 396–400.

43. Baguley C, Brownlow A, Yeung K, et al. The fate of chronic rhinosinusitis sufferers after maximal medical therapy. Int Forum Allergy Rhinol 2014;4(7):525–32.

44. Ramakrishnan VR, Feazel LM, Abrass LJ, et al. Prevalence and abundance of Staphylococcus aureus in the middle meatus of patients with chronic rhinosinusitis, nasal polyps, and asthma. Int Forum Allergy Rhinol 2013;3(4):267–71.

45. Kim YC, Won HK, Lee JW, et al. Staphylococcus aureus nasal colonization and asthma in adults: systematic review and meta-analysis. J Allergy Clin Immunol Pract 2019;7(2):606–15.e9.

46. Pinto Bezerra Soter AC, Pinto Bezerra TF, Pezato R, et al. Prospective open-label evaluation of long-term low-dose doxycycline for difficult-to-treat chronic rhinosinusitis with nasal polyps. Rhinology 2017;55(2):175–80.

47. Van Zele T, Gevaert P, Holtappels G, et al. Oral steroids and doxycycline: two different approaches to treat nasal polyps. J Allergy Clin Immunol 2010;125(5). https://doi.org/10.1016/J.JACI.2010.02.020.

48. Varvyanskaya A, Lopatin A. Efficacy of long-term low-dose macrolide therapy in preventing early recurrence of nasal polyps after endoscopic sinus surgery. Int Forum Allergy Rhinol 2014;4(7):533–41.

49. Wallwork B, Coman W, Mackay-Sim A, et al. A double-blind, randomized, placebo-controlled trial of macrolide in the treatment of chronic rhinosinusitis. Laryngoscope 2006;116(2):189–93.

50. Workstream 2: The MACRO Programme | Workstream 2: The MACRO Programme. Available at: https://workstream2.themacroprogramme.org.uk/. Accessed May 8, 2022.

51. Lourijsen ES, Reitsma S, Vleming M, et al. Endoscopic sinus surgery with medical therapy versus medical therapy for chronic rhinosinusitis with nasal polyps: a multicentre, randomised, controlled trial. Lancet Respir Med 2022;10(4):337–46.

52. Laidlaw TM, Mullol J, Woessner KM, et al. Chronic rhinosinusitis with nasal polyps and asthma. J Allergy Clin Immunol Pract 2021;9(3):1133–41.

53. Nucala | european medicines agency. Available at: https://www.ema.europa.eu/en/medicines/human/EPAR/nucala. Accessed May 1, 2022.

54. Dupixent | european medicines agency. Available at: https://www.ema.europa.eu/en/medicines/human/EPAR/dupixent. Accessed May 1, 2022.

55. Xolair | european medicines agency. Available at: https://www.ema.europa.eu/en/medicines/human/EPAR/xolair. Accessed May 1, 2022.

56. Hopkins C, Wagenmann M, Bachert C, et al. Efficacy of dupilumab in patients with a history of prior sinus surgery for chronic rhinosinusitis with nasal polyps. Int Forum Allergy Rhinol 2021;11(7):1087–101.

57. Bajpai S, Marino MJ, Rank MA, et al. Benefits of biologic therapy administered for asthma on co-existent chronic rhinosinusitis: a real-world study. Int Forum Allergy Rhinol 2021;11(8):1152–61.

58. Chong LY, Piromchai P, Sharp S, et al. Biologics for chronic rhinosinusitis. Cochrane Database Syst Rev 2021;2021(3). https://doi.org/10.1002/14651858. CD013513.PUB3.

59. Hopkins C, Buchheit K, Heffler E, et al. Dupilumab improved health-related quality of life in asthma patients with comorbid chronic rhinosinusitis: QUEST study. Am Thorac Soc Int 2022;A4845. https://doi.org/10.1164/AJRCCM-CONFERENCE.2022.205.1_MEETINGABSTRACTS.A4845.

60. Buchheit KM, Sohail A, Hacker J, et al. Rapid and sustained effect of dupilumab on clinical and mechanistic outcomes in aspirin-exacerbated respiratory disease. J Allergy Clin Immunol 2022. https://doi.org/10.1016/j.jaci.2022.04.007.

61. Lans van der RJL, Fokkens WJ, Adriaensen GFJPM, et al. Real-life observational cohort verifies high efficacy of dupilumab for chronic rhinosinusitis with nasal polyps. Allergy 2022;77(2):670–4.

62. Han JK, Bachert C, Fokkens W, et al. Mepolizumab for chronic rhinosinusitis with nasal polyps (SYNAPSE): a randomised, double-blind, placebo-controlled, phase 3 trial. Lancet Respir Med 2021;9(10):1141–53. https://doi.org/10.1016/S2213-2600(21)00097-7.

63. Weinstein SF, Katial RK, Bardin P, et al. Effects of reslizumab on asthma outcomes in a subgroup of eosinophilic asthma patients with self-reported chronic rhinosinusitis with nasal polyps. J Allergy Clin Immunol Pract 2019;7(2):589–96.e3.

64. Hayashi H, Mitsui C, Fukutomi Y, et al. Efficacy of reslizumab with asthma, chronic sinusitis with nasal polyps and elevated blood eosinophils. J Allergy Clin Immunol 2016;137(2):AB86.

65. Bachert C, Han JK, Desrosiers MY, et al. Efficacy and safety of benralizumab in chronic rhinosinusitis with nasal polyps: a randomized, placebo-controlled trial. J Allergy Clin Immunol 2022;149(4):1309–17.e12.

66. Gevaert P, Omachi TA, Corren J, et al. Efficacy and safety of omalizumab in nasal polyposis: 2 randomized phase 3 trials. J Allergy Clin Immunol 2020;146(3):595–605.

67. Bachert C, Han JK, Wagenmann M, et al. EUFOREA expert board meeting on uncontrolled severe chronic rhinosinusitis with nasal polyps (CRSwNP) and biologics: Definitions and management. J Allergy Clin Immunol 2021;147(1):29–36.

68. Wu Q, Zhang Y, Kong W, et al. Which is the best biologic for nasal polyps: dupilumab, omalizumab, or mepolizumab? A network meta-analysis. Int Arch Allergy Immunol 2022;183(3):279–88.
69. Walter S, Ho J, Alvarado R, et al. Mepolizumab decreases tissue eosinophils while increasing type-2 cytokines in eosinophilic chronic rhinosinusitis. Clin Exp Allergy 2022. https://doi.org/10.1111/cea.14152.
70. van der Lans RJL, Hopkins C, Senior BA, et al. Biologicals and endoscopic sinus surgery for severe uncontrolled chronic rhinosinusitis with nasal polyps: an economic perspective. J Allergy Clin Immunol Pract 2022. https://doi.org/10.1016/j.jaip.2022.02.017.
71. Bachert C, Han JK, Desrosiers M, et al. Efficacy and safety of dupilumab in patients with severe chronic rhinosinusitis with nasal polyps (LIBERTY NP SINUS-24 and LIBERTY NP SINUS-52): results from two multicentre, randomised, double-blind, placebo-controlled, parallel-group phase 3 trials. Lancet (London, England) 2019;394(10209):1638–50.
72. Scangas GA, Wu AW, Ting JY, et al. Cost utility analysis of dupilumab versus endoscopic sinus surgery for chronic rhinosinusitis with nasal polyps. Laryngoscope 2021;131(1):E26–33.
73. Yong M, Wu YQ, Howlett J, et al. Cost-effectiveness analysis comparing dupilumab and aspirin desensitization therapy for chronic rhinosinusitis with nasal polyposis in aspirin-exacerbated respiratory disease. Int Forum Allergy Rhinol 2021;11(12):1626–36.

Unified Airway Disease
Surgical Management

Amar Miglani, MD*, Tripti K. Brar, MD, Devyani Lal, MD

KEYWORDS

- Unified airway • Chronic sinusitis • Aspirin exacerbated respiratory disease
- Asthma • Cystic fibrosis • Endoscopic sinus surgery

KEY POINTS

- There is a strong interplay between the upper and lower airways as evidenced by epidemiologic associations and similarities in inflammatory mediators and transcriptional profiling of the upper and lower airway epithelium.
- Endoscopic sinus surgery (ESS) reduces the inflammatory burden locally in the sinuses and systemically in the serum as measured by immunologic markers. Additionally, ESS improves sinonasal quality-of-life (QoL) and objective measures of chronic rhinosinusitis (CRS).
- Available evidence suggests that ESS improves lower airway symptoms across multiple disease states (e.g. CRS without asthma, CRS with asthma, Aspirin-exacerbated respiratory disease (AERD), Cystic fibrosis (CF) etc). The magnitude of benefit is dependent on multiple factors including the underlying disease state and severity of disease.
- Further high-level controlled trials assessing the impact of ESS on lower respiratory disease are needed. The impact of ESS on non-type 2 lower airway disease has not been studied adequately.
- A multidisciplinary, patient-focused approach that comprehensively manages both upper and lower airway pathology is important to optimize outcomes. In the appropriate setting, surgery may be considered as part of this approach.

INTRODUCTION

The unified airway refers to the interconnectedness between the upper (nose and paranasal sinuses) and lower airways (trachea, bronchi, bronchioles). The unified airway model suggests that diseases of the upper and lower airways are manifestations of a single process.[1,2] Support for this concept is rooted in similarities between upper and lower airway structure (both are lined with respiratory epithelium), similarities in

Disclosures: None.
Department of Otolaryngology-Head & Neck Surgery, Mayo Clinic Arizona, 5777 East Mayo Boulevard, Phoenix, AZ 85054, USA
* Corresponding author.
E-mail address: Miglani.amar@mayo.edu

Otolaryngol Clin N Am 56 (2023) 169–179
https://doi.org/10.1016/j.otc.2022.09.013
0030-6665/23/© 2022 Elsevier Inc. All rights reserved.
oto.theclinics.com

function (both transport oxygen and participate in mucociliary clearance), similarities in cytokine and transcriptional profiling, and the strong associations between upper and lower airway pathology.[2–6] Clinical studies have also demonstrated bidirectional provocation where nasal provocation induces bronchial inflammation and bronchial stimulation induces nasal inflammation.[7,8] Epidemiologically, asthma increases the risk of developing CRS.[6] Conversely, CRS appears to increase the risk of developing asthma and a MarketScan claims database study revealed that in CRS patients without an asthma diagnosis, early ESS may mitigate the risk of developing asthma.[6,9]

OUTCOME ASSESSMENTS

To understand the impact of upper airway surgical intervention on the unified airway, it is first important to understand the assessments employed to study these outcomes. In general, the assessments include subjective and objective measures of disease severity. These outcome assessments may differ when discussing the upper airway versus the lower airway. Subjective measures include patient-reported outcome measures (PROMs), generic health-related quality-of-life symptom scores, and effects on productivity and absenteeism. Generic clinical endpoints include hospitalization rates, emergency department visits, and medications usage. An example of a generic health-related quality-of-life symptoms scores is the Health state utility values (HUV),[10] The HUV ranges from 0, which represents death to 1.0, which represents 'perfect health'. The mean for the US population is 0.81. For CRS patients, the mean preoperative HUV was measured to be 0.65 with and minimal clinically important difference (MCID) of 0.03. For CRS, objective metrics frequently include nasal endoscopy scoring systems, computed tomography scan scores, olfactory testing, nasal airflow measurements, and recurrence/revision surgery rates. For asthma and lower airway assessments, objective testing usually includes pulmonary function testing measurements, measurements of diffusion capacity, body plethysmography, and levels of exhaled nitric oxide. Commonly employed subjective and objective assessments employed in unified airway studies are detailed below, however, it is important to note that this list of assessments is not exhaustive.

a. CRS assessments
   i. Patient reported outcome measures (PROMs): CRS disease specific PROMs include the visual analogue scale, rhinosinusitis outcome measure (RSOM-31),[11,12] rhinosinusitis disability index (RSDI),[12,13] rhinosinusitis quality of life questionnaire (RQLQ),[12,14] chronic sinusitis survey (CSS),[12,15] and Sinonasal Outcome Test 22 (SNOT-22).[12,16] A recent systematic review identified SNOT-22 as the most suitable tool for CRS with a normal range of between 7-9 and the minimum clinically important difference of 8.9 point change.
   ii. Nasal endoscopy scoring systems in the Nasal polyp score (NPS)[17] and the Lund-Kennedy (LK) scoring system.[18] The NPS ranges from 0-4 on each side (0–8 total) with higher scores indicating larger polyps. The LK scoring system grades polyps, discharge, edema, scarring, and crusting on a 0-2 scale with a total score of 0-10 with a higher score indicating more severe pathology.
   iii. CT scoring: The Lund-Mackay CT score[19] is a staging system that measures 6 bilateral areas of sinus opacification from 0 to 2 with a total possible range of scores from 0-24. A higher score indicates more severe disease (i.e. more opacification).
b. Inflammatory Biomarkers (nasal, serum): Inflammatory biomarkers may be assessed pre- and/or postoperatively. Mucosal markers include tumor necrosis factor-a (TNF-a), platelet-derived factor (PDGF), hyaluronic acid (HA). Serum

inflammatory markers include TNF-a, interleukin (IL)-6 (IL-6), and IL-8. Measures of systemic type 2 inflammation include total serum immunoglobulin E (IgE) serum eosinophils, interleukins (IL-4, IL-5, IL-9, II-13), epithelial cell derived cytokines [thymic stromal lymphopoietin (TSLP), IL-25, and IL-33 among others.

c. Ciliary function: The nose and sinuses are lined by pseudostratified ciliated respiratory epithelium. The cilia play an integral part in mucociliary clearance. A common way to test mucociliary clearance in clinical studies is the saccharin method, where 5-10 mg of saccharin is placed on the anterior head of the inferior turbinate. The time taken to experience a sweet taste is measured in minutes where shorter times indicate better mucociliary function.

d. Lower airway assessments

  i. PROMs: Asthma-specific PROMs include the Asthma control questionnaire (ACQ), Asthma control test (ACT), and Asthma quality of life questionnaire (AQLQ), which are detailed below.

    1. Asthma control questionnaire (ACQ)[20]: The ACQ measures the adequacy of clinical asthma control and is intended for adults with asthma. There are 7 items total – 5 items that ask about symptoms, 1 item that asks about B2 rescue inhaler use, and one item that asks about the functional expiratory volume 1 (FEV-1) which clinical staff fills out.

    2. Asthma control test (ACT)[21]: The ACT identifies patients with poorly controlled asthma and the intended population is 12+ years. It is a widely adopted and validated instrument that has even been validated in various ethnic groups. It is an instrument that correlates with physician assessments of asthma control. It is comprised of five questions total.

    3. Asthma quality of life questionnaire (AQLQ)[22]: The AQLQ measures functional problems (i.e. physical, emotional, social, and occupational) that are most bothersome to adults with asthma. There are 32 questions across 4 domains. The domains include symptoms, activity limitations, emotional function, and environmental stimuli.

  ii. Pulmonary function testing (PFT): PFT provides a measure of the objective physiologic status of the lungs. It is gold standard for diagnosis of lower airway pathology. The various measures of pulmonary function assessment include lung volumes/spirometry, diffusion capacity, and body plethysmography. Diffusion capacity is the lungs' ability to transfer gas into blood. This measurement can used to differentiate patients with obstructive disease. For asthmatics, DC is normal, but for patients with emphysema, the DC is impaired (lower). There are various measurements taken during spirometry. The most reported metrics in unified airway studies include:

    1. Forced vital capacity (FVC): The amount of air that can be forcibly exhaled from your lungs after taking the deepest breath possible.

    2. TLC: After a complete exhalation, whatever volume remains n the lung is referred to as the residual volume (RV). Body plethysmography used to assess functional residual volume using Boyles law. The TLC is the sum of the FVC and RV.

    3. Forced expiratory volume 1 (FEV1): The amount of air forcibly exhaled within the first second of expiration.

    4. FEV1/FVC ratio: Is also called Tiffeneau-Pinelli index, is a ratio used in the diagnosis of obstructive and restrictive lung disease. It represents the proportion of a person's vital capacity that they can expire in the first second of forced expiration to the full, forced vital capacity.

    5. Tidal volume is the volume of air movement during quiet breathing

6. Peak expiratory flow (PEF): The highest forced expiratory flow measured with peak flow meter.

iii. Fraction of exhaled nitric oxide (FENO)[23]: Fraction of exhaled nitric oxide is regarded as a noninvasive and reliable marker of lower airway inflammation. It is useful for assessing the clinical status of patients with asthma and predicting the responsiveness to steroids

DISCUSSION

Given the inherent difficulties recruiting for randomized control trials within surgery, there is a paucity of high level 1 evidence looking at the effects of sinus surgery on quality-of-life outcomes. The subsequent discussion will summarize the efficacy of ESS for CRS and its impact on the combined airway. ESS is rarely performed in absence of preoperative or ongoing medical therapy, therefore the subsequent results should be interpreted in this context.

a. *Efficacy of endoscopic sinus surgery for chronic rhinosinusitis*: Much of the highest-level evidence within the CRS literature includes prospective comparative studies. An example of such a study was published by Smith and colleagues which was a multi-institutional prospective cohort study of patients who failed 3 weeks of medical therapy and who elected for either ESS (n = 65) or to continue medical therapy (n = 33). At 12-months follow-up using the RSDI and CSS outcome measures, a significantly greater improvement was found in the surgical group compared to the medical therapy group.[15] A separate longitudinal cross-over study was performed to further compare effectiveness of medical therapy to endoscopic sinus surgery. Patients undergoing medical therapy while awaiting surgical intervention were monitored by tracking their SNOT-22 scores. Similarly, after surgery, their SNOT-22 scores assessed. Following a mean of 7.1 months of continued medical therapy while awaiting surgery, SNOT 22 scores worsened from 57.6 to 66.1. After ESS, SNOT 22 scores improved significantly from 66.1 to 14.6 with 14.6 months of follow-up.[24] A ten-year prospective study more recently demonstrated that the initial clinically significant improvements in QoL seen 6 months postoperatively are durable over the long term with over 75% of patients reporting clinically significant long-term quality of life and HUV improvements. Revision surgery measured approximately 17%.[25] Lourijsen and colleagues recently performed a randomized control trial in adult CRSwNP patients randomizing patients to ESS alongside medical therapy (n = 103) versus medical therapy alone (n = 103). At 12 months follow-up the ESS cohort had greater improvement in SNOT-22 scores compared to medical therapy alone, although the MCID between groups was not met.[26] Patel and colleagues conducted a systematic review and meta-analysis comparing surgical therapy versus continued medical therapy for medically refractory chronic rhinosinusitis. In this review six studies were ultimately included and compared to continued medical therapy, ESS significantly improved patient based QoL scores and nasal endoscopy scores.[27]

b. *Impact of endoscopic sinus surgery on asthma control:* There is mounting evidence supporting the notion that optimization of sinonasal health can improve asthma control. An initial systematic review and meta-analysis reviewed twenty-two studies with mean follow-up across studies of 26.4 months. Patients reported improved asthma control in 76.1% of cases. Additionally, the frequency of asthma attacks decreased in 84.8% and the number of hospitalizations decreased in 64.4%. Medication usage also decreased significantly. Despite improvements in these clinical metrics of asthma control, the mean improvement in FEV1 was not significant.[28] The main limitations of the study were that none of the included studies reported asthma-specific quality-of-life before and after surgery and none of the studies were controlled trials which ultimately limited the strength of conclusions that could be reached. A subsequent study by Schlosser and colleagues followed CRS patients as part of a multi-institutional prospective study and measured AQLQ and ACT at baseline and 6 months postoperatively. The study found that uncontrolled asthma was present in 51% of patients undergoing ESS. Following ESS, significant improvements in AQLQ and ACT were noted with approximately half of patients with uncontrolled asthma improving. Improved asthma outcomes after ESS were associated with lack of corticosteroid dependency, lack of obstructive sleep apnea and large postoperative improvements in SNOT-22 score.[29] Cao et all performed a more recent systematic review and meta-analysis specifically looking at the effects of ESS on pulmonary function in patients with asthma. A total of 13 studies were included and authors concluded that low quality evidence supports the association between ESS and improvements in FEV1 and PEF.[30] Lastly, a recent systematic review focusing on CRSwNP patient with asthma included 3 studies (1 interventional and 2 observational) that demonstrated improvements in asthma control following ESS.[31] One study looked at a prospective cohort and evaluated the impact of ESS in eosinophilic CRSwNP with poorly controlled asthma and assessed ACQ score, blood eosinophil count, FeNO and FEV1 and found improvements across all metrics (ACQ, blood eosinophils, and FeNO decreased and FEV1 increased) at 8 and 52 weeks following ESS.[32] Another study looking at 28 CRSwNP with severe asthma patients found that ESS improved asthma control and decreased pulmonary function decline postoperatively.[33] A separate study looking at effects of ESS on eosinophilic CRS similarly found that ESS improves FeNO and asthma control.[34] Although these studies offer interesting data on the value of ESS in optimizing asthma control, further high-quality studies are needed to identify patients most likely to benefit from this approach, as well as to identify mechanisms through which the beneficial impact might occur.

c. *Timing of endoscopic sinus surgery and the development of asthma:* Perhaps the most impactful study investigating timing of ESS and its impact on the development of asthma was published by Benninger and colleagues[9] who leveraged the Market-Scan claims database and identified CRS without asthma patients undergoing ESS. Patients with a pre-existing asthma diagnosis were excluded. These CRS patients without asthma were grouped based on duration of sinusitis from first diagnosis to surgery and incidence of asthma was determined. Interestingly, the preoperative annual incidence of patients with new asthma diagnosis averaged 4.48%. Postoperatively the yearly incidence of asthma was 0.42%. Patients operated earlier in the disease continuum were therefore at decreased risk of developing asthma. CRS patients with AR were at higher risk of developing asthma as well. In summary, this study revealed a lower incidence of asthma diagnosis in patients that underwent earlier surgical intervention. This suggests that ESS may be disease modulating by mitigating the risk of developing asthma. There is growing evidence that early immunotherapy can reduce risk of development of asthma in allergic and asthma-prone children.[35] A similar relationship between early CRS treatment and asthma may exist. Ultimately, further studies validating these findings are needed.

d. *Impact of ESS on nasal inflammatory markers:* A limited number of studies demonstrate that ESS may reduce nasal inflammatory markers. Wei and colleagues[36] investigated changes in TNF-alpha, platelet-derived factor (PDGF), and hyaluronic acid (HA) in nasal secretions and olfactory function in patients with CRS before and after surgery. Ninety-four patients were divided into the control group receiving extranasal surgery and the observation group receiving ESS. The ESS group resulted in significantly lower levels of TNF-alpha. At one, four, and eight weeks after treatment, the levels of PDGF and HA were significantly higher in ESS group compared to control. Du and colleagues[37] looked at nasal secretions in 30 CRSwNP patients and 10 healthy subjects. Samples were collected 1-day preop and again at 4, 8, and 12 weeks post ESS. Levels of IL-2 and IL-5 in secretions of CRSwNP were significantly higher than their baseline controls. At week 4 and week 8, IL 4 levels in asthmatic group were higher than baseline controls. From the 4th to 12th week after ESS, IL2, IFN-y, IL-4, and IL-17 in nasal secretions of non-asthmatic groups were significantly increased as compared to their baseline controls. There was no significant association between endoscopy and levels of cytokines in postoperative nasal secretions suggesting that postoperative exam may not reflect underlying mucosal inflammation in the early postoperative period while healing might be ongoing.

e. *Impact of ESS on serum inflammatory markers:* In early studies, ESS appears to lower serum and inflammatory markers associated with CRS. Zhao and colleagues[38] retrospectively looked at 120 patients undergoing either ESS alone versus ESS with Budesonide irrigations and found that in both groups, after treatment, the levels of serum TNF-alpha, IL-8, and Il-6 decreased, but the decrease was greater in patients undergoing ESS with Budesonide irrigations. The ESS with Budesonide groups similarly had greater improvements in mucociliary clearance and symptom improvement. Hamada and colleagues[32] looked prospectively looked at 25 CRSwNP subjects with asthma and assessed ACQ, blood eosinophil counts, FEV1, and FeNO at 1 week preoperative, 8 weeks and 52 weeks. Postoperatively, ACQ, blood eosinophil counts, and FeNO significantly decreased (improved) and FEV1 increased (improved). Forty percent of patients sustained improvements out to one year. Interestingly higher baseline total IgE levels predicted improved long-term control. However, in an older study, Lal and colleagues[39] did not find that serum IgE levels changed one year after ESS. Another study looking at CRSwNP and asthma who had undergone ESS found that increased preoperative serum periostin and eosinophils in NP tissue were associated with preventive effects of ESS for asthma exacerbations.[40]

f. *Impact of ESS on ciliary function:* Multiple studies have demonstrated improvements in sinonasal mucociliary function measured via saccharin testing. Zhao and colleagues looked at 120 CRS patients undergoing ESS versus ESS followed by Budesonide irrigations. In both groups, mucociliary clearance improved, but the group treated with Budesonide irrigations following ESS improved to a greater degree.[38] In a separate study, Aroor and colleagues followed 60 patients and measured mucociliary clearance at baselined and then 6 weeks after sinonasal surgery. Overall, mucociliary clearance significantly improved between both time points with patients that received septoplasty and ESS improving to the greatest degree.[41] A study looking specifically at a pediatric population with chronic rhinosinusitis followed 132 patients undergoing ESS.[42] For the first 3 months following surgery, there appeared to be a reduction in mucociliary function, however at 12 months significant improvements over baseline were observed.

g. *Endoscopic sinus surgery and impact on lower airways in CF:* Two meta-analyses (one of which was a systematic review) found that ESS in CF patients produced symptomatic benefits but did not improve pulmonary function.[43,44] Additionally, there were conflicting results with regards to postoperative endoscopy scores, days spent in hospital, and courses of IV antibiotics.[43] More recent literature suggests that there may be specific subgroups of CF patients that may benefit with regards to their pulmonary function. Two studies indicate that post-transplant CF patients may benefit from earlier endoscopic sinus surgery by improving pulmonary function and attenuating pulmonary exacerbations.[45,46] The mechanism for this may have to do with sinus surgery decreasing pseudomonal airway colonization and subsequent bronchiolitis obliterans syndrome. A separate study looked at 181 CF patients undergoing ESS and then tracked postoperative lung function rates. For the entire cohort, lung function did not change following ESS. Among patients with FEV1 <80%, FEV1 declined presurgery by 3.5% per year which halted after surgery with these patients then showing no subsequent change in FEV1. No benefit was identified for patients with baseline FEV1>80%. This study suggested that in CF patients with moderate-to-severe lung disease, ESS can slow the deterioration of pulmonary function.[47] While causality cannot be established with such a study, these finding propose that ESS can lead to improved pulmonary function by reducing upper airway drainage and the mucopurulent secretion burden on the large lower airways. This may ultimately reduce bacterial colonization of the lungs.

h. *Endoscopic sinus surgery and its impact on lower airways in AERD*: Adelman and colleagues performed a systematic review which included eighteen studies investigating sinonasal and asthma symptoms in AERD patients. The evidence demonstrated improvement in sinonasal and asthma symptom severity and frequency, radiographic and endoscopy scores, and QoL after surgery.[48] Two prospective studies challenged AERD patients with ASA before and after surgery and found that after ESS, reactions to ASA were less severe in all patients and many patients had no detectable reaction.[49,50] A lack of clinical reaction ASA was associated with lower blood eosinophilia.

i. *Endoscopic sinus surgery and its impact on lower airways in patients with Bronchiectasis*: Looking specifically at patients with Bronchiectasis, a single retrospective study looking at patients with Bronchiectasis undergoing ESS found that this patient group experienced long-term benefit regarding sinonasal outcomes. However, ESS did not appear to improve pulmonary function.[51]

j. *Turbinate surgery for chronic rhinitis and impacts on lower airway:* There are limited studies investigating asthma control following functional nasal surgery for chronic rhinitis. A study out of the University of Silesa in Poland looked at 47 adults with medically refractory chronic rhinitis and bronchial asthma. These patients underwent argon plasma coagulation turbinectomy and ACT was assessed 3 months postoperative. Subjective nasal congestion and rhinomanometry showed improvements in nasal airflow. Additionally, asthma control improved from 21% to 96%.[52] A separate study conducted by Unsal and colleagues[53] looked at 27 patients with CR undergoing radiofrequency turbinate reduction. FEV1, FVC, and PEF were significantly improved when comparing baseline to 4 months postoperative. Further high-level studies investigating the effects of function nasal surgery for chronic rhinitis on the lower airways are needed.

k. *Prognostication value: Which patients of asthma are most likely to benefit from ESS?* Lee and colleagues investigated nasal Th2 cytokines in patients with CRS and severe Asthma (n = 16) and CRS patients with non-severe asthma (n = 12) and found that Th2 cytokines (IL-4, IL-5, IL-9, and IL-13), thymic stromal lymphopoietin (TSLP), IL-24, and IL-33 demonstrated higher expression in severe asthmatics. Additionally type 2 innate lymphoid cell (ILC2s) counts were higher in nasal tissues of severe asthmatics compared to non-severe asthmatics and correlated with Th2 cytokines. Post-ESS, higher Th2 cytokines and ILC-2 counts had more severe pulmonary decline and these factors may contribute to the recalcitrant status of asthma control.[33]

CLINICS CARE POINTS

- In CRS patients with asthma, ESS improves clinical asthma outcomes measures (decreased asthma exacerbations, hospitalizations, and medication usage) and asthma control. There is emerging support that ESS may improve objective pulmonary function testing measures.
- This impact of ESS may be secondary to a decrease in levels of local and systemic inflammatory mediators in the sinonasal cavities and in the serum, respectively.
- In CRS patients without asthma, early ESS may decrease inflammatory burden and mitigate risk of developing asthma.
- In AERD, endoscopic sinus surgery decreases aspirin sensitivity and may improve asthma control. Therefore, aspirin desensitization should be considered in the postoperative setting.
- In CF, endoscopic sinus surgery improves sinonasal QoL, however it does not improve pulmonary function testing. In select CF patient groups (i.e. moderate/severe obstructive disease and post lung transplant), ESS may slow the deterioration of pulmonary function.
- A multidisciplinary, patient-focused approach that comprehensively manages both upper and lower airway pathology is important to optimize outcomes.
- In the appropriate setting, sinus surgery may be considered as part of a comprehensive approach to managing combined airway disease.

REFERENCES

1. Meena RS, Meena D, Aseri Y, et al. Chronic rhino-sinusitis and asthma: concept of unified airway disease (UAD) and its impact in otolaryngology. Indian J Otolaryngol Head Neck Surg 2013;65(Suppl 2):338–42.
2. Kicic A, de Jong E, Ling K-M, et al. Assessing the unified airway hypothesis in children via transcriptional profiling of the airway epithelium. J Allergy Clin Immunol 2020;145(6):1562–73.
3. Bachert C, Vignola AM, Gevaert P, et al. Allergic rhinitis, rhinosinusitis, and asthma: one airway disease. Immunol Allergy Clin N Am 2004;24(1):19–43.
4. Chanez P, Vignola AM, Vic P, et al. Comparison between nasal and bronchial inflammation in asthmatic and control subjects. Am J Respir Crit Care Med 1999;159(2):588–95.
5. Gaga M, Lambrou P, Papageorgiou N, et al. Eosinophils are a feature of upper and lower airway pathology in non-atopic asthma, irrespective of the presence of rhinitis. Clin Exp Allergy J Br Soc Allergy Clin Immunol 2000;30(5):663–9.
6. Ryu G, Min C, Park B, et al. Bidirectional association between asthma and chronic rhinosinusitis: two longitudinal follow-up studies using a national sample cohort. Sci Rep 2020;10(1):9589.
7. Braunstahl GJ, Kleinjan A, Overbeek SE, et al. Segmental bronchial provocation induces nasal inflammation in allergic rhinitis patients. Am J Respir Crit Care Med 2000;161(6):2051–7.
8. Braunstahl GJ, Overbeek SE, Kleinjan A, et al. Nasal allergen provocation induces adhesion molecule expression and tissue eosinophilia in upper and lower airways. J Allergy Clin Immunol 2001;107(3):469–76.
9. Benninger MS, Sindwani R, Holy CE, et al. Impact of medically recalcitrant chronic rhinosinusitis on incidence of asthma. Int Forum Allergy Rhinol 2016; 6(2):124–9.
10. Soler ZM, Wittenberg E, Schlosser RJ, et al. Health state utility values in patients undergoing endoscopic sinus surgery. Laryngoscope 2011;121(12):2672–8.

11. Piccirillo JF, Edwards D, Haiduk A, et al. Psychometric and clinimetric validity of the 31-item rhinosinusitis outcome measure (RSOM-31). Am J Rhinol 1995;9(6): 297–308.
12. Soler ZM, Smith TL. Quality of life outcomes after functional endoscopic sinus surgery. Otolaryngol Clin North Am 2010;43(3):605–x.
13. Senior BA, Glaze C, Benninger MS. Use of the rhinosinusitis disability index (RSDI) in rhinologic disease. Am J Rhinol 2001;15(1):15–20.
14. Juniper EF, Thompson AK, Ferrie PJ, et al. Validation of the standardized version of the Rhinoconjunctivitis Quality of Life Questionnaire. J Allergy Clin Immunol 1999;104(2 Pt 1):364–9.
15. Smith TL, Kern RC, Palmer JN, et al. Medical therapy vs surgery for chronic rhinosinusitis: a prospective, multi-institutional study. Int Forum Allergy Rhinol 2011; 1(4):235–41.
16. Kennedy JL, Hubbard MA, Huyett P, et al. Sino-nasal outcome test (SNOT-22): a predictor of postsurgical improvement in patients with chronic sinusitis. Ann Allergy Asthma Immunol 2013;111(4):246–51.e2. https://doi.org/10.1016/j.anai. 2013.06.033.
17. Bachert C, Mannent L, Naclerio RM, et al. Effect of subcutaneous dupilumab on nasal polyp burden in patients with chronic sinusitis and nasal polyposis: a randomized clinical trial. JAMA 2016. https://doi.org/10.1001/jama.2015.19330.
18. Psaltis AJ, Li G, Vaezeafshar R, et al. Modification of the Lund-Kennedy endoscopic scoring system improves its reliability and correlation with patient-reported outcome measures. Laryngoscope 2014;124(10):2216–23.
19. Lund VJ, Kennedy DW. Staging for rhinosinusitis. Otolaryngol Neck Surg 1997; 117(3 Pt 2):S35–40.
20. Juniper EF, O'byrne PM, Guyatt GH, et al. Development and validation of a questionnaire to measure asthma control. Eur Respir J 1999;14(4):902–7.
21. Nathan RA, Sorkness CA, Kosinski M, et al. Development of the asthma control test: a survey for assessing asthma control. J Allergy Clin Immunol 2004; 113(1):59–65.
22. Juniper EF, Buist AS, Cox FM, et al. Validation of a standardized version of the Asthma Quality of Life Questionnaire. Chest 1999;115(5):1265–70.
23. van Veen IH, Ten Brinke A, Sterk PJ, et al. Exhaled nitric oxide predicts lung function decline in difficult-to-treat asthma. Eur Respir J 2008;32(2):344–9.
24. Smith KA, Smith TL, Mace JC, et al. Endoscopic sinus surgery compared to continued medical therapy for patients with refractory chronic rhinosinusitis. Int Forum Allergy Rhinol 2014;4(10):823–7.
25. Smith TL, Schlosser RJ, Mace JC, et al. Long-term outcomes of endoscopic sinus surgery in the management of adult chronic rhinosinusitis. Int Forum Allergy Rhinol 2019;9(8):831–41.
26. Lourijsen ES, Reitsma S, Vleming M, et al. Endoscopic sinus surgery with medical therapy versus medical therapy for chronic rhinosinusitis with nasal polyps: a multicentre, randomised, controlled trial. Lancet Respir Med 2022;2600(21):1–10.
27. Patel ZM, Thamboo A, Rudmik L, et al. Surgical therapy vs continued medical therapy for medically refractory chronic rhinosinusitis: a systematic review and meta-analysis. Int Forum Allergy Rhinol 2017;7(2):119–27.
28. Vashishta R, Soler ZM, Nguyen SA, et al. A systematic review and meta-analysis of asthma outcomes following endoscopic sinus surgery for chronic rhinosinusitis. Int Forum Allergy Rhinol 2013;3(10):788–94.
29. Schlosser RJ, Smith TL, Mace J, et al. Asthma quality of life and control after sinus surgery in patients with chronic rhinosinusitis. Allergy 2017;72(3):483–91.

30. Cao Y, Hong H, Sun Y, et al. The effects of endoscopic sinus surgery on pulmonary function in chronic rhinosinusitis patients with asthma: a systematic review and meta-analysis. Eur Arch Otorhinolaryngol 2019;276(5):1405–11.

31. Mullol J, Maldonado M, Castillo JA, et al. Management of United Airway disease focused on patients with asthma and chronic rhinosinusitis with nasal polyps: a systematic review. J Allergy Clin Immunol Pract 2022. https://doi.org/10.1016/j.jaip.2022.04.039.

32. Hamada K, Oishi K, Chikumoto A, et al. Impact of sinus surgery on type 2 airway and systemic inflammation in asthma. J Asthma 2021;58(6):750–8.

33. Lee T-J, Fu C-H, Wang C-H, et al. Impact of chronic rhinosinusitis on severe asthma patients. PLoS One 2017;12(2):e0171047.

34. Terada T, Inui T, Moriyama K, et al. Effects of endoscopic sinus surgery for eosinophilic chronic rhinosinusitis on respiratory functions and FeNO production in the lower respiratory tract. Ear Nose Throat J 2021. https://doi.org/10.1177/01455613211032006. 1455613211032006.

35. Farraia M, Paciência I, Castro Mendes F, et al. Allergen immunotherapy for asthma prevention: a systematic review and meta-analysis of randomized and non-randomized controlled studies. Allergy 2022;77(6):1719–35.

36. Wei L, Zhang Y, Tan H. Changes of TNF-α, PDGF and HA in nasal secretions and olfactory function of patients with chronic sinusitis before and after endoscopic sinus surgery. Exp Ther Med 2018;16(4):3413–8.

37. Du K, Huang Z, Si W, et al. Dynamic change of t-helper cell cytokines in nasal secretions and serum after endoscopic sinus surgery in chronic rhinosinusitis with nasal polyps. ORL J Otorhinolaryngol Relat Spec 2020;82(2):74–85.

38. Zhao Y, Jiang C, Wu Q, et al. Effects of endoscopic sinus surgery combined with budesonide treatment on nasal cavity function and serum inflammatory factors in patients with chronic sinusitis. J Healthc Eng 2022;2022:4140682.

39. Lal D, Baroody FM, Weitzel EK, et al. Total IgE levels do not change 1 year after endoscopic sinus surgery in patients with chronic rhinosinusitis. Int Arch Allergy Immunol 2006;139(2):146–8.

40. Kanemitsu Y, Kurokawa R, Ono J, et al. Increased serum periostin levels and eosinophils in nasal polyps are associated with the preventive effect of endoscopic sinus surgery for asthma exacerbations in chronic rhinosinusitis patients. Int Arch Allergy Immunol 2020;181(11):862–70.

41. Aroor R, Sunu Ali Z, Gangadhara Somayaji KS. Do nasal surgeries affect mucociliary clearance? Indian J Otolaryngol Head Neck Surg 2017;69(1):24–8.

42. Alekseenko S, Karpischenko S, Artyushkin S, et al. Ciliary function and sinonasal mucosal cytology in pediatric patients with chronic rhinosinusitis during a year after functional endoscopic sinus surgery. Rhinology 2021;59(3):319–27.

43. Macdonald KI, Gipsman A, Magit A, et al. Endoscopic sinus surgery in patients with cystic fibrosis: a systematic review and meta-analysis of pulmonary function. Rhinology 2012;50(4):360–9.

44. Yin M, Gao X, Di L, et al. Effect of endoscope sinus surgery on pulmonary function in cystic fibrosis patients: a meta-analysis. Laryngoscope 2021;131(4):720–5.

45. Vital D, Hofer M, Benden C, et al. Impact of sinus surgery on pseudomonal airway colonization, bronchiolitis obliterans syndrome and survival in cystic fibrosis lung transplant recipients. Respiration 2013;86(1):25–31.

46. Johnson JR, Hwang PH, Nayak JV, et al. Comparison of endoscopic sinus surgery timing in lung transplant patients with cystic fibrosis. Int Forum Allergy Rhinol 2022;12(6):821–7.

47. Khalfoun S, Tumin D, Ghossein M, et al. Improved lung function after sinus surgery in cystic fibrosis patients with moderate obstruction. Otolaryngol Neck Surg 2018;158(2):381–5.
48. Adelman J, McLean C, Shaigany K, et al. The role of surgery in management of Samter's triad: a systematic review. Otolaryngol Neck Surg 2016;155(2):220–37.
49. Jerschow E, Edin ML, Chi Y, et al. Sinus surgery is associated with a decrease in aspirin-induced reaction severity in patients with aspirin exacerbated respiratory disease. J Allergy Clin Immunol Pract 2019;7(5):1580–8.
50. Huang GX, Palumbo ML, Singer JI, et al. Sinus surgery improves lower respiratory tract reactivity during aspirin desensitization for AERD. J Allergy Clin Immunol Pract 2019;7(5):1647–9.
51. Kanjanaumporn J, Hwang PH. Effect of endoscopic sinus surgery on bronchiectasis patients with chronic rhinosinusitis. Am J Rhinol Allergy 2018;32(5):432–9.
52. Jura-Szołtys E, Ficek R, Ficek J, et al. Bronchial asthma control after argon plasma coagulation turbinectomy in patients with chronic rhinitis. Eur Arch Otorhinolaryngol 2014;271(6):1581–7.
53. Unsal O, Ozkahraman M, Ozkarafakili MA, et al. Does the reduction of inferior turbinate affect lower airway functions? Braz J Otorhinolaryngol 2019;85:43–9.

Unified Airway Disease
Future Directions

Jumah G. Ahmad, MD[a], Michael J. Marino, MD[b],*,
Amber U. Luong, MD, PhD[a,c]

KEYWORDS

- Unified airway disease • Chronic rhinosinusitis • Allergic rhinitis • Asthma
- Upper airway • Lower airway • Future directions

KEY POINTS

- Investigations that provide a better understanding of the common pathophysiologic mechanisms of airway inflammation will lead to development of novel treatments.
- Urinary leukotriene E4 is a promising biomarker for unified airway disease and a better understanding of how levels are altered by various medications will allow for individualized treatment plans.
- The microbiome is proven to influence airway physiology, but current research is still far from direct patient impact, leaving several exciting opportunities for discovery.
- Targeted therapeutics including biologics, Janus kinase inhibitors, and synthetic peptides have shown promising results, but more research is needed to optimize patient outcomes.

INTRODUCTION

Unified airway disease (UAD) describes the shared epidemiologic and pathophysiologic relationship among the chronic inflammatory diseases of the upper and lower airways including allergic rhinitis (AR), chronic rhinosinusitis (CRS), asthma and chronic otitis media.[1] This concept proposes that these diseases are manifestations of a single inflammatory process and require an integrated diagnostic and therapeutic approach to achieve global disease control.[1] AR is an immunoglobulin E (IgE)-mediated inflammatory process, and several subtypes of CRS are associated with AR, including allergic fungal rhinosinusitis (AFRS).[2,3] Patients with upper airway disease have a higher prevalence of lower airway disease and vice versa. Patients with CRS with

[a] Department of Otorhinolaryngology - Head and Neck Surgery, University of Texas Health Science Center, 6400 Fannin St, #2700, Houston, TX 77030, USA; [b] Department of Otolaryngology – Head and Neck Surgery, Mayo Clinic, Phoenix, AZ, USA; [c] Center for Immunology and Autoimmune Diseases, Institute of Molecular Medicine, McGovern Medical School at The University of Texas Health Science Center, Houston, TX, USA
* Corresponding author. Department of Otorhinolaryngology, Mayo Clinic College of Medicine, 5777 East Mayo Blvd, Phoenix, AZ 85054.
E-mail address: marino.michael@mayo.edu

Otolaryngol Clin N Am 56 (2023) 181–195
https://doi.org/10.1016/j.otc.2022.09.014
0030-6665/23/© 2022 Elsevier Inc. All rights reserved.
oto.theclinics.com

nasal polyposis (CRSwNP) have high prevalence of concomitant asthma, eosinophilia, and IgE-mediated allergic disease.[4] Approximately 10% of patients with CRSwNP experience upper or lower airway reactions after ingestion of nonsteroidal anti-inflammatory drugs (NSAIDs) or aspirin and may be characterized as having NSAID/aspirin-exacerbated respiratory disease (NERD or AERD).[5] Of patients with CRSwNP who have asthma, approximately 30% to 40% will develop aspirin/NSAID sensitivity.[6,7] This interrelationship between inflammatory diseases of the upper and lower airway has supported the concept that the respiratory system functions as an integrated unit.[8,9] In this model, diseases which cause inflammation in one part of the airway will likely stimulate a similar reaction throughout the rest of the airway. Future directions to further establish this entity should focus on pathophysiology, diagnostic markers, flora microbes with particular emphasis on fungi, the role of type 3 inflammation, and targeted therapeutics including biologics, Janus kinase (JAK) inhibitors, and synthetic peptides.

Pathophysiology

For chronic inflammation of both the upper and lower airways, the concept of a single disease has been replaced by syndromes encompassing complex biological network of distinct and interrelating inflammatory pathways. As such, asthma and CRS describe several diseases with distinct mechanistic pathways (endotypes) and variable clinical presentations (phenotypes). The precise definition of these endotypes is central to management due to inherent therapeutic and prognostic implications. The molecular mechanisms behind the heterogeneity of airway inflammation in asthmatic and CRS patients give way to developing management strategies with therapeutics targeted at these specific molecular mechanisms. Collectively, these advances have shifted existing paradigms in the approach to inflammatory airway diseases to tailor novel therapies.[10]

An important consideration in the pathophysiology of airway inflammation is endotyping. A widely accepted categorization of asthma includes two endotypes: those with high (T2-high) and those with low levels (T2-low) of type 2 inflammation. Type 2 inflammation is a distinct immune response characterized by a specific cytokine profile, mainly IL-4, IL-5, and IL-13, and effector cells which include eosinophils, mast cell and basophils. Type 2 inflammation is commonly associated with atopy, eosinophilic disorders, and parasitic infections. Patients with T2-high asthma have eosinophilia, increased number of airway mast cells, and stimulated T helper 2 (Th2) cells.[11] The downstream effects of a type 2 response are the release of histamine and leukotrienes (LTs) causing bronchoconstriction in the lower airway. These inflammatory pathways are perpetuated and maintained by IL-25, IL-33, and thymic stromal lymphopoietin (TSLP) which are produced by dendritic and epithelial cells.[12] The clinical relevance of distinguishing between T2-high and T2-low asthma is the response to certain treatments including inhaled corticosteroids and biologics which are currently targeted against various type 2 cytokines. T2-high asthma generally is responsive to corticosteroids and biologics, whereas T2-low asthma is not.[13] Nevertheless, there are subgroups of patients with T2-high asthma recalcitrant to corticosteroids.[14] Also, with the availability of several biologics targeted at different T2 cytokines, more specific endotyping within T2-high disease is needed. Our understanding of asthma endotypes is still developing, and there are likely several endotypes that have yet to be defined or discovered.

Similarly, the categorization of CRS is evolving toward endotypes. The pathophysiology of CRS is similar to that seen in asthma. About 85% of Western CRSwNP exhibits type 2 inflammation, which explains the effectiveness of corticosteroids for

CRSwNP and the potential benefit of biologics that target elements of this pathway.[15,16] The process begins with epithelial signals (ie, IL-33) that stimulate type 2 innate lymphocytes (ILC2 cells) and Th2 differentiation with the production of cytokines IL-4, IL-5, and IL-13. These invoke a cascade leading to the infiltration and activation of large numbers of eosinophils, mast cells, and basophils. In Asian countries, patients with CRSwNP tend to have a more neutrophilic cellular predominance. Less type 2 inflammation is observed in Asian CRSwNP, which exhibit predominantly type 1 and type 3 inflammation. In parallel, ILC1 and ILC3 cells are activated as well as the corresponding Th1 and Th17 subsets with release of the IFN-γ and IL-17, respectively.[17] Type 2 cytokines influence several biological processes including immunoglobulin class switching to IgE, IgG4 mucous production, inflammatory cell chemotaxis with upregulation of vascular cell adhesion molecule-1 (VCAM-1), and the activation of eosinophils.[18] ILCs in general function as first-line defenders in the airway epithelial barrier. The epithelial signals to ILC2s are well characterized, and these cells are also important sources of type 2 cytokines in CRSwNP, in addition to the Th2 lymphocytes.[19-21]

Although type 2 inflammation has been known to play a role in certain subtypes of airway inflammation, the role of type 3 inflammation characterized by ILC3 and Th17 has been more recently defined. Severe asthma is distinct in that the Th17 signaling pathway mediating neutrophil recruitment into the airways is a key mechanistic contributor as elevated levels of Th17 cytokines have repeatedly been observed in bronchial biopsies from patients with severe asthma.[22-25] IL-17 has thus been established as an independent risk factor for severe asthma.[26,27] Inhibition of IL-17 contributed to decreased inflammation, extracellular matrix remodeling, and oxidative stress in a murine experimental asthma model exacerbated by lipopolysaccharide (LPS).[28] Bromodomain and extraterminal (BET) proteins play an essential role in Th17 differentiation and as such, BET inhibitors are able to abolish Th17-driven neutrophilic inflammation.[29] Dual-positive populations of Th1/Th17 and Th2/Th17 cells accumulating in the airways of patients with asthma are associated with steroid-resistant severe asthma and a predominantly neutrophilic inflammation in the airways.[30] The IL-1β pathway is critical in Th2/Th17-predominant asthma, whereas IL-1α is involved in Th2/Th17-low asthma with neutrophilic inflammation.[31] Th2/Th17-low subtype of asthma demonstrate a mixed inflammatory pattern, with 45% neutrophilic asthma and 55% pauci-inflammatory asthma, in contrast to Th2- predominant and Th2/Th17-predominant asthma.[32] BET inhibition in combination with dexamethasone targeted both Th2 and Th17-driven immune responses in the lung and restored corticosteroid responsiveness in a mixed granulocytic mouse model of asthma.[29] Future directions involve targeting patient endotype and phenotype for therapeutic approaches. These recent efforts to characterize the role of type 3 inflammation in asthma and CRS could identify new therapeutic targets, even among existing medications. For instance, IL-17 inhibitors already have indications for autoimmune disorders such as psoriasis and ankylosing spondylitis.[33]

Leukotriene (LT) dysregulation has classically been associated with NERD/AERD, although this pathway may be more generally implicated in airway disease and can be leveraged as a noninvasive biomarker. The current understanding of the pathophysiologic process involves the LT pathway of arachidonic acid (AA) metabolism, a shared precursor of prostaglandins.[34] LTA4 is the first derivative to be formed via the conversion of AA by 5-lipoxygenase.[35] Subsequently, LTA4 is converted to LTB4 or LTC4 in eosinophils, basophils, and mast cells.[34] LTC4 is secondarily converted to LTD4, followed by conversion to LTE4, which is a stable end-product of this pathway that is measurable in both urine and blood.[36] LTC4, LTD4, and LTE4 all contain cysteine, and are categorized as cysteinyl LTs (cysLTs).[34] These proinflammatory cytokines are known to be potent airway vasoconstrictors and are associated with increased production of IL-5 and reduction in eosinophil apoptosis.[37,38] A fundamental characteristic of patients with AERD is overproduction of cysLTs with ingestion of NSAIDs or aspirin because they inhibit cyclooxygenase 1 and 2 (COX1 and COX2) and shunt AA metabolites toward the leukotriene pathway.[39,40] Similar pathophysiology results in a unified inflammatory response throughout the upper and lower airway. Further advancements in the understanding of the multifaceted pathophysiologic process will continue to allow for development of diagnostic biomarkers and targeted therapeutics.

Given the stability of LTE4 in urine, it has been investigated as a biomarker for diagnostic testing for upper and lower airway inflammatory diseases. Serum levels are too low and up to 5% of airway cysLTs are excreted in the urine with majority being urinary leukotriene E4 (uLTE4).[41] This offers an easy noninvasive method of testing. Currently, spot testing with liquid chromatography mass spectrometry is used with a cutoff of 166 pg/mg creatinine to predict aspirin sensitivity.[36] The utility of uLTE4 as a biomarker continues to be studied and extends to associations with asthma, AERD, CRS, and therapeutic susceptibility.[36] As uLTE4 becomes an important biomarker for linking upper and lower airway pathology, further studies to determine fluctuations in this biomarker over the course of the disease process will be insightful. For instance, a prospective cohort study to examine patients with CRSwNP, asthma, and undiagnosed AERD in evolution before their first episode of NSAID reactivity would help demonstrate the early reliability of uLTE4 to diagnose AERD and better understand its relationship to the overall disease course.[42] Although uLTE4 levels are known to decrease with zileuton use,[43] it has been suggested that uLTE4 levels remain stable despite patient treatment with corticosteroids, adding to its reliability of a disease biomarker.[44,45] However, it is not known how uLTE4 levels may be affected by newer biologic agents such as dupilumab or mepolizumab. A better understanding of how uLTE4 levels are altered by various medications will allow for individualized treatment plans for patients with CRS.

Microbiome

Complex interactions in the microbiome, including those among bacterial, fungal, and viral organisms, may be important for modulating microbiome diversity and host immune interactions in the sinuses and airway. The microbiome influences airway physiology, including both downregulation and activation of inflammatory cascades. Considering the physical connection, similar exposures, cell types, and immune response in airway sites, it is not surprising that microbial communities are similar throughout the whole airway.[46] In fact, these similarities create the foundation for the unified airway hypothesis. Overall, microbiome research is a relatively young field with several exciting opportunities for discovery. Current research is promising but is still far from direct patient impact.[47]

The current focus in this field has been on the role of bacteria, but there is novel research investigating the overall pathobiome: how viruses, fungi, archaea, and other pathogens influence health and disease.[48-51] To better understand host responses to alterations in the microbiome, metagenomic approaches are being used to characterize how functional networks drive chronic airway diseases.[52] Recent translational research has described the use of culture-independent techniques in clinical practice. Some authors have described next-generation sequencing as a complement to traditional microbiology laboratory studies but given the limited understanding of the sinonasal microbiome, advised against its routine use in clinical practice at this time.[53]

Retrospective reviews have reported the use of this technology to characterize acute exacerbations of CRS with more comprehensive identification and quantification of bacteria present, yet the clinical utility of these tests is unclear, in part due to the lack of functional evaluation of antimicrobial susceptibilities.[54] Compared with standard diagnosis with computed tomography scans, DNA sequencing as a biomarker has a high negative predictive value (99.1%) but low positive predictive value (19.4%) of an odontogenic source of CRS.[55] In clinical practice, culture-independent diagnostics identify the same bacteria detected with traditional culture in addition to other predominant organisms that are not found with cultures. Clinical outcomes and utility are yet to be defined, but culture-independent microbiota diagnostics have been suggested as a potential tool for patients with recalcitrant CRS to improve antimicrobial treatment.[56]

Loss of diversity in the bacterial microbiome has been associated with poor respiratory health; and similarly, decreases in fungal diversity may contribute to chronic respiratory disease.[57–60] With this link between fungi and asthma severity, there has been increasing interest in the pulmonary fungal microbiome, or mycobiome. Analysis of lung mycobiome has demonstrated higher fungal loads in patients with asthma subtypes linked to fungal colonization, allergic bronchopulmonary aspergillosis (ABPA) and severe asthma with fungal sensitization (SAFS), when compared with healthy controls.[57,61] Patients with CRS also have distinct features of their microbial community architecture. Increased species in fungal CRS subtypes, such as AFRS, mirrors similar increases in pulmonary conditions such as ABPA (A. fumigatus and A. flavus) and SAFS (Candida, Penicillium, and Cladosporium species).[62] Fungi represent a common trigger for chronic type 2 mediated airway inflammation in asthma and CRS resulting in mucosal barrier dysfunction, respiratory epithelium signaling, innate and adaptive immune responses, microbacterial interactions, and eosinophilic antifungal activity.[63]

Several important research topics in fungi mediated airway inflammation deserve closer attention. Novel pathways activated by fungi such as toll-like receptor 4 have provided a better understanding of the role of fungi in driving type 2 immune response.[64] Additional studies should investigate if these fungi-mediated pathways are fungal species-specific and evaluate the relative contributions of the innate and adaptive immune arms in initiating and maintaining the chronic type 2 airway inflammation. Whether there is redundancy or cross-talk in these pathways that amplify a type 2 inflammatory response is unknown. With regards to innate immunity, AFRS has been found to be associated with downregulated expression of histatin, an antimicrobial peptide with significant antifungal activity.[65–67] The interaction of fungi with bacteria such as Staphylococcus aureus, and the resulting superantigen inflammatory cascade, is another area of investigational interest.[68,69] Of additional interest is gaining an understanding of the molecular environment in the sinuses and lower airway that is permissive for fungus progression through its life cycle, from spore to the generation of fungal hyphae. Furthermore, differences in the immune response at different stages of the fungi's life cycle should be outlined. Given the antifungal activities of eosinophils, their effects on the mycobiome and fungal load associated with therapeutics that lead to depletion of eosinophils, including anti-IL5 biologics, should be explored. The therapeutic role of probiotics on the mycobiome is being actively investigated.[70] In comparison to allergic asthma, there is a relative paucity of animal models available to study CRS.[71–73] A recently described mouse model of fungi-mediated CRS has been reported but additional studies on this model is warranted.[74] With further research, these discoveries may lead to novel therapeutics as well as new applications for existing drugs.

Treatment

Therapeutic options to eliminate and reverse the underlying inflammatory pathophysiologic changes are currently lacking. The goal of management is to maintain control of symptoms over time with the minimal amount of medication.[75] Pharmacologic treatments for asthma are broadly categorized into two groups: control medications used to achieve and maintain baseline control of persistent asthma such as inhaled corticosteroids (ICS) and long-acting beta-2 agonists (LABA), and rescue medications used to treat acute symptoms and exacerbations, namely short-acting beta-2 agonists. ICS have been shown to reduce asthma symptoms, increase lung function, improve quality of life, and reduce the risks of exacerbations, asthma-related hospitalizations, and asthma-related death.[76,77] Patients with persistent symptoms or exacerbations despite optimized regimens can be considered for systemic therapy such as oral corticosteroids and biologics. The medical management of CRS generally includes a combination of nasal saline irrigations, topical steroids, antibiotics, and/or oral corticosteroids depending on the presence of polyps.[78] The use of corticosteroids for the management of CRS is supported by a high level of evidence, with particularly strong evidence for cases of CRSwNP.[79–81] Sinus surgery is generally considered for CRS patients who have failed appropriate medical therapy. Several targeted therapies, initially investigated and used in asthma, have demonstrated efficacy in the management of CRS.[82]

Whether traditional medical treatment of either asthma or CRS impacts the course of the other is unclear. A double-blind placebo-controlled trial of nasal mometasone spray in adults and children with uncontrolled asthma found that there was no improvement in asthma control.[83] The effects of montelukast, an LT receptor antagonist, on patients with nasal polyposis and asthma also have conflicting evidence, with some studies demonstrating significant improvements in nasal symptom score, airflow limitation, and reduction in inflammatory mediators in nasal lavage samples,[84] and others revealing no objective improvement in acoustic rhinometry, nasal inspiratory peak flow, or nitric oxide levels.[85] These discrepancies motivated further investigations and development of targeted treatments based on a deeper understanding of the common pathophysiologic mechanisms. Targeted therapeutics that may represent future research for UAD include biologics, JAK inhibitors, and synthetic peptides **(Table 1)**.

Biologics

Several biologics have been introduced in the treatment of asthma including omalizumab, mepolizumab, reslizumab, benralizumab, and dupilumab.[86] Anti-IgE (omalizumab) therapy has shown benefit for those with severe allergic asthma.[87] Anti-IL-5 (mepolizumab, reslizumab), anti-IL-5 receptor (benralizumab), and anti-IL-4 receptor (dupilumab) therapy can be used for treatment of uncontrolled, severe eosinophilic asthma.[88,89] Tezepelumab, a human monoclonal antibody (mAb) to TSLP (IgG2l) that inhibits TSLP/TSLP receptor interaction, significantly lowers annualized rates of asthma exacerbations among patients whose asthma is uncontrolled on LABAs and medium-to-high doses of ICS.[90] Tezepelumab is currently approved for asthma, but TSLP also plays critical role in driving type 2 inflammation in upper sinonasal airway. Recent immunomodulatory biologics have been demonstrated to improve both asthma and eosinophilic CRS. Dupilumab has been approved for the treatment of both asthma and CRSwNP following phase II and phase III trials, and several other biologics are also being investigated.[91,92] Dupilumab was initially approved in 2017 for the treatment of moderate-to-severe atopic dermatitis and in 2018 for the treatment of

Table 1
Targeted therapeutics for unified airway disease

	Examples	Mechanism of Action	Current Approved Indications
Biologics	Omalizumab	Anti-IgE drug that binds free IgE in the serum, forming trimers and hexamers so IgE bound to drug cannot bind its receptor on mast cells and basophils	Moderate-to-severe persistent asthma; chronic spontaneous urticaria; nasal polyps
	Mepolizumab Reslizumab	Anti-IL5 that prevents receptor binding on the surface of eosinophils	Severe asthma with eosinophilic phenotype; eosinophilic granulomatosis with polyangiitis; hypereosinophilic syndrome; CRSwNP
	Benralizumab	mAb that binds to the alpha subunit of IL-5 receptor on eosinophils, drawing natural killer cells to encourage programmed cell death	Severe asthma with eosinophilic phenotype
	Dupilumab	Human IgG4 mAb directed against the IL4Rα subunit to inhibit the signaling of IL-4 and IL-13	Atopic dermatitis; moderate-to-severe asthma; Severe CRSwNP; eosinophilic esophagitis
	Tezepelumab	mAb to TSLP (IgG2l) that inhibits TSLP/TSLP receptor interaction	Severe asthma
Tyrosine kinase inhibitors	Ruxolitinib	JAK inhibitor that prevents phosphorylating tyrosine residues on themselves blocking pro-inflammatory cytokine receptor chains	Myelofibrosis; polycythemia vera; Acute graft vs host disease; Chronic graft vs host disease
Synthetic peptides	Peptide immunotherapy	T-cell epitope peptides bind to major histocompatibility complexes and induce Th2 anergy, T regulatory cell upregulation, and immune deviation	None; experimental for cat, house dust mites, pollen, and food allergies
	Antimicrobial peptides	Synthetic mimics of antimicrobial peptides applied topically for local/direct effect	None; experimental for treating airway infections and inflammation
	Brensocatib	Dipeptidyl peptidase inhibitor that blocks activation of neutrophil serine proteases, inhibiting neutrophil activity	None; experimental for bronchiectasis

moderate-to-severe refractory eosinophilic or steroid-dependent asthma.[93,94] The biologic is a human IgG4 mAb directed against the IL-4 receptor-α (IL4Rα) subunit to inhibit the signaling of both IL-4 and IL-13, two cytokines in the type 2 inflammatory pathway key to the pathophysiology of atopic dermatitis, asthma, and CRSwNP.

With an increasing number of available biologics, an area of interest will be relative effectiveness and point precision targeting to specific patient populations. There have been several network meta-analyses comparing the currently available biologics. A meta-analysis evaluated the efficacy of monoclonal antibodies to reduce asthma exacerbation rates found mepolizumab, reslizumab and benralizumab reduced exacerbation rates in severe persistent eosinophilic asthma. However, no statistically significant superiority was observed of one biologic over the other in the network meta-analysis.[95] Another study compared the effects of monoclonal antibodies and aspirin desensitization for treatment of CRSwNP. Dupilumab ranked among the most beneficial for all clinically important outcomes studied, followed by omalizumab, and then mepolizumab and aspirin desensitization.[96] Most recently, a study performed a network meta-analysis to compare and rank the efficacy of five treatments (tezepelumab, dupilumab, benralizumab, mepolizumab, and placebo) in overall participants and in subgroups stratified by the thresholds of type 2 inflammatory biomarkers, including peripheral blood eosinophil count (PBEC). In the ranking assessment by annualized exacerbation rate, tezepelumab ranked the highest overall and across subgroups. A significant difference was observed between tezepelumab and dupilumab in the patient subgroup with PBEC less than 150, and between tezepelumab and benralizumab in overall participants and the patient subgroup with PBEC $\geq$ 300 and $\geq$ 150, respectively.[97] These results provide a basis for the development of treatment strategies and may guide basic, clinical, and translational research. More studies with direct head-to-head comparisons and better defined endotypes are needed.

JAK Inhibitors

Another target of interest is the family of JAK proteins, signaling proteins used by many pro-inflammatory cytokine pathways.[98] JAKs are a family of tyrosine kinases that selectively associate with cytokine receptor chains and mediate signaling by phosphorylating tyrosine residues on themselves.[98] Some JAKs play a major role in the signaling of several pro-inflammatory cytokines, often in association with other JAK family members.[98,99] Several JAK inhibitors have been developed for clinical use in inflammatory diseases, including asthma.[99,100] Ruxolitinib is a JAK inhibitor that has been shown to significantly ameliorate all the features of severe asthma, including airway hyperresponsiveness, lung inflammation, and total IgE antibody titers in a murine model.[101] Targeting JAKs is critical for mitigating the hyperinflammation that occurs in severe asthma and provides the framework for their incorporation into future clinical trials for patients that have severe or difficult-to manage airway inflammation.

Synthetic Peptides

Allergen immunotherapy has been known as the only disease-modifying treatment option for patients with chronic AR, typically featuring formulations to promote the development of immune tolerance. Although effective, the use of the whole allergen has been found to promote unintended IgE crosslinking, resulting in local and systemic adverse effects.[102,103] To overcome such limitations, the use of T-cell epitope peptides in allergen immunotherapy, termed peptide immunotherapy (PIT), has been explored with promising outcomes.[104] The T-cell epitope peptides bind to major histocompatibility complexes and induce Th2 anergy, T regulatory cell upregulation, and immune deviation.[105] T-cell epitopes can be derived from a gene sequence to modulate the response to an allergen. Compared with allergen immunotherapy, PIT is quicker, safer and more efficacious.[106] Promising results in cat dander, honeybee venom, Japanese cedar pollen, grass pollens, ragweed and house dust mite clinical trials have shown safety, efficacy and tolerability to PIT.

PIT may hold the potential to change the treatment algorithm for AR, but more extensive research is necessary before widespread use. Within the next decade, PIT is predicted to become more available, following further assessments of its safety and efficacy. Comparative studies will also give insights into the effectiveness of T-cell immunotherapy in relation to pre-existing pharmacologic therapies, differing routes of administration and administration period.

Synthetic peptides have also been designed to mimic antimicrobial peptides. These could potentially be applied topically to the airway for a more local and direct effect, avoiding systemic side effects and addressing antibiotic resistance. Many other small molecules used to provide or block pro-inflammatory activities are being investigated in chronic airway inflammation. One such class of molecules are dipeptidyl peptidase inhibitors (DPP) which block activation of neutrophil serine proteases and hence neutrophil activity. An oral DPP-1 inhibitor, brensocatib, recently reported improved clinical outcomes in patients with bronchiectasis[107] and Phase 2 clinical trials in CRS are being planned. In the future, there is a positive outlook into the development of a greater variety of peptides of better specificities and greater clinical efficacies.

SUMMARY

With the foundation of the UAD hypothesis well established, building on it will require research and efforts to further understand the pathophysiology, identify clinically useful diagnostic markers, define the role of the micro and mycobiome, characterize inflammatory endotypes, and develop targeted therapeutics.

CLINICS CARE POINTS

- In patients presenting with both inflammatory diseases of the upper and lower airway, consider unified airway disease (UAD) on the differential diagnosis.

- When suspecting UAD, consider testing for elevated urinary leukotriene E4, an easy noninvasive method of testing to screen for asthma, aspirin-exacerbated respiratory disease, chronic rhinosinusitis, and therapeutic susceptibility.

- Targeted therapeutics indicated for both upper and lower airway inflammatory diseases can improve UAD control and decrease polypharmacy.

DISCLOSURE

JGA and MJM have no disclosures or conflicts of interest. AUL serves as a consultant for Lyra Therapeutics (Watertown, MA, USA), Medtronic (Dublin, IE), Sanofi (Paris, France), and Stryker (Kalamazoo, MI, USA). AUL serves on the scientific advisory board for ENTvantage Dx (Austin, TX, USA), Maxwell Biosciences (Austin, TX), and Third Wave Therapeutics (San Francisco, CA, USA).

REFERENCES

1. Licari A, Castagnoli R, Denicolò CF, et al. The Nose and the Lung: United Airway Disease? Front Pediatr 2017;5:44.

2. Wise SK, Lin SY, Toskala E, et al. International Consensus Statement on Allergy and Rhinology. Allergic Rhinitis Int Forum Allergy Rhinol 2018;8(2):108–352.

3. Rosenwasser LJ. Current understanding of the pathophysiology of allergic rhinitis. Immunol Allergy Clin N Am 2011;31(3):433–9.

4. Hopkins C. Chronic rhinosinusitis with nasal polyps. N Engl J Med 2019;381(1): 55–63.

5. Laidlaw TM. Clinical updates in aspirin-exacerbated respiratory disease. Allergy Asthma Proc 2019;40(1):4–6.

6. Jenkins C, Costello J, Hodge L. Systematic review of prevalence of aspirin induced asthma and its implications for clinical practice. BMJ 2004; 328(7437):434.

7. Rajan JP, Wineinger NE, Stevenson DD, et al. Prevalence of aspirin-exacerbated respiratory disease among asthmatic patients: a meta-analysis of the literature. J Allergy Clin Immunol 2015;135(3):676–81, e671.

8. Slavin RG. The upper and lower airways: the epidemiological and pathophysiological connection. Allergy Asthma Proc 2008;29:553–6.

9. Krouse JH. The unified airway–conceptual framework. Otolaryngol Clin N Am 2008;41:257–66.

10. Kuruvilla ME, Lee FE, Lee GB. Understanding Asthma Phenotypes, Endotypes, and Mechanisms of Disease. Clin Rev Allergy Immunol 2019;56(2):219–33.

11. Dougherty RH, Sidhu SS, Raman K, et al. Accumulation of intraepithelial mast cells with a unique protease phenotype in T(H)2-high asthma. J Allergy Clin Immunol 2010;125:1046–53, e1048.

12. Gans MD, Gavrilova T. Understanding the immunology of asthma: Pathophysiology, biomarkers, and treatments for asthma endotypes. Paediatr Respir Rev 2019;S1526–0542(19):30081–8.

13. Woodruff PG, Modrek B, Choy DF, et al. T-helper type 2-driven inflammation defines major subphenotypes of asthma. Am J Respir Crit Care Med 2009;180: 388–95.

14. Fahy JV. Type 2 inflammation in asthma–present in most, absent in many. Nat Rev Immunol 2015;15:57–65.

15. Stevens WW, Peters AT, Tan BK, et al. Associations Between Inflammatory Endotypes and Clinical Presentations in Chronic Rhinosinusitis. J Allergy Clin Immunol Pract 2019;7:2812–20, e2813.

16. Tomassen P, Vandeplas G, Van Zele T, et al. Inflammatory endotypes of chronic rhinosinusitis based on cluster analysis of biomarkers. J Allergy Clin Immunol 2016;137:1449–56, e1444.

17. Bachert C, Zhang L, Gevaert P. Current and future treatment options for adult chronic rhinosinusitis: focus on nasal polyposis. J Allergy Clin Immunol 2015; 136:1431–40.

18. Lavigne P, Lee SE. Immunomodulators in chronic rhinosinusitis. World J Otorhinolaryngol Head Neck Surg 2018;4:186–92.

19. Shaw JL, Fakhri S, Citardi MJ, et al. IL-33-responsive innate lymphoid cells are an important source of IL-13 in chronic rhinosinusitis with nasal polyps. Am J Respir Crit Care Med 2013;188:432–9.

20. Mjosberg JM, Trifari S, Crellin NK, et al. Human IL-25- and IL-33-responsive type 2 innate lymphoid cells are defined by expression of CRTH2 and CD161. Nat Immunol 2011;12:1055–62.

21. Nagarkar DR, Poposki JA, Tan BK, et al. Thymic stromal lymphopoietin activity is increased in nasal polyps of patients with chronic rhinosinusitis. J Allergy Clin Immunol 2013;132:593–600, e512.

22. Ramakrishnan RK, Al Heialy S, Hamid Q. Role of IL-17 in asthma pathogenesis and its implications for the clinic. Expert Rev Respir Med 2019;13:1057–68.
23. Al-Ramli W, Prefontaine D, Chouiali F, et al. T(H)17-associated cytokines (IL-17A and IL-17F) in severe asthma. J Allergy Clin Immunol 2009;123:1185–7.
24. Ricciardolo FLM, Sorbello V, Folino A, et al. Identification of IL-17F/frequent exacerbator endotype in asthma. J Allergy Clin Immunol 2017;140:395–406.
25. Sorbello V, Ciprandi G, Di Stefano A, et al. Nasal IL-17F is related to bronchial IL-17F/neutrophilia and exacerbations in stable atopic severe asthma. Allergy 2015;70:236–40.
26. Agache I, Ciobanu C, Agache C, et al. Increased serum IL-17 is an independent risk factor for severe asthma. Respir Med 2010;104:1131–7.
27. Chien JW, Lin CY, Yang KD, et al. Increased IL-17A secreting CD41 T cells, serum IL-17 levels and exhaled nitric oxide are correlated with childhood asthma severity. Clin Exp Allergy 2013;43:1018–26.
28. Camargo LDN, Righetti RF, Aristoteles L, et al. Effects of anti-IL-17 on inflammation, remodeling, and oxidative stress in an experimental model of asthma exacerbated by LPS. Front Immunol 2017;8:1835.
29. Nadeem A, Ahmad SF, Al-Harbi NO, et al. Inhibition of BET bromodomains restores corticosteroid responsiveness in a mixed granulocytic mouse model of asthma. Biochem Pharmacol 2018;154:222–33.
30. Irvin C, Zafar I, Good J, et al. Increased frequency of dual-positive TH2/TH17 cells in bronchoalveolar lavage fluid characterizes a population of patients with severe asthma. J Allergy Clin Immunol 2014;134:1175–86, e7.
31. Cosmi L, Liotta F, Annunziato F. Th17 regulating lower airway disease. Curr Opin Allergy Clin Immunol 2016;16:1–6.
32. Liu W, Liu S, Verma M, et al. Mechanism of T(H)2/T(H)17-predominant and neutrophilic T(H)2/T(H)17-low subtypes of asthma. J Allergy Clin Immunol 2017;139:1548–58, e4.
33. McGonagle DG, McInnes IB, Kirkham BW, et al. The role of IL-17A in axial spondyloarthritis and psoriatic arthritis: recent advances and controversies. Ann Rheum Dis 2019;78(9):1167–78 [published correction appears in Ann Rheum Dis. 2020 Jan;79(1):e12].
34. Rabinovitch N. Urinary leukotriene E4. Immunol Allergy Clin North Am 2007; 27(4):651–64.
35. Rabinovitch N. Urinary leukotriene E4 as a biomarker of exposure, susceptibility and risk in asthma. Immunol Allergy Clin North Am 2012;32(3):433–45.
36. Divekar R, Hagan J, Rank M, et al. Diagnostic utility of urinary LTE4 in asthma, allergic rhinitis, chronic rhinosinusitis, nasal polyps, and aspirin sensitivity. J Allergy Clin Immunol Pract 2016;4(4):665–70.
37. Gyllfors P, Kumlin M, Dahlen SE, et al. Relation between bronchial responsiveness to inhaled leukotriene D4 and markers of leukotriene biosynthesis. Thorax 2005;60(11):902–8.
38. Lee E, Robertson T, Smith J, et al. Leukotriene receptor antagonists and synthesis inhibitors reverse survival in eosinophils of asthmatic individuals. Am J Respir Crit Care Med 2000;161(6):1881–6.
39. Laidlaw TM. Pathogenesis of NSAID-induced reactions in aspirin-exacerbated respiratory disease. World J Otorhinolaryngol Head Neck Surg 2018;4(3):162–8.
40. Laidlaw TM, Levy JM. NSAID-ERD syndrome: the new hope from prevention, early diagnosis, and new therapeutic targets. Curr Allergy Asthma Rep 2020; 20(4):10.

41. Kumlin M, Dahlen B, Bjorck T, et al. Urinary excretion of leukotriene E4 and 11-dehydrothromboxane B2 in response to bronchial provocations with allergen, aspirin, leukotriene D4, and histamine in asthmatics. Am Rev Respir Dis 1992; 146(1):96–103.

42. Choby G, Low CM, Levy JM, et al. Urine Leukotriene E4: Implications as a Biomarker in Chronic Rhinosinusitis. Otolaryngol Head Neck Surg 2022; 166(2):224–32.

43. Mohebati A, Milne GL, Zhou XK, et al. Effect of zileuton and celecoxib on urinary LTE4 and PGE M levels in smokers. Cancer Prev Res (Phila) 2013;6(7):646–55.

44. Hoffman BC, Rabinovitch N. Urinary leukotriene E4 as a biomarker of exposure, susceptibility, and risk in asthma: an update. Immunol Allergy Clin North Am 2018;38(4):599–610.

45. Leigh R, Vethanayagam D, Yoshida M, et al. Effects of montelukast and budesonide on airway responses and airway inflammation in asthma. Am J Respir Crit Caremed 2002;166(9):1212–7.

46. Hanshew AS, Jetté ME, Rosen SP, et al. Integrating the microbiota of the respiratory tract with the unified airway model, 126. Respiratory Medicine WB Saunders Ltd; 2017. p. 68–74.

47. Kumpitsch C, Koskinen K, Schöpf V, et al. The microbiome of the upper respiratory tract in health and disease. BMC Biol [Internet 2019;17(1):87. Available at: https://bmcbiol.biomedcentral.com/articles/10.1186/s12915-019-0703-z.

48. Koskinen K, Pausan MR, Perras AK, et al. First insights into the diverse human archaeome: specific detection of archaea in the gastrointestinal tract, lung, and nose and on skin. MBio 2017;8(6).

49. Zhang I, Pletcher SD, Goldberg AN, et al. Fungal microbiota in chronic airway inflammatory disease and emerging relationships with the host immune response. Front Microbiol 2017;8(DEC).

50. Cleland EJ, Bassioni A, Boase S, et al. The fungal microbiome in chronic rhinosinusitis: richness, diversity, postoperative changes and patient outcomes. Int Forum Allergy Rhinol [Internet] 2014;4(4):259–65. Available at: http://doi.wiley.com/10.1002/alr.21297.

51. Goggin RK, Bennett CA, Bassiouni A, et al. Comparative viral sampling in the sinonasal passages; different viruses at different sites. Front Cell Infect Microbiol 2018;8(SEP).

52. Altman MC, Gill MA, Whalen E, et al. Transcriptome networks identify mechanisms of viral and nonviral asthma exacerbations in children. Nat Immunol 2019;20(5):637–51.

53. Jervis Bardy J, Psaltis AJ. Next generation sequencing and the microbiome of chronic Rhinosinusitis: a primer for clinicians and review of current research, its limitations, and future Directions. Ann Otol Rhinol Laryngol 2016;125(8): 613–21 [cited 2020 Jan 2];Available at: http://www.ncbi.nlm.nih.gov/pubmed/27056556.

54. Vandelaar LJ, Hanson B, Marino M, et al. Analysis of Sinonasal microbiota in exacerbations of chronic Rhinosinusitis subgroups. OTO Open 2019;3(3). 2473974X1987510.

55. Haider AA, Marino MJ, Yao WC, et al. The potential of high-throughput DNA sequencing of the paranasal sinus microbiome in diagnosing odontogenic sinusitis. Otolaryngol Head Neck Surg [Internet] 2019;161(6):1043–7 [cited 2020 Jan 2];Available at: http://www.ncbi.nlm.nih.gov/pubmed/31382814.

56. Rapoport SK, Smith AJ, Bergman M, et al. Determining the utility of standard hospital microbiology testing: comparing standard microbiology cultures with

DNA sequence analysis in patients with chronic sinusitis. World J Otorhinolaryngol – Head Neck Surg 2019;5(2):82–7.

57. Sharma A, Laxman B, Naureckas ET, et al. Associations between fungal and bacterial microbiota of airways and asthma endotypes. J Allergy Clin Immunol 2019;144(5):1214–27, e7.

58. Maiz L, Nieto R, Canton R, et al. Fungi in bronchiectasis: a concise review. Int J Mol Sci 2018;19(1):142.

59. Nguyen LD, Viscogliosi E, Delhaes L. The lung mycobiome: an emerging field of the human respiratory microbiome. Front Microbiol 2015;6:89.

60. Tipton L, Ghedin E, Morris A. The lung mycobiome in the nextgeneration sequencing era. Virulence 2017;8(3):334–41.

61. Fraczek MG, Chishimba L, Niven RM, et al. Corticosteroid treatment is associated with increased filamentous fungal burden in allergic fungal disease. J Allergy Clin Immunol 2018;142(2):407–14.

62. Gelber JT, Cope EK, Goldberg AN, et al. Evaluation of malassezia and common fungal pathogens in subtypes of chronic rhinosinusitis. Int Forum Allergy Rhinol 2016;6(9):950–5.

63. Tyler MA, Lam K, Marino MJ, et al. Revisiting the controversy: The role of fungi in chronic rhinosinusitis. Int Forum Allergy Rhinol 2021;11(11):1577–87.

64. Millien VO, Lu W, Shaw J, et al. Cleavage of fibrinogen by proteinases elicits allergic responses through Toll-like receptor 4. Science 2013;341:792–6.

65. Ooi EH, Wormald PJ, Carney AS, et al. Surfactant protein d expression in chronic rhinosinusitis patients and immune responses in vitro to Aspergillus and Alternaria in a nasal explant model. Laryngoscope 2007;117:51–7.

66. Psaltis AJ, BruhnMA, Ooi EH, et al. Nasal mucosa expression of lactoferrin in patientswith chronic rhinosinusitis. Laryngoscope 2007;117:2030–5.

67. Tyler MA, Padro Dietz CJ, Russell CB, et al. Distinguishing molecular features of allergic fungal rhinosinusitis. Otolaryngol Head Neck Surg 2018;159(1):185–93.

68. Maina IW, Patel NN, Cohen NA. Understanding the role of biofilms and superantigens in chronic rhinosinusitis. Curr Otorhinolaryngol Rep 2018;6(3):253–62.

69. Fraser JD, Proft T. The bacterial superantigen and superantigenlike proteins. Immunol Rev 2008;225:226–43.

70. Nagalingam N, Cope E. microbiology SL-T in, 2013 undefined. Probiotic strategies for treatment of respiratory diseases. Elsevier [Internet] [cited 2019 Dec 18]. Available at: https://www.sciencedirect.com/science/article/pii/S0966842X13000826.

71. Kim JH, Yi JS, Gong CH, et al. Development of Aspergillus protease with ovalbumin-induced allergic chronic rhinosinusitis model in the mouse. Am J Rhinol Allergy 2014;28:465–70.

72. Kim HC, Lim JY, Kim S, et al. Development of a mouse model of eosinophilic chronic rhinosinusitis with nasal polyp by nasal instillation of an Aspergillus protease and ovalbumin. Eur Arch Otorhinolaryngol 2017;274:3899–906.

73. Park SC, Kim SI, Hwang CS, et al. Multiple airborne allergeninduced eosinophilic chronic rhinosinusitis murine model. Eur Arch Otorhinolaryngol 2019; 276:2273–82.

74. Sun H, Damania A, Mair ML, et al. STAT6 Blockade Abrogates Aspergillus-Induced Eosinophilic Chronic Rhinosinusitis and Asthma, A Model of Unified Airway Disease. Front Immunol 2022;13:818017.

75. Krouse JH. Asthma Management for the Otolaryngologist. Otolaryngol Clin N Am 2017;50:1065–76.

76. Pauwels RA, Pedersen S, Busse WW. Early intervention with budesonide in mild persistent asthma: a randomised, double-blind trial. Lancet 2003;361:1071–6.

77. Adams NP, Bestall JB, Malouf R, et al. Inhaled beclomethasone versus placebo for chronic asthma. Cochrane Database Syst Rev 2005;CD002738.

78. Orlandi RR, Kingdom TT, Hwang PH, et al. International consensus statement on allergy and rhinology: Rhinosinusitis. Int Forum Allergy rhinology 2016;6(Suppl 1):S22–209.

79. Snidvongs K, Kalish L, Sacks R, et al. Topical steroid for chronic rhinosinusitis without polyps. Cochrane Database Syst Rev 2011;CD009274.

80. Chong LY, Head K, Hopkins C, et al. Intranasal steroids versus placebo or no intervention for chronic rhinosinusitis. Cochrane Database Syst Rev 2016;4: CD011996.

81. Kalish L, Snidvongs K, Sivasubramaniam R, et al. Topical steroids for nasal polyps. Cochrane Database Syst Rev 2012;12:CD006549.

82. Divekar R, Lal D. Recent advances in biologic therapy of asthma and the role in therapy of chronic rhinosinusitis. F1000Res 2018;7:412. https://doi.org/10.12688/f1000research.13170.1.

83. Dixon AE, Castro M, Cohen RI, et al, American Lung Association–Asthma Clinical Research Centers' Writing Committee. Efficacy of nasal mometasone for the treatment of chronic sinonasal disease in patients with inadequately controlled asthma. J Allergy Clin Immunol 2015;135(3):701–9, e5.

84. Schaper C, Noga O, Koch B, et al. Anti-inflammatory properties of montelukast, a leukotriene receptor antagonist in patients with asthma and nasal polyposis. J Investig Allergol Clin Immunol 2011;21:51–8.

85. Ragab S, Parikh A, Darby YC, et al. An open audit of montelukast, a leukotriene receptor antagonist, in nasal polyposis associated with asthma. Clin Exp Allergy 2001;31:138591.

86. Drazen JM, Harrington D. New biologics for asthma. N Engl J Med 2018;378: 2533–4.

87. Hanania NA, Alpan O, Hamilos DL, et al. Omalizumab in severe allergic asthma inadequately controlled with standard therapy: a randomized trial. Ann Intern Med 2011;154:573–82.

88. Wenzel S, Ford L. Pearlman Det al. Dupilumab in persistent asthma with elevated eosinophil levels. N Engl J Med 2013;368:2455–66.

89. Wang FP, Liu T, Lan Z, et al. Efficacy and safety of anti-Interleukin-5 therapy in patients with asthma: a systematic review and meta-analysis. PLoS One 2016; 11:e0166833.

90. Corren J, Parnes JR, Wang L, et al. Tezepelumab in Adults with Uncontrolled Asthma. N Engl J Med 2017;377(10):936–46 [Erratum in: N Engl J Med. 2019 May 23;380(21):2082. PMID: 28877011].

91. Bachert C, Han JK. Desrosiers met al. Efficacy and safety of dupilumab in patients with severe chronic rhinosinusitis with nasal polyps (LIBERTY NP SINUS-24 and LIBERTY NP SINUS-52): results from two multicentre, randomised, double-blind, placebo-controlled, parallel-group phase 3 trials. Lancet 2019; 394:1638–50.

92. Bachert C, Mannent L, Naclerio RM, et al. Effect of subcutaneous Dupilumab on nasal polyp burden in patients with chronic sinusitis and nasal polyposis: a randomized clinical trial. JAMA 2016;315:469–79.

93. Busse WW, Maspero JF. Rabe KFet al. Liberty asthma QUEST: phase 3 randomized, double blind, placebo-controlled, parallel-group study to evaluate

Dupilumab efficacy/safety in patients with uncontrolled, moderate-to-severe asthma. Adv Ther 2018;35:737–48.

94. Simpson EL, Bieber T, Guttman-Yassky E, et al. Two phase 3 trials of Dupilumab versus placebo in atopic dermatitis. N Engl J Med 2016;375:2335–48.

95. Edris A, De Feyter S, Maes T, et al. Monoclonal antibodies in type 2 asthma: a systematic review and network meta-analysis. Respir Res 2019;20(1):179.

96. Oykhman P, Paramo FA, Bousquet J, et al. Comparative efficacy and safety of monoclonal antibodies and aspirin desensitization for chronic rhinosinusitis with nasal polyposis: A systematic review and network meta-analysis. J Allergy Clin Immunol 2022;149(4):1286–95.

97. Ando K, Fukuda Y, Tanaka A, et al. Comparative Efficacy and Safety of Tezepelumab and Other Biologics in Patients with Inadequately Controlled Asthma According to Thresholds of Type 2 Inflammatory Biomarkers: A Systematic Review and Network Meta-Analysis. Cells 2022;11(5):819.

98. Ghoreschi K, Laurence A, O'Shea JJ. Janus Kinases in Immune Cell Signaling. Immunol Rev 2009;228:273–87.

99. O'Shea JJ, Schwartz DM, Villarino AV, et al. The JAK-STAT Pathway: Impact on Human Disease and Therapeutic Intervention. Annu Rev Med 2015;66:311–28.

100. Pernis AB, Rothman PB. JAK-STAT Signaling in Asthma. J Clin Invest 2002;109: 1279–83.

101. Subramanian H, Hashem T, Bahal D, et al. Ruxolitinib Ameliorates Airway Hyperresponsiveness and Lung Inflammation in a Corticosteroid-Resistant Murine Model of Severe Asthma. Front Immunol 2021;12:786238.

102. Jeannin P, Lecoanet S, Delneste Y, et al. IgE versus IgG4 production can be differentially regulated by IL-10. J Immunol 1998;160(7):3555–61.

103. Smith TRF, Alexander C, Kay AB, et al. Cat allergen peptide immunotherapy reduces CD4+ T cell responses to cat allergen but does not alter suppression by CD4+ CD25+ T cells: a double-blind placebo-controlled study. Allergy 2004; 59(10):1097–101.

104. Calzada D, Cremades-Jimeno L, López-Ramos M, et al. Peptide Allergen Immunotherapy: A New Perspective in Olive-Pollen Allergy. Pharmaceutics 2021; 13(7):1007.

105. Worm M. SPIREs: a new horizon for allergic disease treatment? Expert Rev Clin Immunol 2015;11(11):1173–5.

106. Hafner R, Couroux P, Armstrong K, et al. Two year persistent treatment effect in reducing nasal symptoms of cat allergy after 4 doses of Cat-PAD, the first in a new class of synthetic peptide immuno-regulatory epitopes. Clin Transl Allergy 2013;3(S2):O7.

107. Chalmers JD, Haworth CS, Metersky ML, et al. WILLOW Investigators. Phase 2 Trial of the DPP-1 Inhibitor Brensocatib in Bronchiectasis. N Engl J Med 2020; 383(22):2127–37.

Moving?

Make sure your subscription moves with you!

To notify us of your new address, find your **Clinics Account Number** (located on your mailing label above your name), and contact customer service at:

Email: journalscustomerservice-usa@elsevier.com

800-654-2452 (subscribers in the U.S. & Canada)
314-447-8871 (subscribers outside of the U.S. & Canada)

Fax number: 314-447-8029

Elsevier Health Sciences Division
Subscription Customer Service
3251 Riverport Lane
Maryland Heights, MO 63043

*To ensure uninterrupted delivery of your subscription, please notify us at least 4 weeks in advance of move.

Printed and bound by CPI Group (UK) Ltd, Croydon, CR0 4YY

03/10/2024

01040466-0020